Communication Disorders in Turkish

COMMUNICATION DISORDERS ACROSS LANGUAGES
Series Editors: **Dr Nicole Müller and Dr Martin Ball,** *University of Louisiana at Lafayette, USA*

While the majority of work in communication disorders has focused on English, there has been a growing trend in recent years for the publication of information on languages other than English. However, much of this is scattered through a large number of journals in the field of speech pathology/communication disorders, and therefore, not always readily available to the practitioner, researcher and student. It is the aim of this series to bring together into book form surveys of existing studies on specific languages, together with new materials for the language(s) in question. We also envisage a series of companion volumes dedicated to issues related to the cross-linguistic study of communication disorders. The series will not include English (as so much work is readily available), but will cover a wide number of other languages (usually separately, though sometimes two or more similar languages may be grouped together where warranted by the amount of published work currently available). We envisage being able to solicit volumes on languages such as Norwegian, Swedish, Finnish, German, Dutch, French, Italian, Spanish, Russian, Croatian, Japanese, Cantonese, Mandarin, Thai, North Indian languages in the UK context, Celtic languages, Arabic and Hebrew among others.

Full details of all the books in this series and of all our other publications can be found on http://www.multilingual-matters.com, or by writing to Multilingual Matters, St Nicholas House, 31-34 High Street, Bristol, BS1 2AW, UK.

COMMUNICATION DISORDERS ACROSS LANGUAGES
Series Editors: Dr Nicole Müller and Dr Martin Ball

Communication Disorders in Turkish

Edited by
Seyhun Topbaş and Mehmet Yavaş

MULTILINGUAL MATTERS
Bristol • Buffalo • Toronto

Library of Congress Cataloging in Publication Data
A catalog record for this book is available from the Library of Congress.
Communication Disorders in Turkish/Edited by Seyhun Topbas and Mehmet Yavas.
Communication Disorders Across Languages: 4
Includes bibliographical references and index.
1. Language disorders. 2. Turkish language. I. Topbas, Seyhun. II. Yavas, Mehmet S.
RC423.C6428 2010
401'.9089943–dc22 2010005060

British Library Cataloguing in Publication Data
A catalogue entry for this book is available from the British Library.

ISBN-13: 978-1-84769-246-7 (hbk)

Multilingual Matters
UK: St Nicholas House, 31-34 High Street, Bristol BS1 2AW, UK.
USA: UTP, 2250 Military Road, Tonawanda, NY 14150, USA.
Canada: UTP, 5201 Dufferin Street, North York, Ontario M3H 5T8, Canada.

The policy of Multilingual Matters/Channel View Publications is to use papers that are natural, renewable and recyclable products, made from wood grown in sustainable forests. In the manufacturing process of our books, and to further support our policy, preference is given to printers that have FSC and PEFC Chain of Custody certification. The FSC and/or PEFC logos will appear on those books where full certification has been granted to the printer concerned.

Typeset by Techset Composition Ltd., Salisbury, UK.
Printed and bound in Great Britain by the MPG Books Group.

Contents

List of Figures

Acknowledgments

We express our gratitude to the contributors who made this project possible. Our deep thanks also go to Multilingual Matters and to the series editors Nicole Müller and Martin Ball for their invitation to produce this volume.

Conventions Used within this Book

The following conventions have been used within the book:

ASHA	: American Speech, Language and Hearing Association
AUD	: Audiology
AUDs	: Audiologists
CoHE	: Council of Higher Education of Turkey
CPLOL	: Standing Liaison Committee of Speech and Language Therapists and Logopedists of European Union
DİLKOM	: Education, Research and Training Centre for Speech and Language Pathology
HDI	: Human Development Report
IALP	: International Association of Logopedics and Phoniatrics
ICD-10	: International Classification of Diseases-10
ICF	: International Classification of Functioning, Disability and Health
İÇEM	: Education and Research Centre for Hearing Impaired Children
IPA	: International Phonetic Alphabet
MoH	: Turkish Ministry of Health
MoNE	: Turkish Ministry of National Education
OECD	: Organization for Economic Co-operation and Development
SLD	: Speech and Language Disorders
SLP	: Speech and Language Pathology
SLPs	: Speech and Language Pathologists/Therapists
TÜBİTAK	: The Scientific and Technological Research Council of Turkey
UNESCO	: United Nations Educational, Scientific and Cultural Organization
UNICEF	: United Nations Children's Fund
WHO	: World Health Organization

Contributors

Seyhun Topbaş is Professor of Speech and Language Pathology at Anadolu University, Eskişehir, Turkey. She has a BA in Linguistics and an MA in Applied Language Teaching. She was awarded her second master's degree, an MSc, in Clinical Communication Studies, Speech and Language Therapy at City University of London, England. She is one of the pioneers of the Speech and Language Therapy/Pathology profession in Turkey. She is the founder and director of DİLKOM, a foundation of the Education, Research and Training Centre for Speech and Language Pathology at Anadolu University, and the founder of the graduate (master's and doctorate) program in Speech and Language Therapy. She has authored several articles and chapters in international and national journals, has written and been the editor of three books in language development and disorders, and has developed the first standardized Turkish Articulation and Phonology Test. She is currently on the editorial board of *Clinical Linguistics and Phonetics*. She organized the 12th International Congress of Clinical Linguistics and Phonetics Association in Istanbul.

Mehmet Yavaş is Professor of Linguistics at Florida International University, Miami, Florida. He previously taught at the Catholic University of Porto Alegre, Brazil and was a visiting scholar at the School of Speech Pathology, Leicester Polytechnic (now De Montfort University), UK. His main area is phonology and its application to language acquisition and to speech and language disorders. His numerous articles on applied phonology have appeared in *Clinical Linguistics and Phonetics, Language and Speech, Journal of Multilingual Communication Disorders, Review of Applied Linguistics, Child Language Teaching and Therapy, Journal of Communication Disorders* and *American Journal of Speech and Language Pathology*. He is the principal author of *Avaliaçao Fonologica da Criança* (a phonological assessment procedure for Brazilian Portuguese). His other publications are *Phonological Disorders in Children* (Routledge, 1991), *First and Second Language Phonology* (Singular, 1994), *Phonology: Development and Disorders* (Singular, 1998) and *Applied English Phonology* (Blackwell, 2006).

Funda Acarlar is Associate Professor in the Special Education Department at Ankara University. She received masters and PhD degrees in Child

Health and Education from Hacettepe University. Her clinical and research work has focused on language development and assessment in children with language disorders. acarlar@education.ankara.edu.tr

Ayhan Aksu-Koç is a Professor at Yeditepe University and Boğaziçi University, Istanbul. Her area of specialization is the acquisition of Turkish as a first language, with particular focus on early grammatical and later narrative development, relations between cognition and language, early language support programs and literacy. She has published in various national and international sources. koc@boun.edu.tr

Mehmet Ali Akıncı received a PhD in 1999 (University of Lyon 2). Since 2000, he works as a researcher at CNRS (University of Lyon) and teaches at the University of Rouen. His research fields primarily relate to bilingual language acquisition and currently he is involved in research on biliteracy development in France and Germany. Mehmet-Ali.Akinci@ish-lyon.cnrs.fr

Ezel Babur works as a teacher at a grammar school in Hamburg. Between 2001 and 2007, she worked on the language development of Turkish-German bilingual children at the Collaborative Research Centre on Multilingualism in Hamburg, Germany. Her current research involves Turkish linguistics, acquisition and assessment of (bilingual) Turkish and specific language impairment (SLI) children. ezelbabur@gmx.de

Anne Baker is Professor of Psycholinguistics and Language Pathology and Director of the Amsterdam Centre for Language and Communication at the University of Amsterdam. Her research focuses on variation in language acquisition in a cross-linguistic perspective covering also sign languages and in groups of monolingual and bilingual children with language problems involving the acquisition of morphosyntax and pragmatics. A.E.Baker@uva.nl

Solveig Chilla is a teacher of speech and language pathology and education of the deaf. She currently works as a postdoctoral researcher in the Department for Inclusive and Special Education at the University of Bremen, Germany. Her main research focuses on unimpaired and impaired language development, therapy, and didactics in monolingual and bilingual children, and language acquisition of the deaf. chilla@uni-bremen.de

Nazife Çavuş is a speech therapist with a master's degree in linguistics. She has taught on the role of bilingualism in language diagnosis and intervention. She was involved in a research project on SLI in Turkish-Dutch bilingual children at the University of Amsterdam. Presently she works as a clinical linguist at the Saint Marie Institute in Eindhoven. mail@nazifecavus.nl

Nathalie Decool-Mercier received her MA in 2008 (University of Rouen). She has been a speech therapist since 1994 (diploma from the University of Besançon). Currently, she is involved in a project comparing bilingual Turkish children with monolinguals in France and works on anaphora in oral and written texts of 10-year-olds. natdecool@yahoo.fr

Pınar Ege is at present Associate Professor of Speech and Language Pathology in Special Education Department at Ankara University. She received her MA in Linguistics and her MS in Speech and Language Pathology from Syracuse University in New York and her PhD in Speech and Language Pathology from the University of Texas in Austin, Texas. She also teaches at DİLKOM, located at Anadolu University. pege@hotmail.com

Jan de Jong is a lecturer and senior researcher at the University of Amsterdam (Amsterdam Center of Language and Communication). His previous work concerned the grammatical symptoms of SLI in Dutch children and the linguistic precursors of dyslexia. J.deJong1@uva.nl

Judith R. Johnston is Professor of Audiology and Speech Sciences at the University of British Columbia. She is known internationally for research and teaching on developmental language disorders, especially SLI. In 2003, she was named a Canadian 3M Teaching Fellow for instructional excellence, and in 2004 she was awarded the Honours of the ASHA for her contributions to science and the profession. jrj@audiospeech.ubc.ca

Swathi Kiran is Associate Professor in the Department of Speech, Language and Hearing Sciences at Boston University in Boston, Massachusetts. Her research interests focus on lexical semantic treatment for individuals with aphasia, bilingual aphasia and neuroimaging of brain plasticity following a stroke. kirans@bu.edu

Handan Kopkallı-Yavuz is Associate Professor in the ELT Department at Anadolu University. She received her PhD in Linguistics from the University of Michigan. Her area of research is acoustic phonetics with a special emphasis on the interface between phonetics and phonology in Turkish, and phonological acquisition. She is currently the director of the School of Foreign Languages. hyavuz@anadolu.edu.tr

Theodoros Marinis is Reader in Clinical Linguistics, at the University of Reading, School of Psychology and Clinical Language Sciences, in the UK. He completed his PhD at the University of Potsdam and subsequently worked at the University of Essex, University College London, and the University of Central England. He has published research on first and second language acquisition and processing in adults, typically developing children and children with SLI. His current research focuses on the language abilities and processing of Turkish-English children t.marinis@ reading.ac.uk

İlknur Maviş is Associate Professor in the Centre for Speech and Language Disorders at Anadolu University. Her research focuses on the typological language differences in aphasia and/or bilingual aphasia and its assessment and therapy in Turkish. She has developed an original assessment battery (ADD) for patients with aphasia. She is also interested in language acquisition in Turkish children. imavis@anadolu.edu.tr

Elma Nap-Kolhoff is a PhD candidate at Tilburg University. She studied linguistics at the same university with 'Turkish in Europe' as her specialization. Since 2002 she has been working on her PhD project titled 'Bilingual development of two to four-year-old Turkish children in the Netherlands'. Elma's investigations include early childhood education for a number of educational institutions in the Netherlands. e.m.kolhoff@uvt.nl

Duygu Özge is a research assistant at the School of Psychology and Clinical Language Sciences at the University of Reading and at the Middle East Technical University, Ankara. She is working with Theodoros Marinis on an ESRC-funded project titled 'Real-time processing of syntactic information in children with English as a Second Language and children with Specific Language Impairment'. d.ozge@reading.ac.uk

Umran Tüfekçioğlu is a Professor and the Head of the Teacher Training Program for Hearing Impaired Children at Anadolu University. She received her PhD in Communication Sciences. Since 1979, as the director of İÇEM, she worked closely with overseas advisors in running in-service training programs and founded the four-year degree program for teachers of hearing impaired children. She has publications in this field in Turkish and English. utufekci@anadolu.edu.tr

Kutlay Yagmur is Associate Professor of Multilingualism in the Department of Language and Culture Studies, University of Tilburg. Currently, he is investigating the relationship between the integration ideology of the receiving society and socio-cultural adaptation of immigrants in four national contexts. His publications have appeared in various international journals and concern Turkish immigrants in Australia, Germany, France and The Netherlands; and he has co-edited a book *Urban Multilingualism. Immigrant Minority Languages at Home and School* (2004, Multilingual Matters). K.Yagmur@uvt.nl

Preface

Today, the world is becoming a microcosm. People work and travel all over the globe, and experience immigration and uprooting. In these settings, the need for speech and language professionals becomes ever more important. Individuals, both children and adults, with communicative needs turn to speech–language pathologists (SLPs), who can provide services to enhance their communication skills. The professionals, in turn, are guided by ever-increasing research on language development and disorders in both monolingual and bilingual populations.

While there have been a significant number of publications on several major languages of the world from this perspective, there has not been one on Turkish. Yet, the need for such a book is enormous, as Turkish is used not only by a sizeable population as the native language in Turkey, but also in multilingual settings all around the world, principally in Europe, USA, Canada and Australia.

This volume is exclusively devoted to Turkish communicative development and disorders, and hence the first of its kind. It provides a compendium of information about the profession of speech language pathology, cultural characteristics, assessment materials and research carried out on communication disorders in Turkey. It also covers language acquisition and disorders in multilingual contexts where there is significant Turkish immigration. It comprises a collection of studies on research and clinical practice, including assessment and therapy materials for different communication disorders in Turkish. The diverse experiences and professional backgrounds of the contributors to this volume bring together a wealth of information for those working in the field.

The book is primarily aimed at SLPs who work with Turkish-speaking clients in monolingual and/or multilingual settings and need resources on the language and its assessment. In addition, professionals and researchers from related disciplines such as linguistics, psychology, psycholinguistics, neurolinguistics, audiology and special education will benefit from this book as a resource for understanding typical and atypical language characteristics. Researchers will also find this book relevant to their work as the contents will prove to be useful in understanding the universals and language-specific aspects of speech and language development.

Why this Book was Written

The population of Turkey is approximately 71,5 million, and another five million people of Turkish descent live in Europe, the United States, Australia and other countries of the world. More than four million Turkish speakers live in European Union countries. Over a million speakers of Turkish are found in Bulgaria, Macedonia, and Greece; over 2 million live in Germany (and others in northern European countries, Belgium, France, Denmark, England) where Turks have for many years been "guest workers." Besides, about 200,000 Turkish speakers live in Northern America, 200.000 in Middle East and 150.000 in Australia. Thus, people of Turkish extraction are found throughout the world. Foreign SLP professionals throughout the world work with speakers of Turkish who suffer from communication disorders. There are also Turkish SLPs living outside Turkey. Thus, those SLPs, wishing information pertinent to providing clinical services to Turkish people may find limited resources to guide them to serve both to native or multilingual minority clients. This book wishes to pursue this mission providing information about the professional services and the current research in communication disorders. It also hopes to provide clinicians with some useful information about their client's country, including its language, education system, the current status of the profession and organization of professional services for communication disorders.

Organization of the Book

The book is organized into three parts. Part 1 provides background information. Chapter 1 discusses the development of speech and language pathology profession and its place within the health and education system. The information serves speech–language pathologists in and outside Turkey whose caseloads may include Turkish persons. Chapters 2 and 3 outline the sounds and structural characteristics of the Turkish language. Part 2 is on the typical and atypical acquisition of Turkish. Chapter 4 gives an extensive examination and perhaps the first comprehensive review of the unique features of language acquisition in Turkish. Chapter 5 is about MLU norms in the development of Turkish. Chapter 6 summarizes the Turkish version of SALT and its use for assessment in language disorders, and Chapter 7 focuses on specific language impairment and the adaptation of TELD-3 to Turkish in the identification of language impairments. Chapters 8 and 9 are about the speech and language characteristics of hearing impaired Turkish children. Chapter 10 is a summary of aphasia studies in Turkish, and Chapter 11 examines Turkish-English bilingual adults. Finally, Part 3, brings information from four European Union countries (England, France, Germany, The Netherlands) where Turkish people constitute the majority of minorities, and who are potential candidates for SLP services.

Part 1

Prologue

Chapter 1

A Closer Look at the Developing Profession of Speech and Language Pathology (SLP) in Turkey

SEYHUN TOPBAŞ

Introduction

Speech and language pathology (SLP) in Turkey is a young profession but is growing rapidly. Bleile *et al.* (2007: 1) has stated that 'the amount of attention a country gives to communication disorders depends on its history, cultural ties on language and disability, economics and availability of services; and that the impact of a communication disorder varies depending on where a person is born and lives'. Thus, a glance at the whole system is necessary to visualize the developmental status of SLP within this country. In this chapter, I will first simplify the complicated nature of the Turkish health, education and special education systems and the financing of services, followed by a closer look at the history of the profession and education of speech and language pathologists (SLPs). Finally, I will present the current developments in lieu of my previous report (Topbaş, 2006a), and will articulate the problematic issues in service delivery within this system.

An Overview of the Turkish Health and Education Systems

Turkish health system

The Turkish health care system has a complex structure. To simplify the matter only the basic structure and service delivery will be summarized. Several old laws, although subjected to various changes, still constitute the basis of the practice system. Health policies implemented until 1980 were formed within the Socialization of Health Services Law (1961, No: 224), which attempted to establish a national health service free of charge although this was not achieved until recently. Currently, the health system, including the social insurance system, is undergoing the effects of a reform package, by the *Health Transformation Program* (Akdağ *et al.*, 2007).

Health services in Turkey are supplied by a multitude of public and private providers. The Turkish Ministry of Health (MoH) is the main government body responsible for health sector policy making, implementation of national health strategies and direct provision of primary and secondary health care, maternal health services, children and family planning services and preventive health services. The two key public providers are the MoH and the University hospitals. The MoH operates an extensive network of health facilities through several affiliated public, quasi-public, private and philanthropic organizations, depending on the advocates' concern with policy formulation, provision of health care, finance of health care and whether they have administrative jurisdiction over the delivery of health care (MoH, 2004). Apart from policy making, the provision of health services is supplied by public and private hospitals, outpatient polyclinics, laboratories and diagnostic and rehabilitation centers, providing primary, secondary and specialized inpatient and outpatient care. University (state and foundation) hospitals are under the responsibility of The Council of Higher Education of Turkey (CoHE) as they support medical training. Each medical school has its own university hospital, acting as a main referral hospital as well as providing comprehensive and modern health care.

The MoH also focuses on school health services organized jointly with the Turkish Ministry of National Education (MoNE), which includes vaccination, screening programs (eye, oral and general physical examinations that check height and weight) and primary care services. A recent attempt has been made to implement a health-promoting schools project, in collaboration with the World Health Organization (WHO) and the United Nations Children's Fund (UNICEF), as well as mother and child health centers and family planning centers. Services for those with special needs and necessary rehabilitation services after treatment are also rendered in collaboration with MoNE (MoH, 2004).

Turkish education system

The Turkish National Education System (Act No: 1739) is highly centralized. The MoNE is responsible for all formal and non-formal educational services in the country excluding higher education. Formal regular education includes preschool education, basic education (primary), secondary education and higher education. Both private and public state educational institutions are prominent. Education is free at every level in state institutions. Preschool education is optional for children aged 0–6. These may be infant or nursery schools, or preprimary classes within a primary school. An important step carried out by the MoNE is the mobile kindergarten project for 36–72-month-old children who live in villages and cannot attend preschool and/or for those with a low socioeconomic backgrounds. Primary education, being compulsory, involves the education and training of children in the age group of 6–14 (in total, eight years of education). A national curriculum is implemented across the country. Secondary education, which is not compulsory, consists of four years of education following primary education and includes general, vocational and technical high school training for the 14–16 age group (MoNE, 2007).

In accordance with Law No. 2547 of 1981, the CoHE is the planning, coordinating and policy-making body for higher education cooperating with MoNE to fulfill the principles of national education objectives. Higher education is based on secondary education and comprises a variety of institutions at every level, affiliated with university or non-university institutions, such as police and military academies and colleges. Universities (state or private foundations) consist of two-year vocational schools offering associate's degree (prebachelor's level) programs and four-year faculties and colleges offering bachelor's degree programs. Faculties consist of departments and each department within a faculty is made up of divisions. Distance education is also available from Anadolu University, offering two- and four-year programs. Admission to higher education is based on a very competitive nationwide Student Selection Examination, held every year and administered by the Student Selection and Placement Centre. In addition to formal education, non-formal and other open-education facilities to increase literacy, and/or for other purposes are also available with the objective of national education at all levels of basic and higher education. Graduate-level education is offered by the coordination of graduate institutions affiliated with the universities. Such programs are based on master's and doctoral degrees in education, applied sciences and social and health sciences. The opening of a degree program at any level is subject to ratification by the Council (CoHE, 2008).

Education at all levels is one of the main priorities of state policies, which are based on equal opportunities for every individual as mandated by the Turkish Constitution. However, the impact of rapid population growth, economics and mass internal migration inhibits the expected quality and quantity of services both in urban and rural areas. According to the 2007/2008 Human Development Report (HDI, 2007–2008), the adult literacy rate is 87.4% (% ages 15 and older). The combined primary, secondary and tertiary gross enrollment ratio is shown as 68.7%. The MoNE (2007) statistical report shows that, based on the latest population projections, the percentage of children enrolling in schools increased to 90.13% for primary education, and 56.51% for secondary education in 2006–2007. However, although there seems to be a rapid change, the expected primary school enrollment ratio is 93% for males and 82% for females, and the actual school attendance is lower than this. Thus, nationwide projects, some of which include *Kardelenler* (*Snowdrops*), *Baba Beni Okula Gönder* (*Father, Let Me Attend School*) and the girls' education campaign *Haydi Kızlar Okula* (*Let's Go to School, Girls!*), *Eğitime %100 Destek* (*100% Support for Education*), have been initiated in the 2000s to support the right of access to education as well as financing those individuals, specifically girls, who have not been educated for various reasons (OECD, 2007). These are important steps taken by the collaboration of MoNE, UNICEF, UNESCO, WORLDBANK, universities, volunteer associations, foundations and large companies toward eliminating poverty, advancing sustainable human development and promoting gender equality (MoNE, 2008).

Speech-language disordered individuals (SLDs) in the context of special education legislation

The educational rights of special needs children have been monitored under the MoNE by the National Education Act (No: 2916) since the first special education act came into force in 1983. The Act has been under consideration for considerable change due to accommodation to European Union (EU) regulations (1997, Decree Law: 573). A new reorganized system has recently been put into place by the new Special Education Legislation Act (2005, No: 5378) with the principle of 'Education for All', creating equal opportunities for the disabled. The execution of some articles of the law was implemented in 2006–2007. Accordingly, the public and private schools, and supportive special education and rehabilitation institutions that were previously a part of the health system are now affiliated with the MoNE. Obligations to offer supportive SLP services to individuals with speech-language disorders (SLD) are currently provided under the regulations of the MoNE (MoNE, 2008). This operational definition of people with disabilities is used by authorities in deciding entitlements for people who apply for related benefits and/or pensions with a criterion-based degree of disability based on the International Classification of Functioning, Disability and Health (ICF) (WHO, 2007a).

In Turkey, services for disabled people are provided by both governmental and non-governmental organizations. The MoNE and the General Directorate of Special Education Guidance and Counselling Service Department of MoNE are responsible for implementing educational policies. In provinces and sub-provinces, the Guidance and Research Centres and Special Education Boards affiliated with the General Directorate are responsible for the implementation of policies. The Board defines the principles and procedures of the Guidance and Research Centres, which are responsible for governing evaluation and assessment, placement and supervision for the special needs children. Furthermore, the MoH, the Ministry of Labour and Social Security, the Social Services through the

Turkish Employment Organization, the Social Services and Protection of Children Agency, and the General Directorate of Social Assistance and Solidarity were organized at both central and local levels to serve people with disabilities. To properly coordinate these services, the Prime Ministry Administration for Disabled People was established in 1997.

The new Disability Law has facilitated improvements in the education of disabled people and removed most of the obstacles to their receiving services. All children are covered, whether they have social security or not, and governmental support has been provided to educate all children who are judged by the Special Education Assessment Board to have a need for special education.

According to statistics reported by the General Directorate of Special Education Guidance and Counselling Service Department of the MoNE (2008), about 282,369 school-age children up to the age of 18 years received special education services in both regular and separate education schools in the 2008–2009 academic year. It should be emphasized herein that early childhood and preschool education has become compulsory for special needs children with the new special education act. Thus, 28,252 students are placed into state special education schools, organized mainly for hearing impaired, mentally retarded (educable and trainable), autistic, visually impaired, physically handicapped and gifted children. There are no special schools or classes for SLD. The special education classes under state primary schools serving 9252 children, are mainly for those who are mentally retarded but educable. A total of 4138 students receive services at separate private primary special education schools. The establishment of separate schools differs from the current educational practice in the United States, but may be similar in part to the system in some European countries. The logic underlying the existence of such schools is that they provide education throughout the child's entire curriculum. Integration (mainstreaming) of the disabled is a mandatory principle of the new law, designed to promote a 'least restrictive environment.' A total of 67,756 children receive inclusive education in state primary and secondary schools. The childhood age restriction has also been renewed for those who need lifelong services, and supportive rehabilitation. As a result, 181,665 individuals receive supportive education and/or therapy in private rehabilitation institutions. A related requirement of the law is to provide supportive services such as teacher consultations, in-class support or resource room services whenever necessary. However, the implementation of this aspect lags due to the lack of several support personnel, specifically SLPs and audiologists.

Although there is considerable growing interest in the area, implementation of health and education services in special needs categories (both child and adult) is still inadequate, lacking systematic individualized programs, assessment and intervention materials, due to lack of enough support service personnel. Nevertheless, public awareness is growing on the educational rights of disabled people, and several projects, such as *Umut Adımlar Projesi* (*The Project of Hopeful Steps*) for the counseling of families of special needs children, are in progress through the collaboration of the Prime Ministry Administration for Disabled People, MoNE and some universities. In line with the goals of UNESCO project on 'Education for All', a national action plan was prepared to reach the objectives of providing equality of opportunity at all levels and kinds of education until 2015 (UNESCO, 2008). The implementation of this goal is considered as a priori to reach the European Union indicators as well.

Financing of services

The financing of health services is complicated as well. Turkey has a mixed financing structure based on two main models: One of them is financing from public resources and the other is financing from those who demand the service. Three main sources are the state budget, social security institutions and personal expenses of the individuals. The structure relies heavily on the individuals' employment status subsidized by the social security institutions. The main public social security institutions are affiliated with the Ministry of Labour and Social Security. The coexistence of budgetary and non-budgetary sources of funding in the health sector has resulted in the emergence of a multi-tier health care system in Turkey, defined by who provides health care, who pays for it and how much and the quality of care of that service. The World Bank statistics showed that 30% of the Turkish population is not covered by any social security; hence, they do not have access to any health care systems (Acar, 2008). Thus, the government proposed a reform package to organize a uniform social security institution and a general health care insurance, which the government claim will bring equality and efficiency to the health care system.

The financial support provided by the government (either from MoNE or MoH) for the health care and education of special needs children is free of charge. Thus, the families of the children receive services whether they have social security or not. Up to the present, the social security system has not worked properly for communication disorders; many institutions gave services to SLD by labeling them under mental retardation categories in order to supply financial funding for the families. The cost of speech therapy is now covered to some extent by national insurances after the new legislation was enacted in late 2005. However, there is no well-established coordination among the Social Insurance Institution and hospitals and MoNE; therefore, planning of services and investments cannot be carried out in parallel with the needs of the SLD. As an example, the ICD-10 principles and criteria (WHO, 2007b) are adapted for SLD in order to get financial support. When a client suffers aphasia due to stroke, he or she can receive medical treatment and rehabilitation within a state hospital, or in a private physical rehabilitation center free of charge, if there is an SLP employed there. Likewise, an articulation–phonologically disordered child can be medically diagnosed free of charge; however, she or he cannot get therapy support if the ICD-10 criteria of disability is below 20%. Even if clients' disorder rates exceed this percentage, they can receive support for therapy in special private centers or hospitals only if they have insurance; but they cannot receive financial support if they have to be treated at a university center that is not affiliated with a hospital. Thus, the clients have to pay for their personal expenses. As a result, the implementation of ICF cannot be monitored properly.

History of the Profession of SLP/Speech and Language Therapy

The history of SLP/speech and language therapy in Turkey, as a distinct and independent field, can be analyzed mainly under two developmental roots: the special education root and the medical root.

The history of special education in Turkey goes back to the early 1880s through the efforts of an Austrian, Monsieur Grati (Grati Efendi), who was given permission to open the first school for the deaf-mute in 1881. The Minister of Education of that time, Münif Pasha, approved the opening of the school during the 1891–1892 academic year. The school implemented the French educational program for deaf students adopting sign language. In 1952, some foreign experts in the field of special education, namely Harriot L. Mclaughlin, the Headmaster of the 47th School for the Deaf in New York, and Adolf Fronthaller from Austria, were recruited to train volunteer primary school teachers as teachers of the deaf. At the same time, a teacher training program for Special Education had been initiated at Gazi Educational Institute, but two years later it was closed down (Girgin, 2006). This attempt was a significant step in the history of Turkish special education allowing the graduation of the first special educators in Turkey. Yahya Özsoy was one of those graduates (1954) who worked with deaf children and was interested in the communication development of the hearing impaired. Thus, he was granted an opportunity by MoNE to study at George Peabody College for Teachers, in the United States, and earned bachelor's and master's degrees (Özsoy graduated in 1964). On his return, speech–language services were introduced for the first time under special needs categories with a pedagogical emphasis in collaboration with K. Ingram from America (personal communication with D. Çağlar, November 12, 2003). Özsoy continued his career at the Special Education Department of the Education Faculty at Ankara University, which was founded in 1965. He published his first important book *Speech Disorders* in 1971 (Özsoy, 1971). However, this department also closed down later. The

1960s, also witnessed volunteers from the American Peace Corps and United Nations working as English teachers in schools and/or serving in nursing, child care or agricultural institutions. Very few SLPs among these served children with speech and language difficulties in the areas where they worked (personal communication with K. St. Louis, June 25, 2008). In the following years, MoNE organized 3–4 weeks of in-service training courses to teachers and professionals interested in communication disorders to provide supportive education to the hearing impaired and the mentally retarded. In 1979, the Education and Research Centre for Hearing-Impaired Children (İÇEM) was founded at Anadolu University to enable hearing impaired children to acquire spoken language skills using the auditory/oral approach and to be a model school of its kind. This was followed by the foundation of the Special Education Department. Through this initiative, Anadolu University became a pioneer in teacher training for the hearing impaired, as well as in special education. Thus, the speech and language development of the hearing impaired became the primary focus of the later developments at Anadolu University.

Alongside the above developments, as in all countries, medical doctors were traditionally involved in the diagnosis of hearing impairment. For the hearing impaired, an efficient comprehensive service, encompassing early diagnosis of deafness and hearing aid fitting and maintenance, was needed. Eventually, in 1967, an Audiology Unit was founded by Prof Dr İ Nazmi Hoşal, and in 1968 a master's degree program in Audiology was initiated at Hacettepe University, in Ankara, at the Medicine Faculty within the Ear, Nose and Throat Department, with the collaboration of Dr Richard Israel. This was followed by a doctoral program in 1974 in collaboration with Dr Jack Katz from the United States. Among the first graduates were Erol Belgin, Ferda Akdaş, Soner Yalçın and Nevma Madanoğlu. In 1982, the title and the content of the MS program were revised and changed to *Audiology and Speech Pathology* (Akdaş, 2003; Belgin, 2001). However, the foundation and recognition of Audiology as a formal departmental unit by Higher Education Board was set forth by Ferda Akdaş in 1990 at Marmara University. These clinics, being the pioneer in the field, contributed new developments specifically in audiology. Up to the present, other audiology and speech pathology programs have been established through the efforts of these first graduates. In these programs, as will be seen in the following sections, the students have not been given a choice of speech–language therapy/pathology or audiology separately; rather they were introduced to one dual compact program, with more emphasis on audiology and related auditory processing disorders, although a few speech–language courses were taught as the basis for audiology courses. In sum, the services to SLD were maintained under the special education framework in general with pedagogical emphasis, whereas under audiology there was more clinical emphasis.

Today, SLP is growing away from special education and audiology and forming a 'distinct and independent profession'. This trend has its roots in the 1980s, initiated by Ahmet Konrot, PhD, who was trained in England as a speech–language therapist. On his return in 1982, he set up a small speech therapy unit at the Education Faculty and at the Medico-social Hospital of Anadolu University. His efforts and these units, together with İÇEM, have received national attention as he provided speech therapy services to the first cochlear-implanted adults in Turkey in 1985 (Altay *et al.*, 1989; Konrot, 1994a). In 1988, a second speech therapist, the author of this chapter, who was also trained in England, was employed by the Education Faculty of Anadolu University. In 1990, a doctoral program was initiated for the first time in Turkey in the Education of the Speech Impaired under the sub-department of Special Education, covering both a clinically and linguistically based curriculum. Thus, a curriculum emphasizing the importance of clinical linguistics and phonetics that was similar to those in Europe and the United States was implemented for the first time in Turkey. However, the CoHE soon closed this program in 1996, claiming that Education Faculties be structured only for the teacher training programs (Konrot, 1994b; Topbaş, 2006a).

This situation gave rise to the foundation of the Education, Research and Training Centre for Speech and Language Pathology (DİLKOM) at Anadolu University, approved by the CoHE in 1999, through the collaboration of Dr Ahmet Konrot, Dr Seyhun Topbaş and Dr İlknur Maviş. Pursuant to its mission, DİLKOM established the Department of Speech and Language Therapy and initiated a Master of Science program in *Speech & Language Therapy* in 2000, with the support of two SLPs who were trained in the United States, namely Dr Pınar Ege and Dr Müzeyyen Çiyiltepe, and a doctoral program in 2004 under the *Department of Speech and Language Therapy* coordinated by the Institute of Health Sciences. This program is the first to award its students with a diploma in SLP. It should be kept in mind that 'SLP and audiologist (AUD)' together is an umbrella term to include both twin-sister disciplines belonging to the same family but with a different scope of practice as stated in ASHA (2004, 2007). In this respect, DİLKOM is devoted to training SLPs, acting as a model for the SLP profession in Turkey.

Current Status of Programs in SLP

Programs

Currently, there are no programs at the undergraduate level in Turkey. The programs offered either in SLP or in AUD are at the graduate level and comprise master's degrees and doctoral degrees. The master's degree programs are for at least three years with a thesis (or non-thesis). The doctoral degrees emphasize more specialized courses and have a duration of at least four years consisting of completion of courses, passing an oral and written qualifying examination and defending a doctoral thesis. The programs in general accept graduates of students from related disciplines such as psychology, physiotherapy, special education, nursing, linguistics and the like. All the programs require a predetermined number of hours and cases of supervised practicum and all the programs utilize the European Course Credit System (ECTS) credit system.

As presented in Tables 1.1 and 1.2, there are programs in audiology, audiology and speech pathology and in SLP alone. I will highlight the similarities and differences among programs.

As seen in Table 1.1, four universities offer both master's and doctoral degrees, and six offer master's degrees. Four offer a degree only in audiology and six universities offer a dual degree in audiology and speech pathology. The programs are coordinated by the Graduate Institute of Health Sciences of the related universities. Only two universities (Marmara and Çukurova) have an official Audiology Division under the Department of Ear, Nose and Throat (ENT). Other programs are run under the Department of ENT. However, only a few of them have sustainable and stable programs in continuing graduate education. Some seem to have opened a program but the programs are not in progress, having no students yet enrolled. The reason for not being able to sustain the programs might be attributed to (1) the shortage of audiologists at the doctoral level and (2) the shortage of academic positions as an audiologist (see the section 'Teaching staff at universities'). The Master's Degree Diploma bears the official name of the master's degree completed and the title awarded, where relevant. In some programs the title awarded bears the name of the department as ENT.

The curricula of the audiology programs are designed according to the international standards of audiology. However, analyses of the programs (downloaded from their websites) show that those which advocate running dual programs lack the necessary courses for SLP. Specifically, the programs at the master's level offer only one or two such courses, which, in fact, is compulsory for audiology as stated in ASHA regulations (ASHA, 1990, 2004). Only Hacettepe University has recently renewed its program in the 2008–2009 academic year to include more courses in speech and language. As can be seen in Table 1.1, about 143 audiologists have graduated since their establishment and 53 students are currently enrolled. In this respect, these programs differ from the SLP program run at DİLKOM, at Anadolu University.

As shown in Table 1.2, there are only two programs in SLP, one of which (Gaziantep University) is not available at present. DİLKOM at Anadolu University devoted its mission to training effective therapists; it acts both as a department and as a clinical center affiliated with the University Rectorship. It is a very well equipped center technically, clinically and

Table 1.1 Programs in audiology and in audiology–speech pathology

Institution	*Departmental affiliation*	*Program title*	*Degree*	*Year*	*Graduates by 2008*	*Enrolled in 2008*	*Diploma title awarded*
Hacettepe University	Faculty of Medicine Dept. of ENT	Audiology and Speech Pathology	MSc PhD	1968 1974	55 20	11 3	Audiologist and Speech Pathologist
		Educational Audiology	MSc PhD	1992 1995	20 7	8 1	Educational Audiologist
Marmara University	Faculty of Medicine Dept. of ENT	Audiology and Speech Pathology	MSc PhD	1987 1989	7 7	5 1	Audiologist and Speech Pathologist
Trakya University	Faculty of Medicine Dept. of ENT	Audiology and Speech Pathology	MSc PhD	1988 1993	2 3	0 0	Audiologist and Speech Pathologist
Gazi University	Faculty of Medicine Dept. of ENT	Hearing, Speech and Voice Pathology	MSc	2003	5	12	Hearing, Speech and Voice Pathologist
Başkent University	Faculty of Medicine Dept. of ENT	Audiology, Speech and Voice Pathology	MSc	2005	N/A	N/A	N/A
Dokuz Eylül University	Faculty of Medicine Dept. of ENT	Audiology	MSc	1995	10	6	Audiologist
Çukurova University	Faculty of Medicine Dept. of ENT	Audiology	MSc	1995	1	0	Audiologist
19 Mayıs University	Faculty of Medicine Dept. of ENT	Audiology	MSc	2007	N/A	6	Audiologist
Gaziantep University	Faculty of Medicine Dept. of ENT	Audiology	MSc	2006	1	0	Audiologist

Dept. of ENT = Department of Ear, Nose and Throat; N/A = not applicable.

Table 1.2 Programs only in SLP

Institution	*Departmental affiliation*	*Program title*	*Degree*	*Year*	*Graduates by 2009*	*Enrolled students in 2008*	*Diploma title awarded*
Anadolu University	Dept. of Speech and Language Therapy, DİLKOM	Speech and Language Therapy/Pathology	MSc	2000	53	35	Speech and Language Therapist/ Pathologist
			PhD	2004	1	12	
Gaziantep University	Faculty of Medicine Dept. of ENT	Voice, Speech and Language Therapy (Logopedics)	MSc	2003	N/A	N/A	N/A

Dept. of ENT = Department of Ear, Nose and Throat; N/A = not applicable.

educationally, serving in its own building. The programs are coordinated by the Institute of Health Sciences under the Department of Speech and Language Therapy. Since 2000, approximately 10 students have enrolled each year; 53 students have graduated by 2009, and currently 47 students are enrolled at either the master's or PhD levels.

The standards of IALP News (1998), ASHA (1990, 1994, 2005) and CPLOL (2007) have been instituted at the Department of DİLKOM from the initial step, and competency-based occupational standards are utilized, covering aspects of biomedical, linguistic and professional courses. All students are required to complete the Academic Preparation Program (two semesters) since they hold a bachelor's degree in a field other than SLP. The courses at this level are monitored under the master's degree curriculum. Therefore, the program lasts at least 3–4 years depending on the thesis or non-thesis option. Table 1.3 presents the curriculum of DİLKOM, which is diverse and intensive, combining a strong theoretical and scientific base with extensive clinical practice. The content is similar to that required for the Clinical Competency Certificate (CCC)-SLP in the United States, or its equivalent in the United Kingdom or Australia, leading to a degree that qualifies graduates to practice as SLPs. The students are required to undertake a minimum of 400 h of supervised clinical practicum during their education period. Of this, 80 h includes observation in the Academic Preparation Program. The rest involves client contact hours under the supervision of SLPs at DİLKOM and at hospitals where only DİLKOM graduate SLPs are employed. The doctoral program offers specialization in one sub-area, and involves both research and clinical efficiency skills.

Teaching staff at universities

Both academic and administrative staffs in state universities have civil servant status, and full professors and associate professors have tenure. The numbers of academic and administrative staff posts allocated to each state university are determined by Acts of the Parliament, while staff appointments at all levels are, however, made exclusively by the universities themselves, and are not subject to ratification by any outside authority (CoHE, 2008). In this respect, positional employment is allocated to the occupations as defined by the law. The SLP and AUD professional staffs at universities are presented in Table 1.4.

Currently, in the entire country, eight persons hold advanced degrees in SLP (four of them were trained overseas in the United Kingdom and United States) (Konrot, 2004) and 27 persons hold AUD degrees and act as teaching professors at the universities. About 10 ENT professors also hold master's degrees in audiology. Professors from other disciplines (such as ENT and neurology) also lecture within their area of specialty. All the faculty members work closely with professionals in other countries; and ERASMUS student and staff exchange programs are applicable at all the universities.

Table 1.3 Curriculums at the Department of SLP, DİLKOM, Anadolu University

Master's degree prerequisite courses	*ECTS*	*Master's degree courses*	*ECTS*	*Doctoral degree courses*	*ECTS*
Phonetics and Acoustics of Hearing and Speech	4.0	Research Methods in Speech–Language Therapy	4.5	Advanced Research Methods in Speech and Language Therapy	7.5
Anatomical, Physiological and Neurological Basis of Speech and Language	4.0	Evaluation of Clinical–Educational Research in Assessment and Therapy	5.0	Analysis of Efficacy Research in Speech and Language Therapy	7.5
Developmental Neurology and Childhood Psychiatric Diseases	4.0	Single-Subject Research Design and Case Studies in Speech and Language Disorders	7.5	Special Topics and Current Practice Issues in SLP	7.5
An Overview of Audiology	4.0	Articulation and Phonological Disorders	5.0	Research in Phonology	7.5
Psycholinguistics: Language Development and Language Delay	4.0	Intervention to Cleft Lip Palate: Surgery, Orthodontic and Therapeutic	4.0	Speech and Language Therapy Approaches for Patients with Cleft Palate and Craniofacial Anomalies – Advanced	7.5
ENT; Head and Face Anomalies	3.0	Introduction to Swallowing Disorders	5.0	Advanced Diagnosis and Therapy Methods for Swallowing Disorders	7.5
Child and Adult Audiology	4.0	Developmental Language Disorders: Assessment	4.0	Therapy Approaches for Neuromotor Speech Disorders – Advanced	7.5

Public Health, First Aid and Basic Pharmacology	3.0	Developmental Language Disorders: Therapy	4.0	Aphasia and Contemporary Therapy Approaches	7.5
Speech Pathology and Linguistics	4.0	Voice Disorders	5.0	Advanced Techniques in Diagnosis and Therapy of Voice Disorders	7.5
Clinical Phonology	4.0	Fluency Disorders	5.0	Contemporary and Theories in Speech Fluency	7.5
Speech Science	3.0	Acquired Language Disorders	5.0	Traumatic Brain Injuries (TBI)	7.5
Linguistic Analysis	3.0	Motor Speech Disorders	4.0	Specific Language Impairment in Childhood	7.5
Clinical Neurolinguistics	4.0	Development of Auditory–Verbal Language in the Hearing Impaired	4.0	Speech Therapy for Children and Adults with Cochlear Implants	7.5
Pronunciation and Diction for SLPs	2.0	Speech Therapy for the Hearing Impaired	5.0	Language – Brain Research	7.5
Voice and Music for SLPs	2.0	Alternative Communication and Technologies	4.0	Research in Linguistics	7.5
Introduction to Speech–Language Disorders	4.0	Basic Geriatrics	4.0	Genetics Research in Speech and Language Disorders	7.5
Functional Communication Training	4.0	Family Therapy and Consultation in SLD	3.0	Current Approaches in Language Disorders: Infants and Toddlers	7.5
Developing Therapy Plan and Psychometrics: Observation I	2.0	Basic Instrumentation Methods	2.0	Science Ethics	5.0

(Continued)

Table 1.3 *Continued*

Master's degree prerequisite courses	*ECTS*	*Master's degree courses*	*ECTS*	*Doctoral degree courses*	*ECTS*
Applied Behaviour Analysis: Observation II	2.0	Applied Clinical Studies and Seminar I	2.0	Speech Therapy and Rehabilitation in Laryngectomy	7.5
		Applied Clinical Studies and Seminar II	2.0	Technological Research in Speech Science	7.5
		Applied Clinical Studies and Seminar III	2.0	Experimental Studies in Phonetics Science	7.5
		Applied Clinical Studies and Seminar IV	2.0	Clinical Linguistics	7.5
		Term Project	15.0	Central Auditory Processing Disorders	7.5
		Thesis	30.0	Geriatric Communication Disorders	7.5
				Phoniatrics	7.5
				Clinical Practicum I	2.0
				Clinical Practicum II	2.0
				Clinical Practicum III	2.0
				Clinical Practicum IV	2.0
				Thesis, Proficiency Test and Defense	60.0

Table 1.4 SLP and AUD teaching staff at universities by 2009

Programs	*Teaching staff*
Speech and Language Pathology (PhD)	8
Audiology and Speech Pathology (PhD)	27
ENT doctors who hold a master's degree in AUD	10

Research

All the universities are involved in research with an emphasis on their practical areas. In this respect, Hacettepe University and Marmara University led the research in audiology. Countrywide projects are conducted by these universities in collaboration with MoH on the hearing screening of neonates and on cochlear implantation. Gazi University is conducting a project to standardize and describe the characteristics of Turkish Sign Language. Some ENT doctors conduct research on voice sciences as well.

DİLKOM at Anadolu University fosters research and leads the field in all aspects of SLDs and language acquisition in collaboration with other universities. A number of research studies have been conducted on phonology (an extended summary can be found in Topbaş (2007a) and Topbaş and Yavaş (2006)) and, as reviewed in the chapters of this book, on aphasia, language disorders and the like. Evidence-based practice and efficacy research is one of the priorities at DİLKOM. Thus, single-subject and small-scale group efficacy methodologies in articulation–phonological therapy, stuttering therapy and voice therapy are now in progress. As an example, a countrywide project has been initiated at DİLKOM in 2007 with a grant from TÜBİTAK to provide therapy and self-help for stutterers (*Project e-OZYARDEP: Expanding community-based self-help programs for stuttering through the internet*) to reduce stigma related to stuttering (St. Louis *et al.*, 2008; Topbaş *et al.*, 2009). A special emphasis is given to specific language impairment as this topic is highly underestimated in Turkey, and several tests are being developed.

Current Issues in Service Delivery

SLPs and AUDs are the key professionals in the delivery of services to the communicatively impaired. The professions serve to bridge personnel in the health and education systems. This important duty of the professions, specifically SLP in Turkey, is gradually being recognized.

Clinical populations

In 2002, a countrywide Disability Survey was carried out in Turkey by the State Institute of Statistics in cooperation with the State Planning Organization and The Presidency of Administration of Disabled People (SIS, 2002; MoNE, 2006). According to the results of this report, the total percentage of disability in the overall population was 12.29% based on the 2000 Population Census statistics. The percentage of disabled people, which included physical impairment, visual impairment, hearing impairment, speech–language impairment and mental retardation, was 2.58%, whereas 9.70% had chronic illnesses. Speech and language impairment constituted 0.38% of this number. This did not include the disorders considered secondary to other impairments. The number was even higher (0.89%) for individuals between the ages 0 and 19. The percentage of impairment types within the category was calculated as follows: 25.83% articulation and phonological disorders, 4.03% cluttering, 22.83% stuttering and 4.65% exhibit unknown and/or other types of communication disorders. These numbers were similar to those reported by a study in 1996 and 2001 (Topbaş, 2006a). However, 45.93% of those were detected as *speechless*; and what the term covers was not explicit in the demographics of SIS report. I interpret this as either children who are late talkers or do not talk due to a neurological impairment or adults having aphasia due to stroke or the like.

Staff employment and licensing issues

Currently, staffing and permanent employment in SLP is one of the main problems in both the health and education sectors. The studies reported in Topbaş (2006a), which were carried out in 25 cities of Turkey, revealed tremendous inefficiency in providing services to SLD and poor quality of service due to the shortage of SLPs. It was reported that, unlike in Europe, the United States, or even in developing countries, the treating person for SLD is not an SLP but rather other professionals who may be special education teachers, mainly teachers of the hearing impaired, psychologists, physiotherapists, child care specialists and even doctors. It appeared that intervention was offered to targeted children and/or adults who were of interest to the specialty areas of these professions. That is to say, psychologists and special educators were interested in treating stutterers, articulation impairments and/or language impairments, ENT professionals treated voice disorders and some neurologists and physical therapists worked on aphasia and related neurogenic disorders. The vast majority of direct care providers who were non-SLPs defended their positions by receiving 3–4 weeks of *in-service* training on communication disorders. Yet, the readiness to make a diagnosis and treatment of SLD was reflected in the increased willingness of other professions to provide SLD treatment (Topbaş, 2006a). A search on the internet shows that a lot of centers give SLP services although they do not have any SLPs employed. The predicted danger is that the quality of services is not measured because of the lack of a well-established auditing system in Turkey. This leads to a tremendous scope for practice and ethical issues that have arisen in the implementation of service delivery when SLPs graduate and seek rights to implement services.

In Turkey, a four-year bachelor's degree is considered as a prerequisite for licensing for occupational professionals. To give an example, to be employed as a psychologist, physiotherapist or teacher in a hospital, school or state institution, one has to graduate from a four-year program in psychology, physiotherapy or education, respectively, and have an official bachelor's degree diploma as a psychologist, physiotherapist or teacher. Since the graduate programs are optional or require specialization, positions are not yet recognized at this level.

Considering the health services, allied health professionals constitute a major proportion of the Turkish health care system. However, the professional/occupational definitions for neither SLP nor AUD were included in health policies. Consequently, hospitals cannot directly employ SLPs and AUDs according to their occupational titles but may employ them depending on their undergraduate titles as mentioned above. For example, a few SLPs who are graduates with master's degrees are currently employed in government and private hospital positions as psychologists and physiotherapists. In the educational system, the occupational definitions of SLP and AUD occur within statutory by-laws (2006) of the new special education law. The professionals who could be included in assessment teams, where they can work and their responsibilities are defined by this Regulation. Accordingly, the special education and rehabilitation institutions were obliged to employ an SLP for the provision of SLP services. However, the shortage of SLPs in number currently creates a problem. Many of the institutions try to attract clients pretending they had SLPs, letting other personnel work as SLPs, thus maximizing profit in the sector. It is apparent that the situation may have deleterious effects related to professional ethics and scope of practice, impinging on the rights of the SLP profession. Besides, the quality and efficiency of the services given by non-SLPs are controversial. A recent analysis has shown that a total of 61 SLPs (53 graduates and 8 other SLPs holding CCC-SLP diploma from the United Kingdom and United States) and about 143 AUDs graduated by June 2008 and about 60 candidates from both disciplines are expected to treat people with all types of communication impairments (Topbaş, 2008). There are also a few Bulgarian–Turkish pedagogic speech therapists serving. Due to the scarcity of licensed SLPs and AUDs in a country of 71 million, it is unrealistic to suppose that the profession will be the primary provider of direct services in the near future. A more obtainable goal is to establish undergraduate and graduate programs and train therapists in the future (Konrot, 2004).

Implementation of services

SLP services must be prescribed by a team of medical doctors in the authorized main hospitals depending on the needs of special education, in this case SLD, and the health problem. The special needs individuals are then referred to Psychological Counseling and Guidance Centers affiliated to MoNE within each city where intervention decisions are administered by Special Needs Assessment Boards. The Board's decision in its report is the final process in referring the individuals to special education schools or centers for treatment. If medical treatment is also needed, the services are given within the hospital.

Due to the extreme shortage of staff, each SLP or AUD generally carries a heavy caseload, which consists mostly of preschool and school-age children who exhibit articulation and phonological disorders, fluency disorders, voice disorders, delayed language, specific language impairment and developmental neurogenic language disorders such as cerebral palsy. Clients are often referred by other health professionals or school teachers, or the families seek direct services themselves. One important problem noted is that a physician may not refer a non-speaking child with a developmental communication disability if the etiology is unknown, until the child is 4–5 years of age or older. Thus, functional speech disorders or language impairments with unknown etiologies such as, specific language impairment (SLI) may often go undetected. Cases of laryngectomy, aphasia and voice disorders are referred to an SLP by medical personnel. It is common in Turkey for families to take care of elderly parents; however, as SLDs are accepted as ailments of normal aging, families seldom seek therapy unless they are referred by medical doctors. Whatever be the case, families or parents cannot maintain long-lasting therapy due to many problems, the most important one being financial (Topbaş, 2006a). This was supported by the Disability Survey 2002, which showed that the lowest number of individuals receiving treatment in both health and special education systems were those in the SLD category with 32.92% (Tufan & Arun, 2006).

Assessment and therapy services

At the Department of Speech and Language Therapy, DİLKOM, comprehensive assessments and evaluation procedures are routinely conducted. Thus, candidate therapists learn how to do the procedure during their practicum period and apply their knowledge wherever they work afterwards. Assessment procedure includes taking client and family histories, formal and informal diagnostic assessment, observations and language sampling. Referrals to other professionals, such as occupational therapists and physiotherapists (physical therapists), are made when necessary. Attempts have been made to develop diagnostic and treatment protocols for this specialty area within the last few years (Topbaş, 2006a, 2007). Standardized tests for assessing both articulatory and phonological disorders, aphasia and language disorders have been developed, and some others are still in the process of adaptation and translation. Table 1.5 shows a list of examples. For example, Turkish Articulation-Phonology Test Kit has been developed by Topbaş (2004/5) in collaboration and

Table 1.5 Tests adapted or developed for assessing speech and language

Tool	*Author/s*	*Norms*
Eskisehir Speech Assessment (Eskişehir Konuşma Değerlendirme Takımı)	Özsoy (1982)	–
Ankara Articulation Test (Ankara Artikülasyon Testi-AAT)	Ege *et al.* (2004)	+
Turkish Articulation–Phonology Test (Kit) (Türkçe Sesletim-Sesbilgisi Testi-SST)	Topbaş (2004/5)	+
Test of Early Language Development (TELD-3, Hresko *et al.*, 1999*) Turkish version (Türkçe Erken Dil Gelişim Testi)*	Topbaş and Güven (2007)	+
Test of Language Development (TOLD-4, Newcomer & Hammill, 2008*) Turkish version (Türkçe Özgül Dil Bozuklukları Değerlendirme Testi)*	Topbaş *et al.* (in preparation)	Ongoing
MacArthur Communicative Inventory (CDI- Fenson) Turkish version (TİGE-Türkçe İletişim Gelişim Envanteri)	Aksu-Koç *et al.* (in preparation)	Ongoing
Preschool Language Scale (PLS-3, Zimmerman *et al.*, 2002*) Turkish version*	Yalçınkaya and Belgin (in preparation)	Ongoing
Voice Handicap Index Turkish version	Kılıç *et al.* (2008)	–
Aphasia Language Assessment Test (Afazide Dil Değerlendirme Testi-ADD)	Maviş and Toğram (2009)	+
Gülhane Aphasia Test-2 (Gülhane Afazi Testi-GAT-2)	Maviş *et al.* (2007)	+
Picture Exchange Communication System (PECS-Frost & Bondy, 2002)	Kırcaali-Iftar (2005)	N/A
Systematic Analysis of Language Transcripts – (SALT), Turkish (Version9) [Computer Software]	Acarlar *et al.* (2006)	N/A
TİFALDİ – Turkish Expressive and Receptive Language Test : Expressive Vocabulary Sub-Scale	Güven and Berument (in preparation)	Ongoing
TİFALDİ – Turkish Expressive and Receptive Language Test : Receptive Vocabulary Sub-Scale	Berument and Güven (in preparation)	+
*Maternal Behavior Rating Scale (MBRS-*Mahoney, 2008*) and Child Behavior Rating Scale (CBRS*-Mahoney & Wheedon, 1999)	Diken *et al.* (in press)	N/A
LARSP – Language Assessment, Remediation and Screening Procedure (Crystal, 1982) Turkish version	Topbaş and Ball (in preparation)	Ongoing

support from MoNE under the project titled 'Development of Education Models for Treatment and Inclusion of the Children with Speech-Language Difficulties at the Pre-school Age'. Following this, a series of in-service training has been given to the school psychologists who are responsible from testing at the Guidance and Research Centers (MoNE, 2006).

Treatment sessions are conducted either individually or in small groups depending on the nature of the problem and the individual. Several traditional and current approaches described in the literature are used in treatment. For example, in phonological disorders up to the present, the dominant intervention approach used has been articulation therapy (van Riper, 1963). In the late 1990s, a change from articulation to phonological intervention was introduced through the efforts of Topbaş (1997, 1999, 2004/2005, 2006a, 2006b; Topbaş & Konrot, 1998) based on Dodd (1995), Grunwell (1985) and Ingram (1981). Currently, the Metaphon approach (Howell & Dean, 1995), variations on Minimal Pair Therapy (Gierut, 1989; Saben & Ingham, 1991) and the Cycles Approach (Hudson, 2007) are now in the process of being researched (Topbaş, 2007a; Topbaş & Kopkallı-Yavuz, 1998). Some non-SLPs unconsciously use oral-motor-based therapy techniques to treat articulation–phonological disorders or the like. Thus, special seminars or awareness workshops are given by the professors at DİLKOM to show the negative impact of using such techniques for target disorders. More recently, small steps are being elaborated to improve Turkish mothers' interactional practices with their language-delayed children and milieu teaching strategies are practiced for early childhood impairments (Diken, 2007; Diken *et al.*, in press).

One of the priorities of the new legislation is to develop an individualized education plan (IEP) for every client. In order to achieve this goal, the first formal national individualized education curriculum has been developed very recently by a collaborative team of SLPs, audiologists, educational audiologists, teachers of the hearing impaired and staff of the ministry (MoNE, 2009). The curriculum covers articulation–phonological disorders, fluency disorders, voice disorders and language delay, and gives guidelines and procedures for implementing assessment and therapy through documenting daily or weekly logs. The curriculum program is for use by SLP and AUD professionals employed in public and/or private special education or rehabilitation centers. The program will be a useful tool for those who are working in the hospitals as well.

Professional Associations

There are two associations representing SLPs and audiologists and advocating their rights as a professional body. The Association for Audiologists, Speech and Voice Pathologists (OKSBD) established in 1995 has 115 registered members. The Association for Speech and Language Pathologists (DKBUD) was founded in 2004, with 50 registered members.

The main purposes of DKBUD are as follows:

- to provide unity and support among the members of the association,
- to enhance the field of SLDs and the profession in Turkey,
- to achieve recognition by the government,
- to promote awareness of SLDs, and
- to develop standards for competency, scope of practice, professional ethics and advocate the rights of the profession.

There is now a move to officially register with DKBUD. Professionals who completed an undergraduate degree other than SLP cannot become formal members of DKBUD; they can be related professional members but they cannot vote. Associations in Turkey cannot issue a certification for clinical practice and cannot accredit professional programs either. However, in order to train efficient therapists and convince the government to recognize the profession in the development of health policies and services, DKBUD and DİLKOM are petitioning the government. Through their collaborative efforts, the SLP profession has witnessed an increasing visibility and legitimacy and a growing acceptance of the necessity of employing SLPs in medical and educational settings. A biennial scientific conference is held separately by DKBUD and OKSBD in turn.

Two other non-profit organizations are the Professional Voice Association and The Association of Voice, Speech and Dysphagia (SKYBD). However, these non-profit bodies are formed by several groups of professions, mainly by ENT doctors, singing teachers, as well as SLPs who are interested in and work in voice science.

Working in Turkey

In order to work in Turkey as an SLP, it is not necessary to apply for a certificate that proves one's qualification as an SLP; however, foreigners need a work permit from the Ministry of Foreign Affairs MoFA (2008) and the Ministry of Internal Affairs. An SLP who wishes to work at or be a visiting professor at a university center can also apply to Fulbright (http://www.cies.org/us_scholars) in the United States or similar programs within the European Union such as ERASMUS in accordance with the procedures of the contact university. Similarly, if the foreign SLP already has a fellowship in a university in Turkey, that university may apply to TÜBİTAK (The Scientific and Technological Research Council of Turkey (http://www.tubitak.gov.tr) or Council of Higher Education for a visiting scholar supportive grant for him or her. Currently, there is no institution that is responsible for issuing certificates for SLPs and membership in a professional body is not compulsory (Topbaş, 2006a).

Bringing together the joint efforts of SLPs in Turkey with those in the European Union and the USA in sharing ideas and research in speech therapy activities may further develop the field and aid recognition for the profession.

Useful Websites

Education, Research & Training Centre for Speech and Language Pathology, http://www.dilkom.anadolu.edu.tr

Ministry of International Affairs, http://www.disisleri.gov.tr

Ministry of National Education, http://www.meb.gov.tr

Council of Higher Education of Turkey, http://www.yok.gov.tr

The Scientific and Technological Research Council of Turkey, http://www.tubitak.gov.tr

The Association for Speech and Language Pathologists, http://www.dkbud.org

Türkiye Kekemelik Birliği-Project e-OZYARDEP, http://www.kekemelik.web.tr

The Ministry of Health, http://www.saglik.gov.tr

The Association for Audiologists, Speech and Voice Pathologists, http://www.odyoloji.org.tr

Hacettepe University, ENT Department, http://www.hacettepe.kbb.edu.tr

UNICEF. At a glance: Turkey. http://www.unicef.at

Marmara University, ENT Department, http://www.tip.marmara.edu.tr/kbb

OECD, http://www.oecd.org/edu/reviews/turkey

Chapter 2

The Sound Inventory of Turkish: Consonants and Vowels

HANDAN KOPKALLI-YAVUZ

Introduction

Turkish has 29 letters in the orthography: eight vowels and 21 consonants. In Turkish, one letter corresponds to one sound. The letters and corresponding sounds represented by international phonetic alphabet (IPA) are as follows:

Vowels

Letter	a	e	ı	i	o	ö	u	ü
IPA	ʌ[1]	ɛ	ɯ[2]	i	o	œ	u	y

Consonants

Letter	b	c	ç	d	f	g	ğ	h	j	k	l
IPA	b	dʒ	tʃ	d	f	g	-	h	ʒ	k	l
Letter	m	n	p	r	s	ş	t	v	y	z	
IPA	m	n	p	ɾ	s	ʃ	t	ʋ	j	z	

For the letter 'ğ', no IPA symbol is given because there is a controversy as to which sound it represents. 'ğ' will be discussed in detail in forthcoming subsections.

Consonants

Turkish has 20 consonant phonemes (excluding 'ğ') consisting of stops, nasals, fricatives, approximants, affricates and a flap. Consonants will be discussed in terms of their manner of articulation.

Stops

Turkish uses three places of articulation for stops: bilabial /p, b/, dental/alveolar /t, d/ and velar /k, g/. The place of articulation for /t/ and /d/ is controversial in that some argue that they are dental (Banguoğlu, 1986: 44; Kornfilt, 1997: 484; Underhill, 1980: 6), while others argue that they are alveolar (Aksan, 1980: 35; Demircan, 1979: 67–68, 1996: 45; Ergenç, 1989: 21; Selen, 1979: 75). I argue that /t/ and /d/ are alveolar.

Turkish has a two-way voicing distinction: voiced and voiceless. Voiceless stops are aspirated in word-initial position (Öğüt *et al.*, 2006) and in syllable-initial position (Kopkallı, 1993; Kopkallı-Yavuz, 2000a). Both voiced and voiceless counterparts occur in all three places of articulation as in Example (1).

(1)	*Bilabial*			*Alveolar*			*Velar*	
pas	/pʌs/	'pass'	toz	/toz/	'dust'	kaz	/kʌz/	'goose'
bas	/bʌs/	'step'	doz	/doz/	'dose'	gaz	/gʌz/	'gas'

Velar stops /k/ and /g/ have palatal allophones. When the velar stops occur with front vowels, they surface as palatal stops (Selen, 1979: 85; Underhill, 1980: 8) as in Example (2).

(2)					
kaz	/kʌz/	'goose'	kez	/cɛz/	'times'
koy	/koj/	'bay'	köy	/cœj/	'village'
kır	/kɯɾ̥̌/	'country side'	kir	/cɪɾ̥̌/	'dirt'
kul	/kʊɫ/	'slave'	kül	/cyl/	'ash'
gaz	/gʌz/	'gas'	gez	/ɟɛz/	'(you) travel'
gırtlak	/gɯɾ̥̌tɫʌk/	'throat'	girmek	/ɟɪɾmɛc/	'to enter'
gut	/gʊt/	'gout'	gül	/ɟyl/	'rose'
gonca	/gondʒʌ/	'bud'	göl	/ɟœl/	'lake'

All six stops occur word and syllable initially and intervocalically. The distribution of voiced and voiceless stops within a word, however, is different. While voiceless stops occur in word-final and syllable-final positions, voiced stops cannot occur in word/syllable-final position due to a final devoicing rule (Kopkallı, 1993; Kopkallı-Yavuz, 2003c). The final devoicing rule is reflected in the orthography whereby underlyingly voiced stops are written with letters representing voiceless counterparts when they occur in word- or syllable-final position as can be seen in Example (3).

(3)

Word initial			*Intervocalic*			*Word final*		
pak	/pʌk/	'clean'	kapak	/kʌpʌk/	'cover'	sap	/sʌp/	'stalk'
bak	/bʌk/	'look'	kabak	/kʌbʌk/	'squash'		-------	
tek	/tɛc/	'single'	ata	/ʌtʌ/	'ancestor'	kat	/kʌt/	'story'
dek	/dɛc/	'until'	ada	/ʌdʌ/	'island'		-------	
kök	/cœc/	'root'	ekin	/ɛcɪn/	'crop'	sek	/sɛc/	'dry'
gök	/ɟœc/	'sky'	Ege	/ɛɟɛ/	'Aegean'		-------	

Underlyingly voiced word-final stops surface when a vocalic suffix is attached as illustrated in Example (4). The vocalic suffix changes the syllable structure of the word it attaches to whereby the voiced stop is no longer word/syllable final but becomes syllable initial. ('-' indicates morpheme boundary and '.' indicates syllable boundary.)

(4)

Underlyingly voiced			*Underlyingly voiceless*		
kap	kab-ı	ka.bı	sap	sap-ı	sa.pı
tat	tad-ı	ta.dı	kat	kat-ı	ka.tı
renk	reng-i	ren.gi	fark	fark-ı	far.kı

Nasals

Turkish has two nasal phonemes: bilabial /m/ and alveolar /n/. Both nasals occur in word/syllable-initial and word/syllable-final positions as well as intervocalically as seen in Example (5).

(5)

Bilabial			*Alveolar*		
mine	/mɪnɛ/	'enamel'	nine	/nɪnɛ/	'grandmother'
ham	/hʌm/	'raw'	han	/hʌn/	'inn'
ama	/ʌmʌ/	'but'	ana	/ʌnʌ/	'mother'

The alveolar nasal is prone to place of articulation assimilation. When followed by a velar sound, /n/ is realized as /ŋ/ as illustrated in Example (6) (Kopkallı-Yavuz, 2003a, 2003c).

(6)

denge	/dɛŋɟɛ/	'balance'
denk	/dɛŋc/	'equal'

Place of articulation assimilation is regressive in that the velar sound affects the place of articulation of the preceding nasal and not vice versa.

When /n/ is preceded by a velar sound, the alveolar nasal remains alveolar as in Example (7).

(7) tekne /tɛcnɛ/ 'sailing vessel'

Similarly, when /n/ is followed by a bilabial sound, it surfaces as /m/. In such words, with time the assimilation has been reflected in the orthography as in Example (8).

(8)			
zanbak	→	zambak	'lily'
penbe	→	pembe	'pink'
saklanbaç	→	saklambaç	'hide-and-seek'

'İstanbul' is an exception although it is pronounced as [ɪstʌmbʊɫ]. The letter 'n' is maintained in the orthography perhaps because it is a proper noun.

Fricatives

There are six fricative phonemes in Turkish. The places of articulation for the fricatives are labiodental /f/, alveolar /s, z/, palato-alveolar /ʃ, ʒ/ and glottal /h/. 'v' also occurs in Turkish and is described as a fricative in many sources (e.g. Aksan, 1980; Banguoğlu, 1986; Demircan, 1979, 1996; Ergenç, 1989; Kornfilt, 1997; Selen, 1979). Underhill (1986) states that 'v' is not a fricative, but he is not very clear about the exact description. Kopkallı-Yavuz (2000b) argues that 'v' in Turkish is an approximant. Thus, 'v' is discussed under approximants.

While voicing is distinctive in fricatives, there is a gap in different places of articulation. The labiodental and glottal fricatives have only voiceless counterparts, whereas alveolar and palato-alveolar fricatives have both voiced and voiceless counterparts as exemplified in Example (9).

(9)

Labiodental	*Alveolar*	*Palato-alveolar*	*Glottal*
fare /fʌrɛ/ 'mouse'	sor /sor̥/ 'ask'	şey /ʃɛj/ 'thing'	halı /hʌɫɯ/ 'carpet'
------	zor /zor̥/ 'difficult'	jile /ʒɪlɛ/ 'jumper'	------

Fricatives occur in different positions within a word as in Example (10). Both voiced and voiceless fricatives occur in word/syllable-initial, intervocalic and word/syllable-final positions.

(10)

Word initial			*Intervocalic*			*Word final*		
fil	/fɪl/	'elephant'	sefer	/sɛfɛr̥/	'time'	af	/ʌf/	'forgiveness'
sel	/sɛl/	'flood'	keser	/kɛsɛr̥/	'hammer'	kas	/kʌs/	'muscle'
zil	/zɪl/	'bell'	özet	/œzɛt/	'summary'	az	/ʌz/	'little'
şen	/ʃɛn/	'happy'	eşek	/ɛʃɛc/	'donkey'	kaş	/kʌʃ/	'eyebrow'

jip /ʒɪp/ 'jeep' ajan /ʌʒʌn/ 'agent' bej /beʒ/ 'beige'

hala /hʌɫʌ/ 'aunt' tahıl /tʌhɯɫ/ 'grain' sabah /sʌbʌh/ 'morning'

Although /ʒ/ occurs in different positions within a word in Turkish, the number of words containing /ʒ/ is limited.

Approximants

Turkish has three approximant /ʋ, l, j/ phonemes. Two are central approximants, labiodental /ʋ/ and palatal /j/, while one is an alveolar lateral approximant /l/.

Central approximants

Kopkallı-Yavuz (2000b) investigated the phonetic and phonological properties of Turkish 'v' in different environments in terms of position within a word (word/syllable initial, word/syllable final) and segmental context (intervocalic, before/after consonant). The findings showed that /ʋ/ in Turkish exhibits approximant properties in most environments. Fricative properties are seen only when preceded by voiceless stops and fricatives. Therefore, Kopkallı-Yavuz (2000b) concluded that 'v' in Turkish is a labiodental approximant; thus the phoneme should be represented with the IPA symbol /ʋ/. Selen (1979: 98) and Ergenç (1989: 25) also argue that 'v' is realized as [ʋ] in intervocalic position although they classify it as a fricative. Selen (1979: 98) states that 'v' becomes a 'semi-vowel', represented with [ʋ], in intervocalic position where one of the neighboring vowels is rounded. (When between two unrounded vowels however, Selen argues that 'v' is realized as a fricative /v/.) Ergenç (1989: 25), on the other hand, argues that if preceded or followed by a back vowel, /v/ may be either realized as [ʋ] or deleted.

In the same study, Kopkallı-Yavuz determined the allophones of /ʋ/. Selen (1979: 98) states that /ʋ/ is deleted when in intervocalic position, especially if one of the vowels is rounded and the other is unrounded. Sezer (1986) and van der Hulst and van der Weige (1991: 30), following Sezer (1986) have argued that /ʋ/ drops when preceded by a rounded vowel (11a) or followed by a labial consonant (11b) or a rounded vowel (11c). While /ʋ/ deletion results in vowel lengthening in Examples (11a–b), it does not in Example (11c).

(11)	a. döver	'to beat (aorist)'	/dœʋɛr̥̆/	→ [dœːɛr̥̆]
	b. sevmek	'to love (infinitive)'	/sɛʋmɛc/	→ [sɛːmɛc]
	c. tavuk	'chicken'	/tʌʋʊk/	→ [tʌʊk]

The findings reported by Kopkallı-Yavuz (2000b) showed that, although not always, /ʋ/ dropped when followed by a labial consonant more often than when followed by a non-labial consonant. The allophones of /ʋ/ are described as follows:

(12)

/ʋ/ → [v] after voiceless stops and fricatives
/ʋ/ → [∅] before labial consonants/after labial vowels
/ʋ/ → [ʋ] elsewhere

A number of researchers argue that /ʋ/ becomes /w/ in intervocalic position (Banguoğlu, 1986; Demircan, 1996; Kornfilt, 1997; Underhill, 1976). Kornflilt (1997: 485), for example, states that 'v' becomes /w/ in intervocalic position, but she does not specify the vocalic environment. The only example Kornfilt provides is *kavuk* [kawuk] 'turban', where 'v' is followed by a rounded vowel. Based on this one example, it can be assumed that the rule Kornfilt proposes is: 'v' is realized as [w] when followed by a rounded vowel. Demircan (1996: 43) argues that in vowel+/v/ sequence where the vowel is a back vowel (rounded or unrounded), 'v' is realized as /w/. Banguoğlu (1986) states that /w/ occurred as a phoneme in Old Turkish, but in Modern Turkish /w/ has been either deleted as in /suw/ → /su/ 'water' or has become /v/, /f/, or /p/ as in /sɛwmɛk/ → /sɛvmɛk/ 'to love', /juwga/ → /jufka/ 'fillo', /kœwɾyg/ → /kœpɾy/. He argues that /w/ occurs only as a 'transitional sound' in words such as /kowmʌk/ 'to repel' (Banguoğlu, 1986: 43). Underhill (1980: 4) states that 'v' becomes /w/ between 'a' and 'u'.

The debate as to the realization of /v/ as [w] in Turkish is based on impressionistic rather than phonetic evidence. In the articulation of /ʋ/ in a rounded vowel environment, there is a contact or at least an approximation between the lower teeth and upper lip. Therefore, I argue that /ʋ/ is not realized as a labiovelar central approximant in Turkish; thus [w] does not occur as one of the allophones. However, phonetic studies are needed for conclusive evidence.

The palatal central approximant /j/ in Turkish occurs in word-initial, intervocalic, and word-final positions as in Example (13).

(13)	*Word initial*			*Intervocalic*			*Word final*		
	yel	/jɛl/	'wind'	ayı	/ʌjɯ/	'bear'	ay	/ʌj/	'moon'

Sezer (1986: 231) argues that /j/ is deleted when preceded by a front vowel and followed by a sonorant or [i]. (See also Banguoğlu, 1986: 61; van der Hulst & van der Weige, 1991: 29.) As a result of /j/-deletion, the vowel preceding the /j/ lengthens. Some of the examples he provides are given in Example (14).

(14)	öyle	'thus'	[œjlɛ]	→	[œːlɛ]
	iyi	'good'	[iji]	→	[iː]
	seyret	'watch'	[sɛjɾɛt]	→	[sɛːɾɛt]

There are, however, exceptions to this rule. In the word *keyif* [cɛjɪf] 'joy', for example, /j/ is not deleted although the environment in the rule is satisfied.

Lateral approximant

The only lateral approximant within the Turkish phonemic inventory is /l/. /l/ occurs in word-initial, intervocalic and word-final positions as can be seen in Example (15).

(15)	*Word initial*	*Intervocalic*	*Word final*
	loş /loʃ/ 'dim'	çile /tʃɪlɛ/ 'wide'	sel /sɛl/ 'flood'

/l/ has two allophones: [l] and [ɫ] (Banguoğlu, 1986: 97; Demircan, 1979: 37, 1996: 53; Ergenç, 1989: 23; Kornfilt, 1997: 486; Selen, 1979: 106; Underhill, 1980: 9). [l] occurs with front vowels and in word-initial position regardless of the following vowel. [ɫ] occurs with back vowels. As illustrated in Example (16), [ɫ] does not occur in word-initial position.

(16)	*Word initial*	*Intervocalic*	*Word final*
	lütfen [lytfɛn] 'please'	elin [ɛlɪn] 'your hand'	bel [bɛl] 'waist'
	------	alın [ʌɫɯn] 'forehead'	bal [bʌɫ] 'honey'

There are unpredictable occurrences of [l] with back vowels. For example, /l/ is realized as [l] although it occurs in the back vowel environment in word-final and word-medial positions in borrowed words such as in Example (17).

(17)	a. gol	[gol]	'goal'	hal [hʌl]	'condition'
	b. emlak	[ɛmlʌk]	'real estate'	istiklal [ɪstɪclʌl]	'independence'

Kornfilt (1997: 487) argues that in words such as (17b), in which there is a front vowel in the word, even if it is not tautosyllabic, /l/ will be realized as [l] and not as [ɫ].

Flap

There are a number of different descriptions of Turkish 'r'. It is described as a trill (Demircan, 1979, 1996; Ergenç, 1989; Selen, 1979; Underhill, 1980;

Zeyrek *et al.*, 2007), tap (Kornfilt, 1997; Underhill, 1980) or flap (Kopkallı-Yavuz, 2003a; Kopkallı-Yavuz *et al.*, 2008a). (Here tap and flap are used synonymously. Although Ladefoged and Maddieson (1997: 230–232) distinguish tap and flap based on tongue movement, the distinction is not very clear. Ladefoged (1989: 60) states that '[he] can see no phonological reason for distinguishing the two'. Therefore, I use the term 'flap' based on the tongue movement distinction proposed by Ladefoged and Maddieson (1997) albeit without making any claims.)

The number and manner of allophones of 'r' are also described differently by different researchers. Selen (1979: 93–94) and Ergenç (1989: 24) argue that 'r' has three allophones: a trill word initially, a flap word medially and a fricative word finally. Zeyrek *et al.* (2007) also argue that 'r' has three allophones but the allophones they report are a voiced alveolar trill in word-initial position, a voiced alveolar tap/flap intervocalically and a voiceless alveolar tap/flap in word-final position. Underhill (1980) states that 'r' is a tap or a short trill when before a vowel, fricative when word initial or before a consonant and voiceless when word final. Demircan (1979: 75, 1986: 53), on the other hand, states that 'r' has two allophones – a trill in word-initial and word-medial positions and a voiceless fricative in word-final position. Kornfilt (1997: 484) argues that Turkish 'r' is an alveolar tap that is devoiced in word-final position and thus has two allophones. Kopkallı-Yavuz *et al.* (2008a) investigated the acoustic and articulatory correlates of 'r' in Turkish and found that 'r' is an alveolar flap (/ɾ/) with three allophones based on the position within a word. /ɾ/ is realized as a voiced fricated alveolar flap ([ɾ̌]) word initially, as a voiced alveolar flap ([ɾ]) intervocalically and as a voiceless fricated alveolar flap ([ɾ̥̌]) word finally (18).

(18)

	↗	[ɾ]	intervocalically
/ɾ/	→	[ɾ̌]	word intially
	↘	[ɾ̥̌]	word finally

Affricates

There are two affricates in Turkish: voiced /dʒ/ and voiceless /tʃ/. Both affricates are palato-alveolar (Aksan, 1980; Banguoğlu, 1986; Demircan, 1979, 1996; Ergenç, 1989; Kornfilt, 1997; Selen, 1979; Underhill, 1980). The voiced palato-alveolar affricate behaves similar to stops with respect to the final devoicing rule. While the voiceless counterpart occurs in all positions within a word, the voiced one does not occur in word/syllable-final position as illustrated in Example (19).

(19)		*Word initial*			*Intervocalic*			*Word final*
çam	/tʃʌm/	'pine tree'	açı	/ʌtʃɯ/	'angle'	saç	/sʌtʃ/	'hair'
cam	/dʒʌm/	'glass'	acı	/ʌdʒɯ/	'spicy (hot)'	---		

Soft g (ğ)

In Turkish orthography, there is a letter referred to as soft g: 'ğ'. 'ğ' occurs syllable initially and syllable finally as seen in Example (20) but never word initially.

(20) dağ 'mountain, nominative' da.ğa 'mountain, dative'

The acoustic correlates of 'ğ' are controversial. While some argue that the function of 'ğ' is to lengthen the preceding vowel (Kornflilt, 1997; Selen, 1979; Sezer, 1986; Underhill, 1980), others argue that 'ğ' is realized as a consonant (Banguoğlu, 1986; Konrot, 1981) but the phonetic correlates are not defined. Kopkallı-Yavuz *et al.* (2008b) investigated the acoustic and articulatory correlates of 'ğ'. The results of the acoustic analysis showed that there was no evidence of a segment in the spectrographic representation. The formant frequencies and transition durations and transition frequencies were similar for words with and without 'ğ'. The only difference between the word pairs with and without 'ğ' was vowel duration; the duration of vowels in words with 'ğ' was almost twice as long as words without 'ğ'. The results of the videofluroscopic analysis showed that there was some velar movement and more pharyngeal tension in words containing 'ğ', suggesting that the presence of 'ğ' causes the preceding vowel to be tense. Thus, they concluded that the function of 'ğ' is to lengthen the preceding vowel.

The consonants of Turkish are summarized in Table 2.1.

Vowels

Turkish has eight vowels. Phonologically, Turkish vowels are classified as in Table 2.2 to account for vowel harmony. Phonemically, all eight vowels are short vowels (Kornfilt, 1997: 489).

Although there is agreement about the phonological classification, there is no agreement about the phonetic classification of Turkish vowels. The height and the backness of some vowels are controversial. Selen (1979) and Ergenç (1989) describe /ɯ/ as a central vowel rather than as a back vowel and /a, ɛ, o, œ/ as low vowels. Demircan (1979, 1996) describes /ɛ, o, œ/ as mid-front vowels and /a/ as a low central vowel. Underhill (1980) also describes /a/ as a low central vowel. Kornfilt (1997) describes /a, ɛ, o, œ/ as non-high, /a, o/ as back and /ɛ, œ/ as non-back vowels.

Table 2.1 Consonant chart (phonemic) of Turkish

		Bilabial	*Labiodental*	*Alveolar*	*Palato-alveolar*	*Palatal*	*Velar*	*Glottal*
Stop		p b		t d			k g	
Nasal		m		n				
Fricative			f	s z	ʃ ʒ			h
Approximant	Central		ʋ			j		
	Lateral			l				
Flap				ɾ				
Affricate					tʃ dʒ			

Note: Where symbols appear in pairs, the one to the right represents a voiced consonant.

Table 2.2 Phonological classification of Turkish vowels

	front		*non-front*	
	–round	*+round*	*–round*	*+round*
high	i	y	ɯ	u
non-high	ɛ	œ	a	o

Aksan (1980) and Banguoğlu (1986) classify the vowels as described in Table 2.2.

The differences in phonetic classification are partly due to the limited number of studies investigating phonetic properties of Turkish vowels. Studies that investigate the acoustic correlates of vowels include those by Selen (1979), Ergenç (1989), Kopkallı-Yavuz (2001, 2003b), Kılıç (2003), Kılıç and Öğüt (2004) and Türk *et al.* (2005). The findings reported in these studies show different formant frequency values for the vowels. Thus, different researchers describe the vowels differently and use different IPA symbols to represent them. The reasons for the differences may be because the target vowels are produced in isolation (Kılıç, 2003; Türk *et al.*, 2005) or, if in context, the phonetic context is not the same or similar for all vowels (Ergenç, 1989; Selen, 1979; Türk *et al.*, 2005). Therefore, an experimental study in which the phonetic environment was the same for all the vowels was conducted to determine the acoustic properties of Turkish vowels.

Method

Subjects

Five male and two female adult native speakers of Turkish served as the subjects for this study. All seven subjects were undergraduate students (between the ages of 19 and 25) at Anadolu University. None of the subjects had a known speech and/or hearing impediment. All subjects were phonetically naïve and unaware of the purpose of the study. None had lived outside of Turkey.

Materials and design

The test words consisted of 40 words containing the eight target vowels. The criteria used in the selection of test words were the number of syllables, syllable structure and the consonantal environment (see the appendix). Thus, each of the eight vowels occurred in five different contexts as seen in Example (21).

(21)

Number of syllables	Syllable structure	Consonantal environment		
monosyllabic	closed syllable	/k_p/		
disyllabic	open syllable	/k_tVC/	and	/k_sVC/
disyllabic	closed syllable	/k_tCVC/	and	/k_sCVC/

In monosyllabic words, the target vowel was in the context of /k_p/. In disyllabic words, the first syllable differed only in the target vowel, the consonant preceding and following the target vowel being the same. The second syllable also differed in the vowel due to vowel harmony as well as the final consonant although efforts were made to minimize the differences.

The 40 words were randomized seven times, resulting in seven different lists. The words were embedded in the carrier sentence 'Lütfen ______ der misin?' (Will you please say ____ ?)

Five of the seven lists were analyzed acoustically excluding the first and the last lists. The experiment, therefore, was an 8 (vowels) × 5 (contexts) × 5 (repetitions) × 7 (subjects) experimental design. A total of 1400 tokens were analyzed.

Procedure

Subjects were given the seven randomizations and asked to familiarize themselves with the task. They were instructed to read the lists of words with normal speaking tempo in the carrier sentence. All the instructions were given in Turkish. The recordings were done in an office using TASCAM, a digital tape recorder.

Measurements

Acoustic analyses were done by using Kay Elemetrics CSL Model 4300B. Acoustic measurements were based on wide-band spectrographic and waveform representations. First, the duration of the vowel and its midpoint were determined. The midpoint of the vowel is the least affected part from the neighboring consonants. Then, the formant frequencies (F1, F2, and F3) of the vowel at midpoint were measured. The formant frequencies were determined using FFT Power Spectrum.

Results

The F1 and F2 values of the eight vowels for each token and for each subject were plotted, and for each vowel, an ellipse was drawn to fit the data as seen in Figure 2.1. F1 is a cue to the height, whereas F2 is a cue to the backness of the vowel. Oral constriction lowers F1, whereas

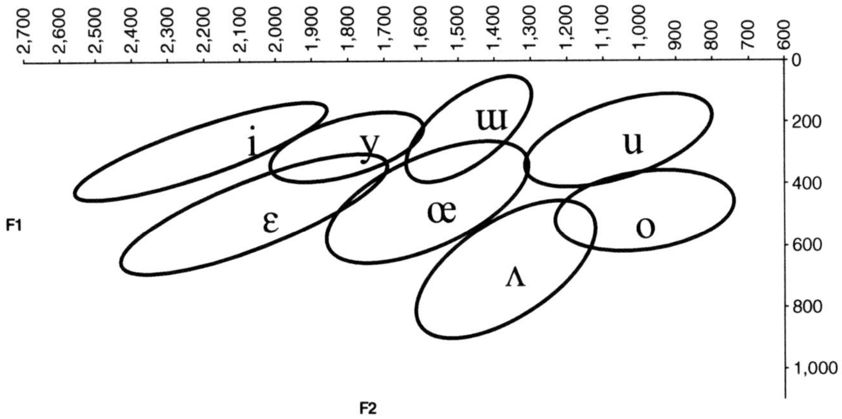

Figure 2.1 Values of F1 and F2 for the eight vowels in all the test words and for all subjects

pharyngeal constriction raises F1. Thus, high vowels have low F1 values, whereas low vowels have high F1 values. As can be seen in Figure 2.1, the F1 values for /i/, /y/, /ɯ/ and /u/ are comparable, which suggests that the heights of these vowels are similar. Again, based on the F1 values, these four vowels are found to be the highest vowels in Turkish. The F1 values for /ɛ/, /œ/ and /o/ are lower than those of high vowels but higher than that of /ʌ/, suggesting that vowels /ɛ/, /œ/ and /o/ are higher than the vowel /ʌ/.

The F2 values determine the backness of vowels. The F2 values are lowest for /u/ and /o/, suggesting that these vowels are the most back vowels in Turkish. /ɯ/ and /ʌ/ have similar F2 values, which are higher than those of /u/ and /o/, suggesting that /ɯ/ and /ʌ/ are not as back as /u/ and /o/. The F2 value for /œ/ is lower than that of /y/, suggesting that /y/ is more front than /œ/. /i/ and /ɛ/ have the highest F2 values and are thus the most front vowels of Turkish. The rounded vowels /y/ and /œ/ exhibit lower F2 values than their unrounded counterparts /i/ and /ɛ/. This is as expected because lip rounding lowers formant frequencies.

The values for F1, F2 and F3 were tabulated and the averages for each context across subjects for each vowel were calculated. Studies have shown that formant frequency values differ according to gender – the formant frequency values are higher for adult females than for adult males (Hillenbrand *et al.*, 1997; Peterson & Barney, 1952). Türk *et al.* (2005) report similar results for Turkish vowels whereby the formant frequency values are higher for women than for men. As the number of male and female subjects is not comparable in this study, the formant frequency values were not calculated separately according to gender. The overall results for each context are given in Table 2.3.

Table 2.3 Mean values of F1, F2 and F3 for each context

Vowel	*Words*	*F1*	*F2*	*F3*
/i/	kitin	235	2018	2897
	kisin	260	1976	2830
	kitler	277	2031	2964
	kistin	251	2023	2778
	kip	315	2052	2752
/y/	kütük	294	1875	2603
	küsün	292	1783	2598
	kütler	314	1830	2531
	küstün	288	1704	2564
	küp	328	1569	2333
/ɯ/	kıtır	327	1581	2719
	kısın	295	1610	2751
	kıtlık	360	1506	2752
	kıstır	308	1585	2750
	kıp	368	1223	2548
/u/	kutup	305	1230	2667
	kusun	298	1234	2637
	kutlar	358	1169	2713
	kustun	312	1247	2717
	kup	317	954	2348
/ɛ/	keten	435	1922	2818
	kesen	439	1868	2837
	ketler	467	1928	2821
	kestin	394	2011	2860
	kep	497	1904	2747
/œ/	kötek	404	1609	2544
	kösen	413	1548	2625
	kötler	441	1527	2523
	köstek	430	1504	2607
	köp	492	1420	2428

(*Continued*)

Table 2.3 *Continued*

Vowel	**Words**	*F1*	*F2*	*F3*
/o/	koton	430	1066	2701
	kosan	433	1090	2740
	kotlar	486	1059	2756
	kostak	459	1061	2588
	kop	535	1012	2658
/ʌ/	katar	644	1451	2771
	kasan	614	1406	2823
	katlar	660	1274	2670
	kastın	652	1287	2802
	kap	716	1294	2596

As seen in Table 2.3, the average values for formant frequencies across disyllabic contexts are comparable. The average F1 values for monosyllabic words are, in general, higher than those of disyllabic words and the F2 values are lower for monosyllabic words than for disyllabic words. As the purpose of this study is to determine the acoustic properties of Turkish vowels, independent of context, the averages of the F1, F2 and F3 values across the five contexts and subjects were calculated for each vowel. The averages are presented in Table 2.4.

The average F1, F2 and F3 values for each vowel across different contexts and subjects are presented schematically in Figure 2.2.

Table 2.4 Average formant frequency values for the eight vowels

Vowel	*F1*	*F2*	*F3*
/i/	276	2025	2829
/y/	307	1719	2493
/ɯ/	338	1455	2678
/u/	318	1031	2571
/ɛ/	455	1923	2805
/œ/	445	1505	2526
/o/	479	1050	2684
/ʌ/	667	1334	2710

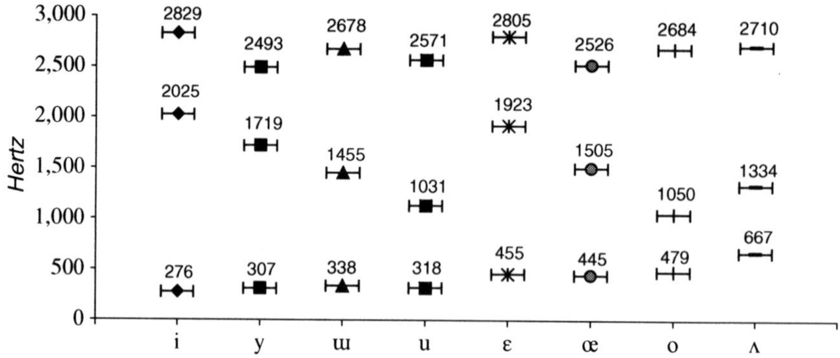

Figure 2.2 The average F1, F2 and F3 values for the eight Turkish vowels

As seen in Figure 2.2, /i/ has the lowest F1 (276 Hz) and the highest F2 (2025 Hz) among the eight vowels and thus is the highest and most front vowel in Turkish. /y/ has a higher F1 (307 Hz) and lower F2 (1719 Hz) relative to /i/; this is as expected because lip rounding lowers formant frequencies and /y/ is the rounded counterpart of /i/. The F1 value for /ɯ/ is low at 338 Hz, suggesting that it is a high vowel. The F2 value for the same vowel is at 1455 Hz, lower than both /i/ and /y/, suggesting that it is further back than these two vowels. The F1 and F2 values (318 and 1031 Hz, respectively) of /u/ are similar to those of /ɯ/, suggesting that /u/ is also a high back vowel. The F1 values rise as vowels lower. The F1 value for /ɛ/ is 455 Hz, suggesting that /ɛ/ is lower than /i/, /y/, /ɯ/ and /u/. The F2 value for the same vowel is high at 1923 Hz, suggesting that it is a front vowel. /œ/, being the rounded counterpart of /ɛ/, has lower F1 and F2 values than that of /ɛ/ at 445 and 1505 Hz, respectively. /o/ also exhibits a similar F1 value to that of /ɛ/ and /œ/ at 479 Hz, suggesting that the heights of the three vowels are similar. The F2 value for /o/, however, is lower (1050 Hz). Thus it is the furthest back of the three vowels. Among the eight vowels, /ʌ/ has the highest F1 value (667 Hz) and thus is the lowest vowel in Turkish. The F2 value (1334 Hz) is higher than that of /o/, suggesting that /ʌ/ is more front than /o/.

The positions of the vowels based on F1 and F2 values are seen in Figure 2.3. Among the eight vowels, /i/, /y/, /ɯ/ and /u/ are the highest vowels. /ɛ/, /œ/ and /o/ are lower than those vowels. Thus they are mid vowels. /ʌ/ is the lowest vowel in Turkish but the F1 value suggests that it is not a low vowel, but rather a mid vowel. In the backness dimension, /i/ and /ɛ/ are the most front vowels. /œ/ is further back than /y/. /ɯ/ is similar to /œ/ in terms of backness, although /ɯ/ is further back than /œ/. /ʌ/ is further back than /ɯ/ and /œ/. The most back vowels are /u/ and /o/, with /o/ being the most back.

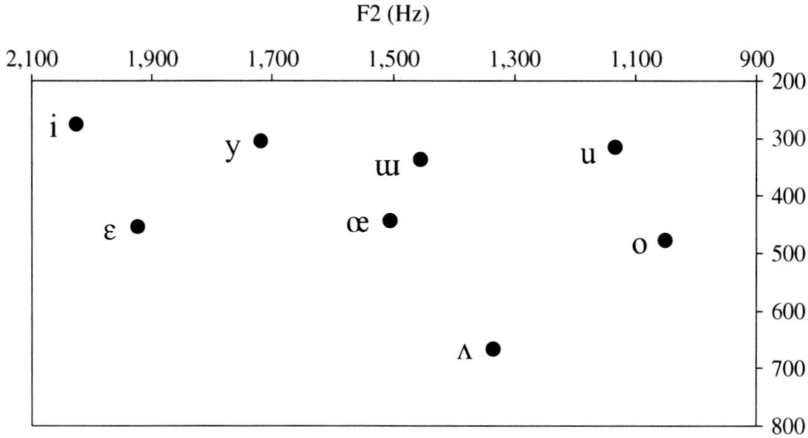

Figure 2.3 Average formant values of Turkish vowels plotted on F1 by F2

Discussion

The findings of this study are compared with those of Selen (1979), Ergenç (1989), Kılıç (2003) and Türk *et al.* (2005). Table 2.5 presents the F1 values reported in different studies.

When the F1 values are compared across studies, the relative height of the vowels shows a difference. Based on the F1 values reported in Selen (1979), /y/ is the highest vowel, followed by /ɯ/, which in turn is followed by /œ/, /ɛ/, /i/ and /u/, all with the same F1 value. The F1 value for /ʌ/ is lower than /o/, suggesting that /ʌ/ is higher than /o/. The order of the vowels from highest to lowest can be summarized as follows: /y/>/ɯ/>/œ/, /ɛ/, /i/, /u/>/ʌ/>/o/. Ergenç (1989) reports two or three F1 values for the vowels based on the position within the word. For five of the vowels, there are two different values as F1 values are reported to be the same in the two contexts. For the remaining three vowels for which there are three F1 values, the lowest and the highest values are given in Table 2.5. The vowels follow a different height order in the study by Ergenç (1989), whereby /i/, /y/, /ɯ/ and /œ/ exhibit the lowest F1 values, suggesting that they are the highest vowels. /ɛ/, /o/ and /u/, with similar F1 values, exhibit a higher F1 value than /i/, /y/, /ɯ/ and /œ/. /ʌ/ has the highest F1 value and is thus the lowest vowel in Turkish. Based on the F1 value (560–600 Hz) reported in the study, however, /ʌ/ cannot be considered a low vowel. The order of the highest to lowest vowels is as follows: /i/, /y/, /ɯ/, /œ/>/ɛ/, /o/, /u/ > /ʌ/.

Based on the findings reported by Kılıç (2003), /i/ and /y/, with almost the same F1 values, are the highest vowels that are followed by /u/. /ɯ/

Table 2.5 F1 values of the eight Turkish vowels reported in different studies

Vowel	*Selen (1979) (Hz)*	*Ergenç (1989)*	*Kılıç (2003) (Hz)*	*Türk et al. (2005)*				*Kopkallı-Yavuz*
				Male		*Female*		
				Isol.	*Cont.*	*Isol.*	*Cont.*	
/i/	400	320–360	278	286	347	423	511	276
/y/	280	320–360	279	372	372	433	433	307
/ɯ/	320	320–400	355	537	537	839	839	338
/u/	400	400–480	295	310	323	477	546	318
/ɛ/	400	400–600	526	486	486	518	508	455
/œ/	400	320–400	427	544	527	523	506	445
/o/	1200	400–440	432	468	468	516	585	479
/ʌ/	800	560–600	664	629	596	778	698	667

also has a relatively low F1, suggesting that it is a high vowel. /œ/ and /o/ have comparable F1 values; thus the height of these two vowels are the same, but /ɛ/, with a higher F1 value, is lower than /œ/ and /o/. As in Ergenç (1989), /ʌ/ is the lowest vowel among the eight vowels.

Türk *et al.* (2005) investigated each vowel produced in isolation and within a word and/or sentence. The results are reported separately for male and female subjects as well as in isolation and context. (Türk *et al.* also included children in their investigation but the results are not reported here.) Based on the relative F1 values, the height order for adult males is the same in both isolation and context although values differ. The order of F1 values from lowest to highest, thus from high to low vowels, is as follows: /i/>/ɛ/>/y/>/ɯ/>/œ/>/ʌ/>/o/>/u/. The order, however, is different for adult females and according to whether the vowels are in isolation or in context. When in isolation, the vowel height order for females is as follows: /i/>/ɯ/>/y/>/ɛ/>/ʌ/>/œ/>/u/>/o/. When in context, the order is as follows: /y/>/œ/>/ɛ/>/i/>/u/>/o/>/ʌ/>/ɯ/.

F2 values, a cue to the backness of vowels, reported in different studies are presented in Table 2.6. Although the F2 values show differences across studies, the relative backness of the vowels show similarities. Based on relative F2 values, Ergenç (1989) and Kılıç (2003) exhibit the same order of backness of the vowels as in this study. From front to back, the order is as follows: /i/>/ɛ/>/y/>/œ/>/ɯ/>/ʌ/>/o/>/u/. The order in Selen (1979) is different and unexpected: /o/>/ɯ/>/ɛ/>/y/>/œ/>/ʌ/>/i/>

Table 2.6 F2 values of the eight Turkish vowels reported in different studies

Vowel	*Selen (1979) (Hz)*	*Ergenç (1989)*	*Kılıç (2003) (Hz)*	*Türk et al. (2005)*				*Kopkallı -Yavuz*
				Male		*Female*		
				Isol.	*Cont.*	*Isol.*	*Cont.*	
/i/	1200	2600–2840	2275	2178	2079	2078	1990	2025
/y/	1700	1560–1880	1715	1633	1633	1729	1729	1719
/ɯ/	2000	1360–1480	1482	1578	1577	1798	1798	1455
/u/	800	800–1120	786	909	955	1192	1292	1031
/ɛ/	1800	1800–2200	1772	1834	1834	1472	1476	1923
/œ/	1400	1440–1520	1548	1517	1526	1220	1222	1505
/o/	2800	1120–1680	811	1065	1065	983	1110	1050
/ʌ/	1400	1360–1520	1081	1259	1382	1415	1464	1334

/u/. In Türk *et al.* (2005), the order of backness differs for male and female subjects as well as for vowels in isolation and in context. For males, the order is as follows: /i/>/ɛ/>/y/>/œ/>/ɯ/>/ʌ/>/o/>/u/ in both contexts, which is the same as the order in this study. For females, vowels in isolation and in context follow a similar order with a difference only in the order of /œ/ and /u/: /i/>/ɯ/>/y/>/ɛ/>/ʌ/>/œ/>/u/>/o/.

There are differences in the F1 and F2 values across studies but there are also similarities. The differences are more evident when the numbers of subjects and tokens are limited as in the studies by Selen (1979) and Ergenç (1989). The study by Selen (1979) had one male and one female subject and each of them was asked to say the words containing the target vowel. As the word list is not given, the environment in which the target vowel occurred is not clear. Ergenç (1989) does not report the number of subjects or repetitions. The target vowels occurred in different positions within a word but the phonetic environments were not considered. The numbers of subjects are increased in Kılıç (2003) and Türk *et al.* (2005), but the contexts in which the target vowels occurred are not comparable across test words. In both studies, the target vowels were produced as isolated sounds – a form not found in natural speech. Nonetheless, as the number of subjects and repetitions of the test words as well as the variety of contexts increase, and when the phonetic contexts are controlled for, the formant frequency values become more comparable. This suggests that the differences in the formant frequency values are due to experimental design.

Conclusion

Based on the findings reported here, Turkish vowels can be classified phonetically as follows. In the height dimension, three levels appear. /i/, /y/, /ɯ/ and /u/ are high vowels with similar F1 values. /ɛ/, /œ/ and /o/ are lower than /i/, /y/, /ɯ/ and /u/ as they have higher F1 values, and /ʌ/ is lower than all the other vowels, with the highest F1 value. /ʌ/, however, cannot be considered a low vowel as the F1 is at 667 Hz. In a study investigating the phonetic properties of Turkish /ʌ/, Kopkallı-Yavuz (2001) also concluded that /ʌ/ in Turkish is an open mid vowel with an F1 at 678 Hz. Therefore, Turkish vowels can be classified into three height levels; /i/, /j/, /ɯ/ and /u/ being high vowels, /ɛ/, /œ/ and /o/ being close-mid vowels, and /ʌ/ being an open-mid vowel.

In the backness dimension, there seems to be a continuum. The F2 value is highest for /i/ at 2025 Hz (suggesting that /i/ is the most front vowel) and lowest for /u/ at 1031 Hz (suggesting that /u/ is the most back vowel). The F2 values from the highest to lowest are /i/>/ɛ/>/y/>/œ/> /ɯ/>/ʌ/>/o/>/u/. /i/ and /ɛ/ are the most front vowels. /y/ is not as front as /i/ but not as back as /œ/. /œ/, /ɯ/ and /ʌ/ are toward the central, and /o/ and /u/ are the most back vowels.

Kılıç and Öğüt (2004) investigated the properties of /ɯ/ to determine whether it is a central or back vowel and found that the average F1 value is 355 Hz and the average F2 value is 1482 Hz. Given the F2 value at 1482 Hz, /ɯ/ is between central and back vowels. When its F2 value is compared to that of /u/, /u/ has a lower F2 value but this is as expected because lip rounding lowers formant frequencies. Thus, they concluded that /ɯ/ should be treated as a back vowel.

The vowel diagram for Turkish, based on the findings of the study presented here, is shown in Figure 2.4.

As seen in Figure 2.4, the vowels /œ/ and /ɯ/ are more centralized than /ɛ/ and /u/. One reason for the tendency to centralize may be that there are no phonemes in that area; thus the movement does not result in a meaning difference. Also, the relative positions of the vowels are more

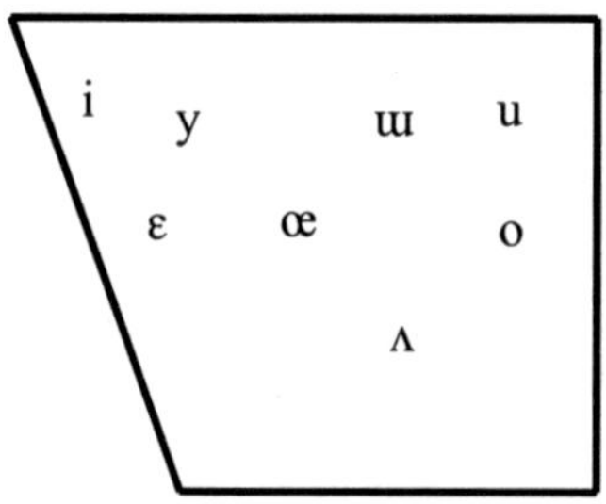

Figure 2.4 Turkish vowels

important than absolute values. Therefore, based on F1 and F2 values, Turkish vowels are classified as follows:

High vowels:	/i/, /y/, /u/, /ɯ/
Mid vowels:	close-mid /ɛ/, /œ/, /o/ open-mid /ʌ/
Front vowels:	/i/, /y/, /ɛ/, /œ/
Back vowels:	/u/, /ɯ/, /o/, /ʌ/

Concluding Remarks

This chapter presented the consonants and vowels of Turkish. The number of studies investigating the phonetic properties of Turkish, although limited at the moment, is increasing. The findings of such studies provide an insight into the characteristics of Turkish sounds. The conclusions drawn here are based on the studies available at the moment. As the number of acoustic studies increases, the properties of Turkish sounds will become more accurate.

Notes

1. This vowel has also often been transcribed as /a/ (see Chapter 2).
2. This vowel has also been transcribed as /ɨ/.

Appendix

Test words

Monosyllabic
/k_p/
1. kap
2. kep
3. kip
4. kıp
5. kop
6. köp
7. kup
8. küp

disyllabic:open
/k_tVC/
9. katar
10. keten
11. kitin
12. kıtır
13. koton
14. kötek
15. kutup
16. kütük

disyllabic:open
/k_sVC/
17. kasan
18. kesen
19. kisin
20. kısın
21. kosan
22. kösen
23. kusun
24. küsün

disyllabic:closed
/k_tCVC/
25. katlar
26. ketler
27. kitler
28. kıtlık
29. kotlar
30. kötler
31. kutlar
32. kütlen

disyllabic:closed
/k_sCVC/
33. kastın
34. kestin
35. kistin
36. kıstır
37. kostak
38. köstek
39. kustun
40. küstün

Chapter 3

Some Structural Characteristics of Turkish

MEHMET YAVAŞ

General

Turkish belongs to the Southwestern subgroup of Turkic languages, which are part of a larger Altaic language family. It is the official language of Turkey and is one of the official languages of Cyprus. It is also spoken by Turkish-speaking minorities in countries that formerly belonged (in whole or in part) to the Ottoman Empire, such as Bulgaria, Greece, Macedonia, Romania and Serbia. Additionally, a significant number of Turkish speakers (mainly *guestworkers*) are found in several European countries, such as Germany, France, the Netherlands, Switzerland, Austria, Belgium and the United Kingdom.

The Turks of Anatolia originally came from central Asia. Starting from the 10th century, with the spread of Islam among Turks, Turkish vocabulary was influenced considerably by Arabic and Persian words. The 15th and 16th centuries show the climactic example of Arabic and Persian influences via 'Divan literature', whose sole purpose was to serve the elite. This tendency also quickly influenced the folk literature and also spread into the scientific writings in the 16th century. The prestige and dominance of Arabic and Persian vocabulary continued uninterruptedly until the second half of the 19th century, when the 'Beneficial Reforms' of Sultan Abdulmejid introduced a shift from Islamic cultures to Western cultures. While this movement stopped new imports from Arabic and Persian, it introduced many French words as a result of contact with the Western world. Although the year 1908 (the beginning of the nationalistic 'Young Turk' movement) is frequently cited as the beginning of the conscious effort to replace foreign vocabulary with native Turkish words, the most intensive efforts in this domain were launched after the proclamation of the Turkish Republic in 1923. Turkish was written in the Arabic script until the Latin script was adopted via the writing reform of 1928. This was one of the reforms introduced after the establishment of the Turkish Republic.

What follows in this chapter is a brief account of some of the structural characteristics of Turkish phonology, morphology and syntax.

Phonology

In this section, we will describe certain aspects of Turkish phonology that were not dealt with in Chapter 2. Specifically, we will look at syllable structure, stress and vowel harmony.

Syllable structure

The syllable structure of Turkish can be described as (C) V (C) (C), because the vowel nucleus is the only obligatory element. There are no onset clusters. Borrowings with initial consonant clusters are broken up by an epenthetic high vowel, which is in agreement with the following vowel in backness and rounding (e.g. [gurup] 'group' and [tirɛn] 'train').

Certain double codas, which can be described in the following way, are allowed.

(1) Sonorant C + obstruent (e.g. [faɾk] 'difference' and [ilk] 'first')
(2) Voiceless fricative + stop (e.g. [tʃift] 'couple' and [yst] 'top')

An additional minor pattern (from borrowings) can be observed in a combination of ks#, as in [boks] 'box'.

Sequences of two consonants that are not tautosyllabic, which are permissible in Turkish, have to split up into different syllables following the maximum onset principle (Clements & Keyser, 1983), as in [san.ki] 'as if', [sal.kɯm] 'bunch/cluster' and so on. By the same token, an intervocalic consonant is always assigned to the following syllable and there is no question of ambisyllabicity (e.g. [sa.kat] 'injured' and [ka.lɛm] 'pencil').

Stress

Turkish is said to be a syllable-timed language in that all syllables, stressed or unstressed, have more or less equal duration. Stress, which has the phonetic correlates of loudness and higher pitch in Turkish, in general, falls on the last syllable. The weight of the syllable is irrelevant for the stress; the final stressed syllable can be light (i.e. open syllable with no coda) as in [a.ɾa.bá] 'car' or heavy (i.e. closed with a coda) as in [ka.pák] 'lid'. Suffixation does not affect this pattern either, and the final stress continues on words with a stem combined with suffixes (e.g. [a.ɾa.ba.já] 'to the car', [a.ɾa.ba.mɯ.zá] 'to our car' and [a.ɾa.ba.la.ɾɯ.mɯ.zá] 'to our cars').

However, there are a number of exceptions to the final stress rule. Place names constitute the most significant group (Sezer, 1991). In such words, stress falls on the penultimate syllable (syllable before the last) as in [is. tám.bul], [sám.sun], [an.tál.ja] and [va.ʃíŋk.ton]. If the penultimate syllable is light and the antepenultimate syllable is heavy, then the stress falls on the antepenult (e.g. [áŋ.ka.ɾa] and [ɛ́ɾ.zu.ɾum]). If, on the other hand, both the penult and the antepenult are light, the stress falls on the default that is the penult, as in [a.dá.na], [gi.ɾɛ́.sun] and [ka.ná.da]. Besides place names, the final stress rule is violated in many (but not all) adverbs (e.g. [já.zɯn] 'in summer' and [hɛ́.mɛn] 'right now'), in interjections and vocatives (e.g. [háj.di] 'let's, come on') and in reduplication (e.g. [tɛmíz] 'clean'→[tɛ́ɾtɛmiz] 'very clean' and [kojú] 'dark' [kópkoju] 'very dark').

In compounds, the first element retains its stress, while the second element loses its stress (e.g. [báʃkent] 'capital' (from [baʃ] 'head' and [kɛnt] 'city'), [kytʃýkdil] 'uvula' (from [kytʃýk] 'small' and [dil] 'tongue').

Vowel harmony

Although eight Turkish vowels have, phonetically, three degrees of height (high, mid and low), phonologically, the system is usually defined with two degrees of height, as shown in the following matrix:

	a	*ɛ*	*o*	*œ*	*u*	*y*	*ɯ*	*i*
Back	+	–	+	–	+	–	+	–
High	–	–	–	–	+	+	+	+
Round	–	–	+	+	+	+	–	–

Traditionally, a rule of vowel harmony makes all vowels in the same phonological word agree in the feature [back], whereas another rule applies only to high vowels making them agree in rounding. The two rules are sometimes written in the following collapsed form and apply iteratively left to right:

$$\begin{bmatrix} +\text{syl} \\ \langle +\text{high} \rangle \end{bmatrix} \rightarrow \begin{bmatrix} \alpha\text{back} \\ \langle \beta\text{round} \rangle \end{bmatrix} \Big/ \begin{bmatrix} +\text{syl} \\ \alpha\text{back} \\ \langle \beta\text{round} \rangle \end{bmatrix} \; C_0 \_\_\_\_$$

(is assimilated to the backness of the previous vowel irrespective of the number of intervening consonants, and in addition, a high vowel also assimilates to the rounding of the previous vowel).

The harmony rule is strong in native stems but has many exceptions due to numerous borrowings from the several languages mentioned in the introduction. The following common words make this point well: [ʃɛftali] 'peach', [fiyat] 'price', [kalɛm] 'pencil' and [inat] 'obstinacy'.

On the other hand, the rule is very productive in suffixes.

[okul – lar - ɯn - ɯz – dan] 'from your school'
school-plu.-pos.-your-from
[gɛl - ɛ - mɛ – miʃ – ti – k] 'we hadn't been able to come'
come-be able-neg.-perf.-past-we
[oyun – dʒu- mu – sun]? 'Are you a player?'
play - er- quest.- you

As we see, a word generally contains only vowels with the same value in the feature [back]. Also, a high vowel in the non-initial syllable has the same value in the feature [round] as that of the preceding syllable. If the vowel is not [high], then the only assimilation it will undergo is in backness, as demonstrated in the first example above. The plural ending *–lEr*[1] (lɛr/lar) with its non-high vowel follows the harmony only in backness, not in rounding. In such a situation, that is, when a non-round vowel follows a round vowel, all vowels following the non-round vowel will be non-round, regardless of their height.

Although the suffix harmony in backness is very strong, it is not exceptionless. The progressive marker *–Iyor* has the harmonizing first vowel 'I' (high vowel) followed by the non-alternating second vowel, which can create violations to the backness harmony, as in [gel-iyor-um] 'I am coming'; the word has two initial front vowels followed by two back vowels. The non-alternating /o/ creates its own harmony for the following vowels:

[gɛl – mi – yor – mu – sun]? 'Aren't you coming?'
come-neg.-prog.-ques.-you
[gɛl – mi – yor – lar – mɯ]? 'Aren't they coming?'
come – neg – prog – 3rdpl – ques

In the first example, the non-alternating /o/ is followed by the two high vowels of the 'interrogative' and 'second singular' endings, which harmonize with /o/ both in backness and in rounding. In the second example, the 'plural' ending has a non-high vowel and thus harmonizes with /o/ only in backness. The last suffix, 'interrogative', has a high vowel and harmonizes with the previous 'plural' vowel both in backness and in rounding.

There are some other apparent violations to the harmony in backness that are explainable through consonantal influence. These are manifested when a stem-final palatal lateral (clear-l) unpredictably follows a tautosyllabic back vowel. In such cases, the suffix harmony is regulated by the consonant rather than the stem-final vowel. See

[hol] 'hall' → [hol – y – myz - yn] 'of our hall'
Hall- acc.- our – of
as compared to [ampul - lɛɾ - imiz - dɛn] 'from our lamps'
lamp – plu.- our – from

Although traditional harmony is progressive (i.e. left-to-right), some instances of borrowing assimilations with double onsets reveal a regressive (right-to-left) harmony too. As mentioned earlier, Turkish does not have initial clusters and inserts an epenthetic vowel to break the disallowed double onset in the borrowings: [pɯɾoʒɛ] 'project' (from French *projet* [prɔʒe]) and [fiɾɛn] 'brake' (from French *frein* [frɛ]). In these examples, the epenthetic vowel harmonizes regressively with the second vowel (the original first vowel of the borrowing). However, there are other instances where this is not the case: [pilaʒ] 'beach' (from French *plage* [plaʒ]) and [pilatin] 'platinum' (from French *platine* [platin]). Such examples all have the palatal lateral as the second consonant, which determines the backness of the epenthetic vowel.[2]

Morphology

Turkish is one of the best examples of an agglutinating language. It is basically a suffixing language with one exceptional prefix (reduplication).

Derivational suffixes, as expected, are closer to the root than inflectional suffixes. Among the suffixes that derive nominals, the ones that attach to verbal stems come before the ones that attach to nominal stems.

The sequences of nominal inflectional suffixes, which follow derivational morphemes, start with the plural marker -lEɾ: *giriş-**ler***[3] (enter+act. n+pl) 'entrances' and *kuş-**lar*** (bird + pl.) 'birds'. After the plural, we have the agreement suffixes that express the person and number of their possessors and thus are sometimes called 'possessive' suffixes. Case morphemes come last in this category. The following is a brief account of the cases in Turkish. The *Nominative*, which does not require any elaboration, is not marked overtly.

The *Accusative* (or objective) ending *–(y)I* is used if a definite noun is the object of the verb. It is not used if the object is indefinite. The contrast can be shown in the following:

Ahmet mektup yaz-dı 'Ahmet wrote a letter' versus Ahmet mektub-**u** yazdı 'Ahmet wrote the letter'.

The *Dative* case suffix *-(y)E* indicates

(1) the place to or toward which the motion is directed.
Ahmet Istanbul-**a** gitti 'Ahmet went to Istanbul'
Ahmet Istanbul-to go-past
(2) the person (or thing) to or for whom the action is directed (i.e. English indirect object).
Kuş - **a** yem ver –di -m 'I gave food to the bird'
(bird-to food give-past-1st sg.)

In addition to these, some Turkish intransitive verbs (e.g. *başlamak* 'to start' and *bakmak* 'to look') take the dative.

Ders-**e** erken başla-dı-m 'I started the lesson early'
Lesson-to early start-past-1st sg.

Ablative case suffix *–DEn*, which corresponds to English 'from', indicates

(1) The place from which motion proceeds
Ahmet Izmir-**den** dön - dü 'Ahmet returned from Izmir'
from return-past

(2) The person (or thing) from whom the action proceeds.
Mektub-u Ahmet-**ten** al-dı-m 'I took (got) the letter from Ahmet'
Letter-acc. Ahmet-from take-past-1st sg.

Locative suffix *–DE* indicates the place at which an action occurs, or the place at, in or on which an object is located.

Araba ev – in ön – ün – **de** dur - du 'The car stopped in front of the house'
Car house-gen. front-of-loc. stop-past

In the string of verbal suffixes, the first one after verb is *voice*. In this group, we have the *reciprocal –(I)ş* (*yaz-**ış**-tı-k* 'we wrote to each other'), the *passive –Il/n* (*-Il* after consonants, -and *–n* after vowels) *yaz-**ıl**-dı* 'it was written' and the *causative –Dir/t* (*t* is added after polysyllabic stems ending in a vowel or a liquid) *yap-**tır**-dı-k* (do-caus.past-3rd pl.) 'we caused it to be done'. There are some co-occurrence and/or ordering statements to be made in relation to these suffixes. The reflexive and the reciprocal cannot co-occur. The passive can co-occur with either one of these voices, and when it does, it has to follow them.

gör- **üş** – **ül** – dü 'It was negotiated'
see-recip.-pas.-past

The causative can co-occur with the passive and precedes it.

aç – **tır** – **ıl** – dı 'It was made to be opened'
open– caus.-pas.- past

The causative can (rarely) co-occur with the reciprocal, and in such cases, it will follow it.

iki taraf – ı gör- **üş** – **tür** – dük 'We had the two sides negotiated'
two side-acc. see-recip-caus-3rd pl.

The suffixes of *voice* can be followed by the verbal negation marker *–mE*, which is unstressed (even in final position) and moves the stress to the preceding syllable, as in *konuş-**ma*** 'don't talk'. This suffix is followed by *mood* markers. These are the *desiderative –sE*, (e.g. *konuş-ma-**sa*** 'wish s/he doesn't speak'), the *necessitative -mEll* (e.g. *konuş-ma-**malı*** 's/he must not speak') and the *optative -y(E)*(e.g. gid-*e*-yim 'let me go'). These suffixes are mutually exclusive.

Five *tense* suffixes are next in order. These are the *progressive*, the *future*, the *present* (aorist), the *definite past* and the *narrative past*.

The *progressive*, which is marked by suffix *–(I)yor*, is used when the subject is in the process of performing some action or when the action is going on at the time of the utterance.

Hasan mektup yaz-**ıyor** 'Hasan is writing a letter'
letter write-prog.

As mentioned in the section on phonology, *-Iyor* is a non-harmonic suffix in that the second vowel *o* does not change (the first vowel, I, changes). When another suffix follows the progressive, it harmonizes with *o*.

The suffix *–EcEk* marks the future tense. When the verb stem ends in a vowel, this suffix is preceded by a *y*, linking consonant, which has the effect of raising the preceding vowel.

dön-me–di–ler 'they didn't return' BUT dön-mi–**yecek**–ler 'they are not going to return'
return-neg.-past-3rd pl. return-neg.-fut.- 3rd pl.

Note that the vowel raised because of *y* is not subject to high vowel rounding harmony, and thus the form does not become *dönmüyecek* [dœnmyjɛdʒɛk].

The *present* (aorist) tense, which is used to indicate the habitual, or repeated actions, or to make statements regarding timeless truths, uses two endings: *-(I)r* or *–(E)r*. *–Er* is used with monosyllabic verbs that do not end in a liquid:

git-mek 'to go' gid-**er** 's/he goes' uç-mak 'to fly' uç-**ar** 's/he flies'

-Ir is used with verbs of more than one syllable:

çalış-mak 'to work' çalış-**ır** 's/he works' ısır-mak 'to bite' ısır-**ır** 's/he bites'

And it is also used as well with monosyllabic verbs that end in a liquid:

gel-mek 'to come' gel-**ir** 's/he comes' var-mak 'to arrive' var-**ır** 's/he arrives'

There are some exceptions to this last generalization, as *gir-mek* 'to enter' becomes *gir**er*** (not *girir*) and *gül-mek* 'to smile' becomes *gül**er*** (not *gül**ür***).

If the verb ends in a vowel, the E or I of the suffix is dropped, and the ending is *–r.*

oku-mak 'to read' becomes *oku-r* 's/he reads'.

Turkish has two past tenses. The suffix ***–DI*** is used for the *definite past tense*, and ***–mIş*** is used for the *narrative (reported) past tense.*

Ahmet dün Istanbul-dan gel-**di** 'Ahmet came from Istanbul yesterday'
yesterday from come-past
Ahmet dün Istanbul-dan gel-**miş** 'Ahmet reportedly came from Istanbul yesterday'
yesterday -from come-nar.past

In *–DI* past, we have the commitment of the speaker, whereas in *–mIş* past this is not so; the implication is that whatever is stated has been reported to the speaker. These two past tenses are sometimes known as 'witnessed' versus 'unwitnessed' past tenses.

Although, in general, only one *tense* or *mood* marker can occur at a time, there are instances where two tense markers (or a tense marker and a mood marker) can co-occur.

yürüyüş-üm-e başla-**yacak-tı**-m 'I was going to start my walk'
walk- pos.-dat. Start-**fut.-past**-1st sg.
ders – i bitir – me – **mel**iy – **di** - n 'you shouldn't have finished the lesson'
lesson-acc. finish-neg.-necess.-past-2nd sg.

Agreement markers that indicate the agreement of the verbal or nominal head of a construction with its subject in terms of person and number are as follows:

	1st sg.	2nd sg.	3rd sg.	1st pl.	2nd pl.	3rd pl.
Nominal	-(I)m	-(I)n	-(s)I(n)	-(I)mIz	-(I)nIz	-lErI(n)
Verbal	-Im	-sIn	∅	-Iz	-sInIz	-lEr

The suffix-initial vowels in parentheses are used only after stems ending in consonants; the suffix-initial consonant in parenthesis is deleted after a stem ending in consonants. The suffix-final consonant in parenthesis is deleted in word-final position.

Nominal agreement is used in

(1) a possessive noun phrase
Ahmet - **in** elbise -**si** 'Ahmet's dress'
Ahmet-gen. dress-pos.3rd sg.
In Turkish, possession is expressed by *two* suffixes. Genitive case suffix is attached to Ahmet, and the possessive suffix *(s)*I is attached to *elbise*. The possessive suffix indicates that the noun to which it is attached is possessed by some other noun.
(2) a gerundive complement
Ahmet biz – im Hasan - ı gör – düğ[4] – ümüz – ü söyle – miş
we- gen. acc. see- ger- 1st pl. – acc say – nar. Past
'Ahmet said (reportedly) that we saw Hasan'

Verbal agreement is used with

(1) a main clause predicative verb
(ben) bu kitab - ı gelecek hafta oku – yacağ - ım
I this book-acc. next week read – future- 1st sg.
(2) a main clause predicative adjective
(siz) bugün çok yorgun – sunuz 'you are very tired today'
you today very tired – 2nd pl.

The pronouns *ben, siz* can be omitted since *ım, -sunuz* indicate the person and number of the subject adequately.

Gender is not expressed in nouns or pronouns; it does not affect agreement.

Syntax

The basic word order of transitive sentences in Turkish is that of subject–object–verb. If the sentence has more than one object, and if one of them is a direct object, the order in which direct object is closer to the verb is more common.

Ahmet Ali – ye kitab – ı gönder - di 'Ahmet sent the book to Ali'
-to book-acc. send – past

Basic simple sentences are of two types:

(1) sentences with verbal predicates
adam elma ye-di 'The man ate apple(s)'
man apple eat-past

(2) sentences with non-verbal predicates. In this group, there are two possibilities:
(a) with nominal or adjectival predicates
bu kalem Ahmed-in 'This pencil is Ahmet's'
this pencil Ahmet-gen.
bu ev küçük 'This house is small'
this house small
(b) with existential predicates
bu ev - de bir köpek **var** 'There is a dog in this house'
this house-loc. one dog exist.

Sentences with verbal predicates and with non-verbal predicates maintain the distinction when embedded:

Adam – in elma – yı ye – diğ – in – i gör – dü – m
man – gen. apple-acc. eat- fact.N-gen.-pos. see – past- 1st sg.
'I saw the man eating the apple'
bu ev – in küçük ol – duğ – un – u gör – dü – m
this house-gen. small be – fact. N –gen.-pos. see-past-1st sg.
'I saw that the house is small'
bu ev – de bir köpek ol – duğ – un – u gör – dü – m
this house-loc a dog be – fact. N-gen-pos. see-past-1st sg.
'I saw that there is a dog in this house'

While sentences with verbal predicates (i.e. the first one) take the factive nominalizer suffix *-Dik*, sentences with non-verbal predicates (nominal or adjectival predicates), and those with existential predicates (as exemplified in the last two sentences), require the verb *ol-* 'be/become' when embedded.

Since the grammatical roles of the noun phrases (NPs) are made transparent via case marking, word-order variation becomes permissible. In general, the divergences from the pragmatically neutral canonical SVO order are associated with certain semantic or pragmatic distinctions. Sentence-initial position is the topic position, whereas preverbal position is the focus position. Material of importance (high information value) is found in preverbal (focus) position and is also accompanied by a major pitch change in intonation.

Ahmet mektub – u **dün** gönder – di 'Ahmet sent the letter **yesterday**'
Ahmet dün **mektub – u** gönder – di 'Ahmet sent **the letter** yesterday'
Mektub – u dün **Ahmet** gönder – di '**Ahmet** sent the letter yesterday'

One of the notable things that word order can mark is definiteness. Turkish does not have a definite article. Although accusative case marking has a definitizing effect, as shown in the section on morphology, subject NPs do not carry any case marking, and mass nouns and abstract nouns, which do not take an indefinite article, may be ambiguous between definite and indefinite readings when they are the subject of a sentence. In such cases, word order distinguishes between definite and indefinite readings of the subject.

yağmur halı – yı ıslat –tı 'The rain made the carpet wet'
rain carpet-acc. wet-past
as opposed to
halı – yı yağmur ıslat – tı 'Some rain made the carpet wet'

As we can see, the sentence-initial position gives a definite reading on a subject NP, and the preverbal position imposes an indefinite reading.

In some cases, word order signals the definite and indefinite readings for animate subjects with no number distinction.

köpek bahçe – de uyu – yor 'The dog is sleeping in the garden'
dog garden-loc. sleep-prog.
contrasting with
bahçe – de köpek uyu – yor 'A/some dog is sleeping in the garden'

The relative order of subject NP and the nominal predicate is semantically important in "equational" sentences. Thus, while

Hasan öğretmen – miş 'Hasan, reportedly, is a teacher'
teacher- rep.past
öğretmen Hasan – mış 'The teacher, reportedly, is Hasan'

In the first sentence, 'teacher' is the predicate and has an indefinite reading; while in the second sentence, it is the topic and has a definite reading.

Word order also differentiates the sentences known as 'clefts' (e.g. 'It is Ahmet who asked the question') from 'pseudo-clefts' (e.g. 'What surprised me was your invitation'). Pseudo-clefts in Turkish are made with a headless relative clause (in the form of a participial construction) and a nominal predicate.

(1) bu soru–yu sor-an kimse Ahmet – tir 'The person who asked this question is Ahmet'
This question-acc. ask-part. person Ahmet- pred. mar.
(2) bu soru – yu sor – an Ahmet - tir

(1) beni şaşırt – an şey sen – in davet – in – dir 'What surprises me is your invitation'
(2) beni şaşırt –an sen – in davet – in - dir

I-acc. Surprise- thing you-gen. invitation-gen-pred. mar.

The (1) sentences in each pair above have a lexical head noun for the relative clause. In the second sentence of these pairs, there is no head noun. A difference in the order of the nominal predicate and the headless relative clause results in the cleft sentence, as shown below:

Ahmet – tir bu soru – yu sor – an 'It is Ahmet who asked this question'
pred. mar. this question-acc. ask-part.
sen – in davet – in – dir ben – i şaşırt – an 'It is your invitation that surprises me'
you-gen. invit.-pos.-pred. m. I-acc. surprise-part.

The change in the word order for cleft sentences is an indication that pragmatically they are more marked than pseudo-clefts.

As a typical OV language (head final), Turkish follows the implicational relations for the order of elements in many structures. Verb-final languages have a strong tendency to have 'postpositions' instead of 'prepositions', and Turkish follows suit.

Ahmet okul – a git – ti 'Ahmet went to school'
school-to go-past
Ahmet okul – da 'Ahmet is at school'
school -at
Ahmet okul – dan gel – di 'Ahmet came from school'

Here, 'to', 'at' and 'from' of English are represented by the 'dative' *–a*, 'locative' *–da* and 'ablative' *-dan*. And as seen in the last example, prepositional phrases come before the verb.

Manner adverbs precede the verb:
Ahmet **hızlı** koş – uyor 'Ahmet is running fast'
fast run – prog.

In possessive structures, genitive comes before the noun:

Hasan – **ın** kitab – ı 'Hasan's book'

Auxiliaries come after the main verb:

Ahmet git – **meli** 'Ahmet must go'
go – must

Adjectives precede the nouns:

küçük çocuk 'small child'

If there is an article (Turkish only has the indefinite article), then the adjective precedes it:

küçük bir çocuk (small + a + child) 'a small child'.
When there is a numeral, however, that precedes the adjective:
iki küçük çocuk (two + small + child) 'two small children'

We can see, as a left-branching language, the governed elements precede their governors. We can also show this in 'recursion' whereby sentences can show up within larger sentences, which in turn can be part of still larger sentences. One way of this expansion is embedding. A VO language such as English employs 'right-branching embedding' (e.g. a relative clause that modifies the head-noun comes to the right of it), as exemplified via the familiar nursery-rhyme 'The house that Jack built'. The first sentence begins with 'This is the house', which is expanded by a *that*-clause to its right and becomes 'This is the house that Jack built'. In Turkish, branching goes in the opposite direction from English, that is to the left of the head-noun. Thus, the translation of the English sentence would be

bu Jack – in yap – tığ – ı ev 'This is the house that Jack built'
this Jack-gen. build-part.-pos house

Relative clauses in Turkish are formed in the following way: first, we move the head noun to the end of the sentence, and then select the appropriate form of participle and replace the tense suffix with a participle suffix (subject participle is *-(y)En* and object participles are *–Dik* for 'non-future' or *-(y)EcEk* for future).

adam yemeğ – e gel – di 'The man came to dinner'
man dinner – to come-past
yemeğ – e gel-di adam (The head noun is moved to the end)
yemeğ – e gel –**en** adam 'The man who came to dinner'
Ahmed – in gönder – **diğ** – i mektup … 'The letter that Ahmet sent/is sending …'
gen. send – part.-acc. Letter
Ahmed – in gönder – **eceğ** – i mektup … 'The letter that Ahmet is going to send …'

Another point that should be made in relation to word order in Turkish is the direction of verb phrase deletion. In English, for instance, there is a process of deleting all but the first one of a series of identical verbs or verb phrases in coordinate sentences. Thus, the sentence, 'Ahmet read a newspaper, and Hasan read a magazine', can be simplified to 'Ahmet read a newspaper, and Hasan a magazine'. This operation, which is called *gapping*, has a forward direction in English. In Turkish, gapping can work in either direction. Thus, the Turkish translation of the sentence above would be either:

Ahmet bir gazete, Hasan bir dergi oku - du.
Ahmet a newspaper, Hasan a magazine read-past

or,

Ahmet bir gazete oku-du, Hasan da bir dergi
Ahmet a newspaper read-past Hasan too a magazine

However, in embedded sentences, only backward gapping is allowed. Thus,

Ben Ahmed-in bir gazete Hasan-ın da bir dergi oku-duğ-un-u gör-dü-m
I Ahmet-gen. a paper and Hasan-gen.too a magazine read-fa.N-gen.-pos. see-past-1st sg.
'I saw that Ahmet read a paper and Hasan a magazine'

It is not possible with a forward gapping

*Ben Ahmed-in bir gazete oku-duğ-un-u Hasan-ın da bir dergi gör-dü-m.

Questions

Wh questions in Turkish are formed with the following particles: *ne* 'what', *neden/niye/niçin* 'why', *hangi* 'which', *kim* 'who' and *nerede* 'where'. While it is possible to find these particles in two positions – namely, preverbal or sentence-initial – the former is the more preferred order. Thus,

bu- nu arkadaş – ın – a **kim** söyle-di? 'Who told this to your friend?'
this-acc. friend-gen.- dat. who say-past
is preferred over
kim bu-nu arkadaş – ı – na söyle – di?

Yes–no questions are signaled by an interrogative particle *–mI*. The location of *–mI* is at the end of the constituent questioned. If the constituent is a whole sentence, *-mI* goes to the end of the sentence.

Ahmet Istanbul-dan gel-di-**mi**? 'Did Ahmet come from Istanbul?'
from come-past-mI

If the constituent is a different one, then *–mI* is found at the end of that constituent.

Ahmet Istanbul-dan-**mı** gel-di? 'Was it Istanbul where Ahmet came from?'
from-mI come-past

or

Ahmet-**mi** Istanbul-dan gel-di? 'Was it Ahmet who came from Istanbul?'

As the translations make obvious, such questions correspond to clefted questions in English.

If the predicate is non-verbal, *-mI* follows the predicate but precedes the personal ending.

siz öğretmen – **mi** – siniz? 'Are you a teacher?'

Notes

1. Capital letters I, for /i, ɯ, u, y/ (high vowels), and E, for /E, a/, are used for suffix vowels, and their phonetic shape is determined by the vowel harmony rule, as detailed in the chapter. Capital D represents /d/ or /t/, dependent on the context.

   gel-miş [gɛlmiʃ] 'Reportedly, s/he has come'
   gör-müş [gœɾmyʃ] 'Reportedly, s/he has seen'

2. There are other examples where the consonantal influence over the epenthetic vowel is different. If a velar stop is the first consonant of the cluster, then its backness [+back], rather than the following lateral, is the dominant factor. [kɯlinik] 'clinic' (from French *clinique* [klinik]), [kɯliʃɛ] 'cliché' (from French *cliché* [kliʃe]).
3. In this chapter, with the exception of the section on phonology, the Turkish data are given in the national orthography. Most of the letters of the Turkish alphabet correspond to the conventional phonetic symbols. The differences are given below:

Letter	*Phoneme*
ç	/tʃ/
c	/dʒ/
ş	/ʃ/
j	/ʒ/
ı	/ɯ/
ö	/œ/
ü	/y/

4. The letter ğ (soft-g) deserves a special comment:
   In between vowels, ğ is not pronounced, but the two vowels before and after it remain in separate syllables (in some dialects, this is restricted to back vowels; ğ between and after front vowels is pronounced as [j]).

   ağaç 'tree' [aatʃ] eğer 'if' [ɛɛɾ] or [ɛjɛɾ]

Morpheme internally: after a back vowel, before a consonant or at the end of a word, its realization is zero, and the preceding vowel is lengthened.

dağ 'mountain' [da:] tuğla 'brick' [tu:la]

Many examples in the text show that letters *k* and *g* alternate for the same form. This is due to the following *k-deletion* rule:

k → ∅ / V C V ___ + V

(/k/ is deleted in the non-initial syllable when in between vowels at a morpheme boundary) where ∅ is the phonetic realization of the letter ğ.

gel-ecek	's/he will come'	[gɛlɛdʒɛk]
gel-eceğ-im	'I will come'	[gɛlɛdʒɛim]

Part 2

Communication Development and Disorders in Monolingual Settings

Chapter 4

The Course of Normal Language Development in Turkish

AYHAN AKSU-KOÇ

Introduction

Language acquisition is a complex process determined by the interaction of multiple factors and its course follows both a universal sequence and a language-specific one. The aim of this chapter is to describe the patterns of acquisition displayed by normally developing monolingual Turkish children in order to provide a basis for comparison with patterns of deviant or delayed development.

Most studies of acquisition accept the premise that development is a function of the reciprocal interactions between cognitive and linguistic changes that take place within a social-interactional context. Among the processing and cognitive capacities that acquisition and use rest on are attention, auditory and visual perception, working memory and related executive functions, long-term memory, abstraction, generalization, concept formation and representation. Among the social-interactional skills are joint attention, ability to take perspectives and ability to read others' minds. The present overview is situated within the framework of this premise although detailed contributions of each process will not be taken up unless they are within the scope of the research reported.

Since a detailed description of Turkish is given in Chapter 3, a brief characterization will suffice here. Turkish is an agglutinative language of the Turkic family. The neutral word order is SOV, with concomitant properties of suffixed inflections, postpositions and preposed demonstratives, numerals, possessives, adjectives and relative clauses (Aksu-Koç & Slobin, 1985). Word order is flexible; order of constituents may shift for pragmatic purposes of signaling topic-focus (Erguvanlı, 1984). Hence the expression of basic grammatical relations depends on the use of inflectional marking on verbs and nouns. Verbs are marked for voice, negation, modality, aspect–tense–mood and person–number. Nouns, pronouns, question words and nominalized forms of the verb or the adjective are marked for number, possession and case. Nominative case and singular are unmarked base forms that have no phonological realization. Since person–number is marked on predicates, subject nouns are typically omitted. Object nouns may also be omitted depending on the context of utterance. Turkish thus presents the learner with a rich morphology, much variation in word order and much ellipsis of nominal arguments. It may therefore be expected that symptoms of deviance or disorder in linguistic functioning will be reflected in different parts of the grammatical system than in the more often studied typologically different Indo-European languages.

The chapter is organized as follows: the section 'Phonological Development'presents a summary of research on phonological development and the section 'Input' on input. The section 'Early Grammatical Competence' discusses evidence on the acquisition of word order, noun and verb inflections and the section 'Interface of morphology, syntax, semantics and pragmatics' discusses changes at the interface of morphosyntax, semantics and pragmatics. The section 'Developments in the Lexicon' summarizes research on lexical development and the section 'Later Grammatical Competence: Complex Sentences' discusses research on the acquisition of complex sentences. With this overview, I aim to show that frequency of the structures in the input, their degree of complexity, their communicative functions and the level of social-cognitive development of the child interact in the gradual but active construction of grammar. I conclude by considering some of the implications of the patterns and processes observed in normal development for delayed or deviant acquisition.

Phonological Development

Turkish words undergo allophonic variation subject to rules of vowel and/or consonant harmony: all grammatical suffixes harmonize with the last vowel of the lexical stem. Each morpheme is syllabic and stress is typically word final. Each morpheme retains its phonological and semantic identity as well as its relative position in the string.

Phonological acquisition in Turkish has been most extensively studied by Topbaş. Reporting on data from normally developing children, Topbaş (1989) points to the significance of input by noting reliable correlations between the frequency of phonemes /k/, /t/ and /tʃ/ in child speech (CS) and child-directed speech (CDS). She observes that between ages 1 and 3, children engage in both syntagmatic simplification (syllable elision and reduplication, consonant elision and assimilation, vowel lengthening and consonant cluster simplification) and paradigmatic simplification (fronting, palatalization, plosivization, gliding and voicing/devoicing) (Topbaş,

1996). She attributes the early and nonproblematic progress of phonological acquisition in Turkish to the perceptually and productively simple nature of phonotactic processes and syllable templates in the language.

In more recent work, Topbaş surveys the research on the acquisition of phonology by language disordered as well as normally developing children and observes that acquisition proceeds rapidly following paths similar to those in other languages while displaying language-specific differences and error patterns (Kopkallı-Yavuz & Topbaş, 2000; Topbaş, 2006b, 2007a; Topbaş & Kopkallı-Yavuz, 1998; Topbaş & Yavaş, 2006; Yavaş & Topbaş, 2004). Data from a normative sample of 665 children show that, by age 3;6, nearly all sounds are established at syllable-initial and final positions. The order of acquisition of consonants is stops > nasals > affricates > glide/ liquids > fricatives > flaps. Errors are most frequent around age 2;0 when there is a growth spurt in vocabulary. While labial, alveolar and velar plosives, nasals and the glide /j/ are established between 13 and 15 months, the voiced fricative /z/, the glottal fricative /h/ and the flap /r/ and its allophonic variations emerge around age 2;6 and do not stabilize until around four years. Liquids occur earlier but are subject to deletion when they are in clusters. The various processes of structural and systemic simplification occur until ages 3;6–4;0. The processes of reduplication, consonant voicing, fronting and assimilatory substitutions are suppressed early, whereas liquid deviation and consonant cluster reduction are suppressed late. The early acquisition of nasals and stops fits the universal pattern, but Turkish affricates are acquired earlier than fricatives in contrast to English, and consonant deletion in pre- and postconsonantal positions is much more common in Turkish than in many other languages. Compared to this normative sample, phonologically disordered children start correct pronunciation later, make more consonant errors, have difficulty producing the sounds acquired late by normally developing children and display some unusual error patterns that are consistent and systematic and some errors that are inconsistent and idiosyncratic. Nevertheless, they also display the same universal and language-specific tendencies.

Other examples of sensitivity to language-specific phonological structures are given by Kopkallı-Yavuz and Topbaş (2000). They report that contrary to the generalization across languages that children prefer monosyllabic to multisyllabic words and open over closed syllables, Turkish children attempt to produce disyllabic words more frequently than other types and closed syllables more often than open syllables. Even when they apply phonological processes, they observe language-specific constraints as demonstrated by Ketrez (2007) in her analyses of metathesis in the speech of a girl between ages 1;5 and 1;7 who moves sounds in words with labial consonants (e.g. *kitap* → *cipat*) however, only in those phonological environments where the syntactic requirement for adherence to morpheme order in Turkish is not violated, overriding the universal tendency to produce bilabials in prominent position. Her analysis shows how the phonological and morphosyntactic components of language begin to form an interface from the earliest phases of acquisition onwards.

Children acquire vowels early and make few errors in vowel harmony given the extreme regularity of the system (Aksu-Koç & Slobin, 1985; Topbaş, 2007a). An analysis by Altan (2009a) of spontaneous speech data from children between ages 2;0 and 4;8 shows that children observe the harmony rules except when they (1) inflect a mispronounced word to fit the mispronounced form, (2) regularize words that behave irregularly to fit the rules and (3) regularize the irregular aorist. Experimental tests with 2–6-year-olds, of production, grammaticality judgments, and elicited imitation using novel and regular words indicate that in adding the plural, possessive or case inflections to irregular words, 2–4-year-olds make increasing errors of regularization, which decrease around ages 5–6, but no errors on words that fit the harmony rules. Altan concludes that children learning Turkish learn the vowel harmony rules very early but the exceptions take a long time to master.

Nakipoğlu-Demiralp and Ketrez (2007) studied the aorist *-Ir*, which presents a case of morphophonemic nonuniformity. Any vowel-ending verb regardless of its syllable structure takes *-r*; consonant ending verbs take a variant of *-Ir* if multisyllabic and *-Ar* if monosyllabic except for a small subset that ends in sonorants that take *-Ir* (*al-ır, dur-ur, san-ır, kal-ır, vur-ur, bil-ir, gel-ir, ol-ur, var-ır, bul-ur, gör-ür, ver-ir*). However, there are 70 more sonorant-ending monosyllabic verbs that require *-Ar* (e.g. *böl-er, don-ar, çal-ar, gir-er, del-er, gül-er*). Nakipoğlu-Demiralp and Ketrez (2007) showed that children make both overregularization and irregularization errors depending on the dominant form in their system. At younger ages, when monosyllabic verbs are more numerous in CDS and CS, children make *-Ar* overregularizations with monosyllabic verbs ending in sonorants (e.g. *al-ar, vur-ar*). At later ages, as multisyllabic verbs increase in number and passivization and causativization change their syllabic and phonological structure, *-Ir* examples become more frequent in CDS and CS and children make *-Ir* irregularization errors (e.g. *böl-ür, çal-ır*). Again, the mastery of the aorist inflectional paradigm takes a long time, extending as far as age 7. Both the input and consequently the child's own system constitute the context for the observed patterns of development.

Input

The argument that in distinguishing lexical categories children must be attending to how members of the same class behave in the input with respect to combinatorial as well as to semantic properties was first made by Maratsos (1982) and has found support in ensuing research (Aksu-Koç, 1998a; Brodsky *et al.*, 2007; Ketrez, 2003; Küntay & Slobin, 1996, 2001; Tardiff, 1994, among others). Characteristics of CDS in Turkish are particularly interesting given the flexible word order, rich noun and verb morphology and high rate of nominal ellipsis. Analyzing Turkish CDS in this light, Küntay and Slobin (1994, 1996, 2001) identified partial repetitious clusters of maternal utterances that change in lexical items, grammatical morphology and word order while maintaining a constant communicative intention, as exemplified in Example (1) directed to a child at age 1;10 (Küntay & Slobin, 2001: 929–930).[1]

(1)	MOT:	*Bana*	*oda-n-dan*	*bi tane*	*bebek*	*getir-ebil-ir mi-sin?*
		PRO&DAT&1S	room-POSS2S-ABL	INDEF	doll	bring-POT-AOR QUE-2S
		Can you bring me a doll from your room?				
		Getir.				
		bring				
		Bring				
		Getir	*bebeğ-in-i*			
		bring	doll-POSS2S-ACC			
		Bring your doll.				

These clusters, which they call 'variation sets', constitute a discourse context in which the patterns of distribution of nominal and verbal categories are displayed transparently. Küntay and Slobin (1994) found that about 20% of the maternal utterances are made up of variation sets and that the core of a variation set consists of a verb with optionally expressed arguments. They observe that the distribution of nouns and verbs in utterance-initial versus utterance-final positions is about equal and does not render one category perceptually more salient than the other. Due to variations in word order and patterns of nominal addition and deletion, position is only a weak cue for the abstraction of lexical categories, and morphological form is the only other source of information. Nouns and verbs differ because (1) they take a different set of suffixes, and (2) verbs, where many different types of notions are marked, display greater inflectional diversity, whereas nouns just take case, number and possession. Most variation sets have the verb repeated, but about 40% of these show a change in form, while the invariant word-initial position of the verb stem and the consistent pattern of suffixation remain constant. Nouns that can stand alone as bare forms are repeated less frequently because of ellipsis or being replaced by a pronoun, but if repeated, they change form only about 25% of time (Küntay & Slobin, 1994, 2001). This higher rate of repetition of verbs that display greater inflectional variety suggests a verb dominant pattern in Turkish CDS; verbs in CS appear as morphologically complex as in CDS, but nouns are less complex than in CDS.

These patterns are corroborated by CS and CDS from children between ages 2;0 and 4;8 of the Berkeley Crosslinguistic Acquisition Project and suggest an early verb-learning bias in Turkish. Küntay and Slobin report that for all ages, verbs exceed nouns in number of morphemes added to the root: children's average mean length of utterance (MLU) equals 2.60 for verbs and 1.67 for nouns; and the adults' average MLU equals 2.18 for verbs (lower than children's because of a high number of imperatives) and 1.96 for nouns. Similar values were obtained by Aksu-Koç *et al.* (2007): in CDS from a child between ages 1;3 and 2;0, the average MLU for verbs equals 2.43 and for nouns 1.70 and there are as many as 17 different noun affixes and 37 different verb affixes, if not more. These patterns in the input reflect the morphological richness of the Turkish verb compared to the noun and are mirrored in the children's output by a faster rate of development for verbs than for nouns (Xanthos *et al.*, in press). It appears that frequency and complexity balance out in favoring the two categories for the child's attention and result in their simultaneous emergence. Verbs that display more complexity in the form of morphological richness are more frequent in the input; nouns that are less frequent have less morphological complexity.

Input also guides the child in carving the semantic domains represented by the formal means. As will be discussed in the section 'Input', the distribution of the tense–aspect–mood inflections with different types of verbs in CS closely mirrors their distribution in CDS, although at first the child's use of a given inflection is restricted to specific types of verbs (e.g. the past inflection *-DI* is used exclusively with achievement verbs that refer to telic events) and only later generalizes to other types. Such restricted use might be the result of a processing strategy that helps focus on specific morphosyntactic patterns in relation to specific event structures, yielding underlying semantic configurations (Aksu-Koç, 1998a).

The nature of the input also changes as the child's system develops. Ketrez (2003) found a significant increase between ages 1;3 and 2;0 in the morphosyntactic complexity of CDS as measured by MLU and a parallel increase in CS for three mother–child pairs, indicating that mothers tailor their speech according to their addressee. Similarly, Küntay and Slobin (2002) observed a striking drop in the number of variation sets in CDS from 80 at age 1;3 to 36 at age 2;0 with a concomitant change in their interactive functions from information querying to control orientation, indicating that as children's linguistic and social-cognitive skills change, the pragmatic functions of parental talk change as well. Parents of language-delayed children are also reported to adjust their intentional communicative language to the level and response capacities of their children (Topbaş *et al.*, 2003).

However, it is not only the child's level of linguistic competence that determines the nature of input. Quality of CDS is also a function of the mother's level of education. Küntay and Ahtam (2004) report that in talking to their 3–4-year-olds, highly educated mothers avoid frequent topic shifts and elaborate on the same topic with more utterances and more descriptive information, whereas mothers with low level of education ask more close-ended repetitive questions. The importance of parental education for the development of children's vocabulary, syntactic competence and narrative skills is also observed in the significantly higher level of performance of preschoolers whose mothers are well educated as compared to their agemates whose mothers have only a few years of schooling (Aksu-Koç, 2004; Aksu-Koç *et al.*, 1999, 2002; Sofu, 1995).

Early Grammatical Competence

Word order

The neutral word order in Turkish is SOV, but it can be varied for pragmatic purposes. In the absence of case markers, only SOV and OVS orders are grammatical. The sentence-initial position is for subject/topic, preverbal position is for direct objects when they are unmarked (i.e. indefinite and nonreferential) and postverbal position is for backgrounded, old information (Erguvanlı, 1984; Kornfilt, 1997).

Turkish children show early sensitivity to the standard word order as well as to these restrictions. Slobin and Bever (1982) asked 2–4-year-olds to act out reversible transitive sentences for the six possible word orders with inflected object nouns. Children relied on inflection rather than word order in identifying agent–patient relations, displaying 75–95% correct performance over all types. Younger children changed nonstandard to standard SOV order. Trials with unmarked noun, noun, verb (NNV) sequences yielded either random performance or a preference to pick the first noun as an agent. These findings indicate that Turkish children correctly assign grammatical roles to sentence constituents when these are case marked, and follow closely the relative frequency of word orders used by adults.

Batman-Ratyosyan and Stromswold (2002) replicated these findings testing 3–5-year-olds with different word orders in the absence of case marking. Children correctly imitated the grammatical SOV and OVS orders but not the ungrammatical ones, with three-year-olds displaying a preference for the standard SOV order. Similar results were obtained using grammaticality judgments. In a set of comprehension experiments that juxtaposed the roles of word order, case marking and pragmatic context in assigning grammatical roles to constituents in reversible sentences, all children did well on SOV sentences. On OVS sentences, case marking but not pragmatic context helped interpretation, and compared with older children, younger children relied more on the morphological cues.

Exploring the role of syntactic frames in sentence comprehension, Göksun *et al.* (2008) also found that young children attend to case marking and to the most frequent SOV order. Two-to-five-year-olds and adults were asked to act out with toys sentences with familiar transitive and intransitive verbs in novel syntactic frames, with or without the accusative marker. All children acted out canonical sentences correctly. In interpreting noncanonical sentences, children relied on their knowledge of the usual argument structure of the verb rather than an abstract syntactic frame construed in terms of number (and configuration) of arguments. Critically, in enacting transitive sentences with one noun phrase (NP), both children and adults made more causative than noncausative interpretations, revealing more attention to the verb than the novel frame it appeared in. Similarly, in response to intransitive sentences with two NPs, noncausative responses were more frequent than causative ones. In all cases the presence of the accusative increased causative responses although it did not take priority over verb knowledge. Two-year-olds responded more to case morphology and 3–4-year-olds responded more in terms of the syntactic frame, but this trend declined for older children who acted more like adults who used both morphology and verb knowledge, repairing the syntactic frame to fit the restrictions of the verb. Göksun *et al.*'s (2008) findings thus show that Turkish children learn very early to rely on the verb to infer meaning in novel syntactic environments. They propose several reasons for this: (1) case morphology makes it easier to acquire verb-argument structures, (2) frequent noun ellipsis in input makes 1-argument frames for transitive verbs familiar and easily interpretable and (3) syntactic frames may be interpreted differently depending on constraints of flexible word order. The primacy of the verb compliance pattern is not surprising given the dominance of verbs in the input. It is also in line with Tomasello's (1992; Tomasello & Brooks, 1999) proposal that verb learning is at first item based and that general transitive and intransitive schemas develop only after children encounter many examples of different frames.

Evidence for attention to restrictions on the syntactic positions of constituents within sentences and phrases is provided by Ekmekçi (1986) and Ekmekçi and Can (2000) from the period between 1;7 and 2;4, indicating an early awareness of the head-final property of Turkish. In noun phrases, modifiers precede the head noun (e.g. Adj+N = *mai sabun* 'blue soap' (1;8); Relative Clause+N = *ağla-yan bebek* 'cry-PRES.PART baby' (2;3)), complements are positioned before the verb both in verb phrases (e.g. *yüz-ünü kapat-mış* 'face-ACC cover-EVID' (1;11)) and in adjunct phrases (e.g. N+ABL = *elin-den ye-di* 'hand-ABL eat-PAST' (1;11)). Deviations from these orders that are grammatical are also observed before age 2;0. For example, unmarked indefinite and nonreferential noun phrases restricted to the preverbal position (*Kaem getir* 'pencil bring' 'Bring me a pencil' at 1;10) are case marked for definiteness when moved to the postverbal position (*Getir kaem-i* pencil-ACC bring 'Bring me the pencil' at 1;10). In question answers, noun phrases are correctly placed in the preverbal position if they give new information, but in postverbal position if they refer to what is already given in the discourse, as in Example (2):

(2) MOT: *Bacağ-ın-ı* *ne* *yap-acak-lar?*
leg-POSS:3S-ACC what do-FUT-3P
What will they do to his leg?
CHI: *Kes-eceğ-le* *bacağ-ın-ı*
do-FUT-3P leg-POSS:3S-ACC
They will cut his leg off.

Pronoun use in Turkish is a marked option since the subject is indicated by agreement marking on the verb (Enç, 1986). It is restricted to contexts of emphasis or contrast concerning the agent of action: the pronoun is placed postverbally if the speaker wants to focus on the object or the action. Children initially indicate the subject by marking agreement on the verb in accordance with the null-subject rule. Then they use full NPs in subject position for purposes of switching reference; pronouns are used for reference continuity, even as early as 15 months (Altan, 2009b; Topbaş & Özcan, 1997). Children between ages 2 and 4 follow the same restrictions as adults although they tend to overuse pronouns in comparison (Slobin & Talay, 1986). They can pre- and postpose pronouns for pragmatic functions such as contrasting agents or objects (*Çay iç-er-im ben.* Tea drink-AOR-1S I 'I drink tea (not water)' (2;0)), or shifting perspectives, for example from the object to the self, as in Example (3).

(3) CHI: *Aç-ıl-ıyor,* *aç-ıl-ıyor.*
open-PASS-PROG, open-PASS-PROG
It is opening, it is opening.

Ben *aç-ar-ım,* *aç-ıl-ır.*
I open-AOR-1S open-PASS-PROG
I (will) open it, it (will) open.

Such examples show that pragmatically motivated shifts in word order occur very early and do not wait upon developments in the theory of the mind as suggested by Batman-Ratrosyan and Stromswold (2002). Two-to-three-year-olds are good at shifting perspectives in discourse and reading adult intentions in contexts of joint attention (Meltzoff, 2002; O'Neill, 2005; Tomasello, 2003; Tomasello *et al.*, 1993; Rollins & Snow, 1998), both abilities being sufficient to support such pragmatic use.

The use of different word orders for pragmatic purposes has also been observed in narratives of three-, five- and nine-year-olds and adults elicited by use of a wordless picture book '*Frog Where Are You?*' (Aksu-Koç, 1994). In their stories, children reserved the sentence-initial position for topic, preverbal position for focus and postverbal position for background information, in line with the adult grammar. The percentage of (S)OV orders was higher than verb medial orders because in their effort to carry a complex storyline forward, children tended to maintain the perspective of the major protagonist and avoided topic shifts. Four- and five-year-olds kept him as the topic and in the agentive role, whereas after this age they could use passive and intransitive constructions for topic maintenance (Aksu-Koç & Tekdemir, 2004). The high percentages of verb-final orders also contrast with that observed in conversation (Slobin, 1982), suggesting that the two genres have different demands for information structuring.

Morphological development: Verb and noun inflections

Given the pragmatic variations in word order, position cannot serve as a cue for syntactic relations in Turkish. Children, therefore, have to attend to patterns of inflectional marking in order to differentiate nouns and verbs and to mark grammatical relations. We traced the emergence of tense–aspect–mood and person–number inflections on verbs and case and number marking on nouns in Aksu-Koç and Ketrez (2003) and Ketrez and Aksu-Koç (2009) in longitudinal spontaneous speech data from four girls, daughters of university educated urban parents, overlapping in age between 1;3 and 3;3,[2] with MLUs in morphemes ranging between 1.0–1.4 and 4.32–5.75.[3] Some of the more detailed analyses below are based on Deniz's corpus, but the children go through similar developmental phases and experience difficulty on similar structures albeit with different rates of development.

Taking inflectional development as a process of paradigm building, we determined three phases: *premorphology, proto-morphology* and *morphology proper* (Dressler & Peltzer-Karpf, 1995). We adopted the following criteria for productivity (Ketrez & Aksu-Koç, 2009): (1) Use of each verb/noun inflection contrastively with different verbs/nouns (e.g. *git-ti* go-PAST versus *gel-di* come-PAST) or in different verb/noun+inflection combinations (e.g. *gid-iyor-du* go-PROG-PAST). (2) Use of each verb/noun as a bare form contrastively with inflected forms (e.g. *git* go versus *git-ti* go-PAST versus *gid-iyor* go-PROG) yielding different inflectional types. Each distinct verb+inflection combination is taken as an inflectional type (e.g. *git-ti* go-PAST and *gid-iyor* go-PROG represent two inflectional types for *git* 'go'). (3) Lower number of omission or commission errors than number of grammatical productions of the inflection. (4) Consistency in use as reflected in the presence of the inflection in consecutive samples (Allen, 1996; Brown, 1973; Kilani-Schoch & Dressler, 2002 discuss similar criteria).

Phase I. Premorphology: MLU (range: 1.20–1.34)[4]

In this early phase, children produce monosyllabic or bisyllabic words, forms created by onomatopoeia, reduplication (e.g. *da-da* [:ayı] 'teddy bear') and analogy (e.g. *maa-am* [:maymun] 'monkey'), but with the correct intonation and stress pattern (Aksu-Koç, 1997; Baykoç-Dönmez & Arı, 1992; Çapan, 1988; Özcan & Topbaş, 2000).

There is no evidence for verb or noun inflections that meet the criteria for productivity. Inflectional complexes consisting of an undecipherable syllable (&) as the verb plus a sequence of unanalyzed morphemes (e.g. child form: *&ınmaz &-PASS-NEG-AOR*; adult form: *kaşı-n-m-az* scratch-PASS-NEG-AOR 'one does not scratch'), or alternatively, verbs with meaningless extra syllables (e.g. *gel-bi-&-yiz* come-&-AOR:1P?) modeled on adult utterances constitute predecessors of verbs. Such structures that have phonological form but no real morphological content reflect sensitivity to patterns of the input, but lack a full analysis of words into combinable units (Aksu-Koç, 1997; Peters & Menn, 1993). Since there is no inflectional marking, there is no evidence for the lexical categories of nouns and verbs either. For example, *da:at* (:kağsıt 'paper') is used to both request a piece of paper and as a proto-imperative to mean 'draw a picture' (Deniz, 1;3). Similarly, *at-tı* (throw-PAST 'threw') is used at times as a verb to mean 'I threw', at times as a noun to mean 'ball' (TT, 1;5). This period provides evidence on the fact that Turkish children also go through a precategorical period like that observed in the case of children acquiring English as claimed by Radford (1990).

Phase II. Proto-morphology: MLU (range: 1.58–3.42)

This period is marked by an increase in the number of words and the productive use of verbal and nominal inflections, which provide evidence for the emergence of the two lexical categories. Paradigm building starts: about 60% of utterances have a verb and about 60% of both verbs and nominals are produced in more than one form.

Verb inflections: Verbs are marked for voice, modality, negation, tense–aspect–mood and person–number. The tense–aspect–mood markers are multifunctional and their exact value depends on context. The negative marker *-mA* is always after the verb stem and precedes the inflectional markers but follow the voice suffixes. Person/number suffixes mark subject–verb agreement and have four paradigms depending on the tense–aspect–mood inflection they are appended to. To illustrate, for the verb *gel-*, the first plural is *gel-iyor-uz* in Paradigm I, *gel-di-k*, in paradigm II and *gel-e-lim* in Paradigm III. The third person plural agreement marker is *-lEr/lAr*, which is also the plural marker for nouns. The question particle *mI* appears in two different positions: between the t-a-m markers and the agreement marker in paradigm I, and after the agreement markers at the end of the word in the other paradigms.

The following order of emergence of tense–aspect–mood inflections is generalizable across children (see also Aksu-Koç, 1988a; Boeschoten, 1990; Çapan, 1988; Ekmekçi, 1987; Sofu, 1998). The past tense/perfective aspect marker -*DI* is used first, to comment on changes of state experienced in the immediate context. In Example (4) the verb is produced first in bare form, then with past tense and then with tense plus first person marking.

(4) CHI: *anne ga:k (kalk) anne* (Deniz, 1;6)
mother get:up mother
Mother get up mother
CHI: *ka:k-ti [kalktim]*
get:up-PAST-0*1sg
Got up
CHI: *ga-di-m [kalktim]*
get:up-PAST-1sg
I got up

Next, the present/progressive -*Iyor* for talk about ongoing events and the optative -*(y)A* for invitations to joint attention are acquired. The negative marker -*mA* also appears at this point. Then the future -*(y)AcAk* is used to express intention for action, the past/perfect/evidential -*mIş* to comment on states that constitute new information, and the habitual/possible marker aorist -*Ir* to refer to norms sanctioning or prohibiting behavior. Example (5) shows the increase in grammatical complexity between 1;6 and 1;8.

(5) CHI: *ben* *badi [pazil]* *yap-iyo-m* (Deniz, 1;8)
I puzzle make-PROG-1S
I am making a puzzle.

Individual agreement paradigms emerge together with the associated t-a-m markers. First person singular and plural are the earliest and most frequent, and third plural appears about a month later. Errors consist mainly of omissions; there are also occasional substitutions of the second person singular for the first, which suggests that children at first take the second person singular they hear in speech addressed to them as a morpheme that makes absolute reference rather than a relational one that shifts in discourse. Errors of omission of the third person plural, which is ungrammatical with [– animate] subjects, optional with [+ animate] subjects and preferred only with [+ definite] ones (Sezer, 1978), are not uncommon and show the difficulties children have in figuring out the restrictions on its use. The production of a given inflection may also be affected by phonological factors. Ketrez (1999b) has observed that at the time she is correctly marking first and third person plural correctly (-*Iz*/-*Ik* and -*lAr*, respectively), Mine omits the /-*m*/ representing the first singular just as she omits the final sound of words that end in /-*m*/, such as *lokum, kalem* (reported by Arslan (1996) who described her phonological development), indicating that the problem arises from the difficulty she has in producing sonorant sounds.

Negation is marked morphologically from the beginning; however, children have also been reported to make substitution errors where the lexical negatives *yok* 'not exist' and *değil* 'not the case' applicable to substantive predicates are used instead (Aksu-Koç & Slobin, 1985; Çapan, 1988). The question particle *mI* is acquired without error; however, it appears last in Paradigm I where it has to be inserted between the t-a-m and agreement markers, which require the interruption of a meaningful inflectional sequence (Slobin, 1985).

Building verbal paradigms: Increasing complexity is reflected in the growth of paradigms that display the distinct inflectional types for a specific verb at a given point in development. For example, in Deniz's corpora, the first two-member paradigms are observed at 1;6 when only four of her 22 verbs are used contrastively in bare versus inflected form, yielding eight different inflectional types. At 1;7 when she has 33 verbs, she displays a growth spurt with three- and four-member paradigms, but with a high rate of substitution and omission errors. At 1;8, both the number of verbs and the number of paradigm members increase, yielding as many as 79 inflectional types and a significant drop in errors at 1;9. Table 4.1 presents examples from different points in development.

Table 4.1 shows that some verbs such as *gel* 'come' and *yap* 'do/make' appear in successive sessions as bearers of new inflection types, suggesting that new forms first appear on verbs that have achieved productivity with other inflections already having been analyzed into root/stem versus inflectional segments (Aksu-Koç & Ketrez, 2003a).

In summary, emergence of inflections waits upon the acquisition of a minimum number of verbs and the verbal complex gets constructed gradually. To figure out how the system works, the child zeroes in on one inflectional form and uses it with several verbs and its associated agreement markers before generalizing to new inflections. Such a strategy is in line with the hypotheses that a critical mass of words is needed for the emergence of syntax (Marchman & Bates, 1994) and that lexical development and grammatical development are highly correlated early in development (Bates & Goodman, 1999; Marchman *et al.*, 2004). The rich productive morphology appears to induce the child to acquire inflections early on (Aksu-Koç & Slobin, 1985; Xanthos *et al.*, in press). Where there are deviations from regularity as in the case of the aorist inflection *-Ir* however, mastery is a protracted process that may last throughout the preschool years.

Nominal Inflections: are number, possessive, and case, which occur in that order when all three are present, as in *kedi-(ler)-(im)-(de)* cat-PL-POSS:1S-LOC 'at my cats'. The case system consists of a single paradigm that is fully productive and regular. The accusative, dative, genitive,

Table 4.1 Sample verbal paradigms in Deniz Phase II (1;6–1;9)

Age	*Lexical item*	*Translation*	*Inflectional type*	*Category*
1;6 Two-member	ol	be	ol-du	PAST
			ol-du mu?	PAST QUE
	gel	come	gel	Imp.
			gel-di-m	PAST-1S
1;8 Three-member	gel	come	Gel-di-m	PAST-1S
			Gel-iyor-um	PROG-1S
			Gel-di-k	PAST-1P
Five-member	yap	do/make	yap	Imp.
			yap-ma	(Imp.)-NEG
			yap-ma-m	NEG.AORIST-1S
			yap-ıyor-um	PROG-1S
			yap-acağ-ım	FUT-1S
1;9 Nine-member	yap	do/make	yap	Imp.
			yap-ma	(Imp.)-NEG
			yap-ıyor	PROG
			yap-ıyor-um	PROG-1S
			yap-ıyor-sun	PROG-2S
			Yap-mı-yı-m	NEG-OPT-1S
			Yap-tı	PAST
			Yap-tı-n	PAST-2S
			Yap-mış	EVID

Source: Adapted from Aksu-Koç and Ketrez (2003).

locative, ablative and comitative/instrumental are applied to nouns, pronouns, demonstratives, question words, and derived nouns. The word-final position of the suffixes reinforced by word-final stress renders case markers perceptually salient (Aksu-Koç & Slobin, 1985). The control of the nominative, which designates the subject, can be inferred from the use of agreement markers on the verb and from its contrastive use with the accusative and the dative in transitive sentence frames.

Nominal inflections emerge at the same time as verbal inflections in the proto-morphological phase. The accusative *-(y)I*[5] for direct objects and the dative_*-(y)A* for oblique objects are the most frequent, and show a rapid increase in the subsequent months. Accusative marking on nouns is obligatory when the object is referential and specific (definite or indefinite); it is always obligatory on pronouns and nouns that have possessive morphology. Example (6) illustrates the appropriate use of the two cases with *tak* 'attach', a ditransitive verb, despite the child's difficulty in producing both arguments and the verb in a single utterance.

(6)	MOT:	*bu-nu*	*san-a mı*	*tak-a-yım?*	(Deniz, 1;7)
		this-ACC	you-DAT QUE	attach-OPT-1S	
		Shall I attach this on you?			
	CHI:	*gat [:tak].*			
		attach&IMP			
		Attach.			
		(...)			
	CHI:	*bu-nu*	*ban-a [=! cries]!*		
		this-ACC	I-DAT		
		This to me.			
		(...)			
	CHI:	*bu-nu*	*gat!*		
		this-ACC	attach		
		Attach this.			

The dative emerges in responses to *nere-ye* 'where-to' and *kim-e* 'who-to' questions and may express direction, goal or beneficiary of an action. By the end of the proto-morphological period, it is one of the contrastive forms that a given noun/pronoun appears in (e.g. *ben-i* 'I-ACC' versus *bana* 'I-DAT' versus *ben-im* 'I-GEN'). The accusative and dative are earlier and more frequent than the other cases but they are also produced with more errors. This may be because as core cases functional in syntactic relations, they are subject to constraints that arise from the particular properties of the verbs that select them as arguments. Other factors that may cause difficulty are the multidimensional semantics of the dative, the complex interaction of the syntactic function of the accusative as a direct object marker with the pragmatic functions of word order, and the semantic features of objects such as specificity and referentiality. Errors of omission are more frequent than errors of substitution.

The locative *-DA* emerges as early as the accusative, and the dative, possibly because it indicates general rather than specific location (e.g. 'at' versus 'in' or 'on'), is obligatory even with indefinite nouns and is the word- or sentence-final salient element when the nominal it is attached to functions predicatively (Ketrez & Aksu-Koç, 2009). The ablative *-DAn* expresses locative source or a partitive relation. Deniz, for example, uses at 1;8, the same noun contrastively in the dative, the locative and the ablative as in the following three-member paradigm: *araba-dan* 'car-ABL', *araba-da* 'car-LOC' and *araba-ya* 'car-DAT', which suggests that the semantics of space is differentiated into source, goal and static location. The instrumental and the commutative *-(y)lA* are rare both in CDS and in CS.

The genitive *-(n)In* case specifies the possessor and the possessive morpheme *–(s)I(m/n)* marks agreement on the possessed. In early proto-morphology there are many instances of the genitive missing in obligatory contexts.

(7)	CHI:	*dede (/2) &de.*		(Deniz, 1;6)
		grandfather-*0GEN		
	MOT:	evet	dede-nin	teyb-i.
		yes	grandfather-GEN	tape-recorder-POSS&3S
		Yes, grandfather's tape-recorder.		

Correct use emerges in response to adult questions that require the specification of the possessor. The possessive, which is more frequent than the genitive, both in CDS and in CS, is earlier than the genitive.

Number is indicated with the plural morpheme *-lEr/lAr* suffixed to nouns, demonstrative pronouns and question words after the stem and before the possessive and case markers. In personal pronouns, number and plural are fused (*ben* 'I' versus *biz* 'we'), except in the case of the third person plural (*o* 's/he, it' versus *o-nlar* it-3P 'they'). Plurality is not marked when there is a numeral or quantifier preceding the noun (e.g. *iki kedi-Ø* (two cat) 'two cats'). The plural suffix *-lEr/-lAr* appears when case marking gets relatively consolidated and the child can add different nominal inflections to the same form as in *ayak-**lar**-ı-nı* foot-PL-POSS&3S-ACC 'his feet' (Deniz, 1;8). Plural morphology occurs in such multi-inflection combinations as soon as it emerges. There are also early examples of its use in constructions with correct noncanonical morpheme order. In *üt-te-ki-ye:* [: *üst-te-ki-ler*] top-LOC-*ki*-PL 'the ones on the top' (Deniz, 1;9), the plural morpheme follows the case marker, whereas it precedes case in nominal structures without *ki*.

Number marking on nominals is also later than the use of the same morpheme as the third person plural marker on verbs where it becomes fusional, deviating from the general typological features of Turkish. This, however, does not appear to be problematic since children acquire the fusional first person plural slightly before the third, and before plural marking on nouns. We explained this (Ketrez & Aksu-Koç, 2009) by noting that (1) person–number marking on verbs has high frequency in CDS because it is syntactically obligatory due to the null-subject property of Turkish, and (2) number marking on nouns has low frequency in CDS because the 'singular' form of the noun is numerically neutral, denoting either a category or an individual member of a category (Lewis, 1967).

Table 4.2 presents examples of multimember paradigms with increasing number of inflectional types per word form in Deniz's speech. The few inflections observed until 1;6 do not reach productivity but from then onwards both the number of paradigms and the number of members of the individual paradigms increase. At 1;9 for example, there are 38 nominals that present multimember paradigms, one with as many as nine

Table 4.2 Sample nominal paradigms in Deniz Phase I and II (1;6–1;9)

Age	*Lexical item*	*Inflectional type*	*Category*
1;3–1;5	*a:bi* 'brother'	*A:bi*	N
		A:bi-ye	N-DAT
		*A:bi-*0ye*	N-*0DAT
		*A:bi-*0nin*	N-*0GEN
	anne 'mother'	*Anne*	N
		*anne-*0si-yi*	N-*0POSS-ACC
		*anne-*0si-*0ni*	N-*0POSS-*0ACC
1;6 (Two-member)	*bu* 'this'	*bu*	PRO
		bu-nu	PRO-ACC
1;7 (Five-member)	*bura* 'here'	*bura-dan*	PRO-ABL
		bura-ya	PRO-DAT
		bura-da	PRO-LOC
		bura-da-yım	PRO-LOC-1S
		bura-da-ymış	PRO-LOC-EID
1;8 (Six-member)	*ayakkabı* 'shoe'	*ayakkabı*	N
		*ayakkabı-*0sı-nı*	N-*POSS&3S-ACC
		ayakkabı-yla	N-COM
		ayakkabı-lar-ı-nı	N-PL-POSS&3S-ACC
		ayakkabı-sı-nı	N-POSS&2S-ACC
		ayakkabı-sı	N-POSS&3S
1;9 (Nine-member)	*bu* 'this'	*bu*	PRO
		bu-nu	PRO-ACC
		bu-na	PRO-DAT
		bu-ndan	PRO-ABL
		bu-nun-la	PRO-GEN-INS
		bu-nlar	PRO-PL
		bu-nlar-ı	PRO-PL-ACC
		bu-nun	PRO-GEN
		bu-nlar-dan	PRO-PL-ACC

Source: Adapted from Ketrez and Aksu-Koç (2009).

members. These figures show that all nominal inflections have emerged and are being used at some level of productivity at the end of the proto-morphological stage.

Table 4.2 also shows that pronouns (e.g. the demonstrative *bu* 'this') reach productivity earlier than nouns. This is because there are more occasions for using them with different cases: they replace nouns, they are obligatorily case-marked even in immediately preverbal position and are used more frequently.

In summary, by the end of proto-morphology, case, possessive and plural markers achieve productivity, and multiple marking on a single form becomes common. After 1;9 there are no new structures and what has emerged gets to be used with a greater number of word forms and in more diverse constructions. Ekmekçi (1987), Özcan (1996) and Topbaş *et al.* (1997) similarly report the presence of all forms of case marking and the use of multiple markers on nouns by 23 months.

Our findings, which show the simultaneous emergence of verb and noun inflections, contrast, however, with acquisition data from second language acquisition by adults and children. Both Haznedar (2003) and Gürel (2000) report that their subjects acquire t-a-m and agreement morphology with ease and almost no error, whereas they make many case omissions during the same period. Reporting on data from two suspected SLI and two normally developing Turkish children growing up bilingual in the German immigrant context, Bernreuter (2005) also states that nominal inflections emerge as a more vulnerable domain subject to more errors than verb inflections.

Phase III. Morphology-proper: MLU (range: 3.17–4.06)

The third phase is characterized by the relative consolidation and generalization of nominal and verbal morphology. Case, plural and possessive marking are extended to indefinite, reflexive and reciprocal pronouns, adjectives and cardinals. The accusative and the dative are used with arguments of novel verbs. Multiple marking on the same form becomes frequent and derivational morphology begins. In the verbal system, development involves voice alternations by inserting the causative, passive, reflexive or reciprocal affixes into the verb complex and making the associated syntactic operations of adding or deleting subjects/objects with correct case marking. These developments at the interface of morphology, syntax, semantics and pragmatics result in reorganizations at a more complex level. Below, I give some examples of these interactions.

Interface of morphology, syntax, semantics and pragmatics

Tense–aspect–modality

To illustrate the gradual construction of a complex semantic domain, let me summarize the developments in the expression of tense–aspect–mood as observed in two longitudinal (seven children between 1;1 and 3;3) and two cross-sectional studies (90 children between 3;0– and 6;6) (Aksu-Koç, 1988a, 1998a, 1998b; Aksu-Koç & Alıcı, 2000; see also Küntay & Slobin, 1999).

As noted in the section 'Input', in the early phases there is a very close correspondence between CS and CDS regarding the frequency of use of specific inflections with specific types of verbs depending on their inherent aspectual characteristics (Aksu-Koç, 1998a). *-DI* occurs at highest frequency for achievement and accomplishment verbs in the mother's speech and almost exclusively with achievement verbs in the child's speech (e.g. *aç-tı-m* open-PAST-1S 'I opened (it)'). In the next few months, this initial use became limited in scope to comments on the completion of immediate changes of state with observable results, generalized to a past-tense marker as the child starts taking the past process into account. *-Iyor* emerges with state and activity verbs, again following the frequency pattern in the mother's speech; its use is extended to achievement and accomplishment verbs only weeks later. Although *-Iyor* is more frequent in the input than *-DI*, it is not the first marker children pick up because *–Iyor* expresses a variety of aspectual–temporal (e.g. commenting on ongoing activities and existing states) and modal functions (e.g. questioning intentions and talking about norms of behavior), whereas *-DI* is limited to reference to the expression of perfective aspect – past tense.

Initial uses of *–Ir* are with activity and state verbs, partially mapping onto the most frequent use with activity and achievement verbs in CDS. These utterances first express notions of deontic modality related to prohibitions (e.g. *bi daha yap-ma-m* again do-NEG:AOR-1S 'I won't do it again') or sanctions (e.g. ye-ri-m 'I'll eat'), then notions of epistemic possibility (e.g. *el-in sıkış-ır* hand-POSS get.stuck-AOR 'your hand will get stuck'), and finally habitual aspect (e.g. behavioral routines). The modal uses of *–Ir*, the future *-AcAk* and the negative abilitative *-AmA* as early as age 2;0 are also reported by Ekmekçi (1987) and Savaşır (1986). Boeschoten who compared Turkish-Dutch bilingual with monolingual 4–8-year-olds similarly found the earlier and more frequent use of these inflections to express deontic notions than epistemic notions. *-MAlI*, which expresses the semantically stronger notion of necessity, is observed to be acquired the latest (Boeschoten, 1990; Taylan & Aksu-Koç, 2003).

–MIş is a very common feature of CDS; caregivers mark with *-mIş* those utterances that invite the child to notice some state or change of state as 'new information'. It first appears in CS to comment on newly encountered (*burda-y-mış* here-EVID 'it is here') or changed states of objects (*patla-mIş* pop-EVID 'it's popped'), indicating perfect aspect. Its contrastive use with *-DI* marks a differentiation between old/assimilated versus new information, that is, between a shared versus an unshared perspective on events. Evidence for the inferential/past function is observed a few months later when *–mIş* is used in reference to present

states resultant from nonwitnessed past processes and *-DI* in reference to directly perceived events.

A further distinction is marked within indirect experience with the modal clitics *-ImIş* and *-DIr* from the inflectional paradigm of substantive predicates. *-ImIş* is first observed around two years, in rote picture description and story telling frames in line with its narrative function in adult language. Its use to indicate knowledge acquired through language, that is, for reported speech, is observed sometime between 2;6 and 3;0. *-DIr* marks assertions based on well assimilated knowledge. It indicates factivity (e.g. categorical assertions) or nonfactivity (presumptive or deductive statements) depending on context. Its first uses in spontaneous speech are for requesting categorical information within a question format (*Bu nedir?* 'What is this?), and later, around age 3, for making assertions with less than full certainty in the absence of available evidence (e.g. to suggest the possible location of a toy: *yatağ-ın-da-dır* bed-*POSS-LOC-DIr* 'it must be in its bed') (Aksu-Koç, 1998b; Aksu-Koç & Alıcı, 2000).

These reorganizations that result from differentiation and consolidation of the t-a-m system involve changes in the interface of conceptual, semantic and pragmatic development. They also reflect the role of input in guiding this process, lending support to a distributional bias hypothesis (Shirai & Andersen, 1995). Children pattern their use of the different forms following their distribution in adult speech, which is itself shaped by the constraints imposed by the child's cognitive processing strategies and by the social-interactional formats of mother–child discourse (Aksu-Koç, 1998a; Ketrez, 2003). Similar patterns in tense–aspect acquisition have been reported for German by Behrens (2001) and in the acquisition of evidential modality for Korean by Choi (1995) and for Cantonese by Lee and Law (2000).

Marking reference in discourse

Turkish does not have an article system for marking referents as definite or indefinite. Instead it orchestrates a number of devices such as case marking, word order, the numeral *bir* 'one', which functions like an indefinite article, and contextual cues.

As already discussed, children know very early that indefinite objects can only occupy the preverbal position, whereas accusative marked definite objects can be shifted around. Omissions of the accusative are not many but the majority occur in the preverbal position that allows unmarked objects with nonreferential and nonspecific reading in the adult language. Ketrez (2004) carried out a detailed analysis of these errors in the speech of Deniz and observed that they increase in Phase III when her morphosyntax gets consolidated and errors of omission for the other cases decrease. She found that 8% of the preverbal omissions are clearly ungrammatical since they were missing on either a pronoun, proper noun or a specific object, as in Example (8):

(8) CHI: *ayı-cık* *bu-*0* *deyre-iyo* *[:seyir ed-iyor]*
bear-DIM this-*0ACC watch-PROG
The little bear is watching this

At this point in development, there are no ungrammatical case omissions in any position besides the preverbal one and objects in postverbal position are all case marked, suggesting that the child already has an adult-like rule that unmarked objects are allowed only in the preverbal position. However, the fact that she omits marking from specific objects shows that she has not yet learned fully the language-specific constraint, which requires specific objects to be case marked, and that the accusative is not yet a 'specifity marker' for her. In a further study, Ketrez (2005) presents experimental evidence from older children that shows that adult-like use of the accusative rests upon the understanding of the information structure of the language and advances in discourse pragmatics at the interface of different components of grammar.

Developments in children's expression of information structure are revealed by studies of narrative discourse. Analyzing picture book elicited narratives, Dasinger and Küntay (1998) found that three-year-olds achieve referential continuity using null subjects carried by person markers on the verb but scarcely use the indefinite marker *bir* 'one' to introduce characters into discourse before age 7. Özcan (1997) similarly observed that referential continuity is achieved by the null-subject strategy whereas the use of third person pronouns (*o/onlar*) is not frequent. Küntay (1999, 2002) also investigated the introduction of referents in spontaneously occasioned narratives, lists, and picture elicited narratives. She found that for first mentions, preschoolers use presentational constructions with the indefinite *bir* 'one' (*bir X var* 'there:exists one X') and with a possessive pronoun (*benim var* POSS:PRO exist 'mine exists' [:I have]) but not explicit indefinite noun phrases. In picture elicited narratives, first mention of the main animate character was realized by the use of a bare NP by 3–6-year-olds, with the use of indefinite NPs increasing after age 7. Küntay's studies reveal that children's referential strategies are dependent on genre; they are more sophisticated in spontaneous narratives and lists than in picture elicited ones where shared information between the teller and the listener can be assumed. Özcan's (1998) findings similarly show that 3–7-year-olds and most adults prefer definite NPs, null subjects and demonstratives when referents are available in context for both participants and that indefinite constructions increase after age 7 when only the speaker has the relevant knowledge.

Voice alternations

The passive, causative, reflexive or reciprocal affixes are interposed between the verb and the t-a-m markers and change the argument structure of the verb. Early acquisition data show that children start using these constructions around age 2;0 (Aksu-Koç & Slobin, 1985; Özcan & Topbaş, 2000; Savaşır & Gee, 1982; Slobin, 1994; Sofu, 1995). In our data, passive and causative verbs emerge between 1;6 and 2;0 and development continues until 3;0. During this period about 10% of the verbs bear passive morphology and 10% of the verbs causative morphology. The reflexive emerges between 1;9 and 2;1 on less than 5% of verbs, whereas the reciprocal is not observed (Ketrez, 1999b).

The passive is used most often from a nonagentive perspective, when a desired action does not occur because objects resist, when a past resultant state is under focus or when habitual activities or norms of behavior are talked about. Slobin (1994) reports the use of such agentless passives in spontaneous speech as early as age 2;0–2;6. In our data, children produce the passive form of a verb in the same session with its active form (e.g. *aç-ıl-* 'open-PASS' versus *aç-* 'open') sometime between ages 1;8 and 2;0, making errors only when there is a specific agent involved. In the case of these occasional errors, the verb is marked with the passive morpheme; however, the agent, which is the child herself, is incorrectly mapped onto the surface subject with first person marking on the verb or with the pronoun *ben* 'I', or both, as in Example (9).

(9) CHI: *yap-a-mi-yoy-um [=! tries to close something]* (Deniz-1;11)
do-POT-NEG-PROG-1S
I cannot do it.
CHI: *kapa-n-ma-z,* <u>ben</u> **kapa-n-dı-m.*
close-PASS-NEG-AOR I close-PASS-PAST-1S
It does not close, I am closed (it). [uttered upon success]

Ketrez (2000) argues that such errors illustrate the difficulties children have in suppressing the agent rather than in moving the theme argument to subject position since they occur neither in passives that do not involve an agent (e.g. referring to diapers that spontaneously get undone: *adı:-dı [aç-ıl-dı]* open-PASS-PAST (Deniz, 1;8)) nor in passives that refer to habitual or normative activities that lack specific agents (e.g. referring to the right time to read a book: *oku-n-u:r* read-PASS-AOR 'it is read' (Mine, 1;11)). That is, children can move the theme argument to subject position and insert the passive morphology, but have difficulty in suppressing the agent only in passives that describe an action/state brought about by a specific agent, typically the child herself. Thus the errors in mapping semantic roles onto syntactic positions do not seem to result from a lack in syntactic knowledge but from a conflict at the discourse–pragmatic level that 'arise from an attempt to talk about an action performed by the self, but from the point of view of the object that is undergoing the action' (Ketrez, 1999a).

The causative particle transitivizes intransitive verbs or adds an instigative meaning to already transitive verbs. Syntactically, an agent/instigator argument is inserted into the sentence frame to occupy the subject role together with associated changes in case marking; however, this argument does not necessarily appear in the surface due to nominal ellipsis. Early errors display an inability to attach the suffix to the stem, which results in an ungrammatical construction, as exemplified with a transitive verb in Example (10).

(10)	CHI:	**gi:-di-m [giy-di-m].*			(Deniz-1;6)
		put+on-PAST-2S			
	MOT:	*ama*	*sen*	*onu*	*giydirdin.*
		But	you	it-ACC	put+on-CAUS-PAST-2S
		But you dressed it			

The error of undermarking in Example (10) is similar to the passive errors discussed above since the child fails to suppress the self as the real agent and marks the verb for first person, although the subject of the sentence is the argument that is affected by her action (i.e. her doll). But at this age she does not have the morphology either.

To explain the causative errors due to overmarking of intransitive verbs that have lexically transitive counterparts, we suggested in Aksu-Koç and Slobin (1985) that children might be assigning a general causative meaning to the morpheme, and not having yet learned which verbs are lexically causative (e.g. *yan-* 'burn' versus *yak-* 'cause to burn'; *gir-* 'enter' versus *sok-* 'make enter') and which allow for productive causative derivation, they add the affix that is the dominant productive pattern in the language, yielding errors such as **yan-dır-ıyor* 'burn-CAUS-PROG' and **gir-dir-* 'enter-CAUS'. Cases of undermarking as in **üt-tü-nü çık-yo* [çık-arı-ıyor] cloth-POSS&3S-ACC come:out-PROG 'he is coming out his clothes' [= taking off his clothes] (Deniz 1;9) can also be explained in the same way. In short, learning this part of Turkish morphology which presents irregularities is open to competition between overgeneralization by analogy versus rote learning. The fact that the addition of the causative morpheme does not always result in the presence of an additional argument due to the high frequency nominal ellipsis in CDS may also slow down sorting out the irregularities.

Despite these errors, correct use of causative morphology in proper syntactic structures, with shifts between causative and noncausative forms of the verb, is observed starting around 2;0 (e.g. *dat-ın-ı düse:-t-iyoy-um* hair-POSS&2S-ACC fix-CAUS-PROG-1S 'I am fixing your hair' and *düde:-di* fix-PAST 'it is fixed' (Deniz 1;9)). Such examples show how children can alternate between two morphological forms of the verb and appropriate case markers when they want to stress different perspectives and thus different arguments (Ketrez, 1999a).

Participial constructions

Participial adjectives produced by derivational processes provide additional evidence for the phenomena discussed above. In a study using pictures for elicitation (Aksu-Koç, 1988a), 3–4-year-olds produced errors such as **ısır-mış elma* (bite-PAST.PART apple 'apple that has bitten', resulting from undermarking with the passive particle. Adjectives derived with *-mIş* focus on the end state achieved by the undergoer of a change of state verb. For intransitives such as *patla-* 'blow up/pop' that have a single argument which is the undergoer, the participial form directly expresses this focus as in *patla-mış balon* pop-PAST.PART 'popped baloon'. For transitive verbs such as *ısır-* 'bite', the passive particle must be included to suppress the agent, yielding *ısır-ıl-mış* elma (bite-PASS-PAST.PART apple 'apple that has been bitten'), because it is the resultant state of the patient and not the agent that is being encoded. Errors such as **ısır-an elma* (bite-PRES.PART apple 'apple that bites') instead of *ısır-ıl-an elma* (bite-PASS-PRES.PART apple 'apple that is bitten') are similarly due to the undermarking of the passive, which the present participle requires when used to modify an inanimate patient noun rather than an agent. These errors show that derivational morphology that changes verb argument structures present difficulties at the interface of morphology, syntax and semantics because they require knowledge about the semantics of the participial suffixes, a proper analysis of verb argument structures, and their correct alignment.

Summary

In summary, developments at the interface of morphosyntax, semantics and pragmatics are gradual. While construction of inflectional paradigms does not pose a learning problem given their extreme regularity, using these in appropriate sentence frames in appropriate contexts rests on a more protracted process of learning. Paradigm building can be explained by rule learning but learning the argument structures requires experience with individual verbs (Tomasello, 1992). Morphological processes involved in voice alternations present irregularities that call for rote learning, which again implies item-based learning. Mastery of all the functions of nominal and verbal inflections waits upon further developments in complex syntax and semantics in the following years, examples of which are discussed below.

Developments in the Lexicon

Developmental trends in English (Fenson *et al.*, 1994) indicate that productive vocabulary around 16 months is about 50 words, reaching 320 around age 2. As yet, we do not have approximations of productive vocabularies based on large samples, but small sample studies indicate that the early vocabularies of Turkish children are balanced between nouns and verbs. For example, Sofu's (1995) study with four girls between 2;0 and 3;6 shows that children's noun vocabulary increases from an average of 30 at 2;0 to 300 at 3;6, and verb vocabulary from an average of 30 to 255. These figures indicate that nouns and verbs start off equal but there is a greater increase in the number of nouns with age. Küntay and Slobin (2001) also report a noun bias in terms of variety but a verb bias in terms of frequency.

Nouns

Sofu (1995) reports that the majority of the nouns children use are simple. At 3;6 only 6–12% of all nouns used are derived and 2–3% are compounds, indicating that derivational strategies are preferred over compounding in line with the typological characteristics of the language. Early examples of contrastive pairs with productive suffixes start around 2;6 (e.g. *ev* 'house' versus *ev-cik* 'house-DIM', *halı* 'rug' versus *halı-cı* 'rug-AGENTİVE'). Nouns are derived more often from verbs than from other nouns. Interestingly the diminutive is used with very low frequency both on nouns (6% of total derived nouns) or adjectives (8.5% of total derived adjectives). We did not find the diminutive to be very frequent either in Deniz's or her mother's speech (Ketrez & Aksu-Koç, 2007). Although diminutives are a functional strategy for simplifying the inflectional system in languages such as Italian and Dutch in the early stages (Kempe *et al.*, 2007), diminutives in Turkish, rather than simplifying inflectional morphology that is very regular to begin with, seem to introduce phonological, morphological, lexical and pragmatic complexity.

Verbs

Up to age 2, root verbs are the most frequent; after age 3, the proportion of simple inflected verbs is 50–65%, of derived verbs 30–45% and of compound verbs 5–6% (Özcan & Topbaş, 2000; Sofu, 1995). Creative examples from children between ages 3 and 7 (Ekmekçi, 1988) show the productive use of both word formation processes. Verbs are derived either by means of voice particles or by suffixation on nouns, verbs or adjectives. A common strategy is to use the suffix *-lI* to derive a new verb from an adjective (*saçımı güzel-le* 'make my hair beautiful' (3;7)) or a noun (e.g. *dondurma *dil-li-yorum* 'I'm tonguing ice cream' instead of *yala* 'lick' (3;6). Derivational errors involve redundantly nominalizing a verb already derived from a noun (using *kir-len-ti oldu* 'got dirty' instead of *kir-li oldu*). Compounding with *ol-* 'be/become, *et-* 'make/do' and *yap-* 'make/do' yields either structures that exist in the adult language (e.g. *banyo yap-* 'take a bath') or creative structures for which adults have a specific lexical verb or a different compound from that the child has not acquired yet (e.g. *gül:çene oldum* (laugh:chin be-PAST-1Sg to mean 'I got (chin):tired of laughing'). Compounding also results in new NPs in line with Clark's (1993) 'principle of contrast' (e.g. *saplı et* 'meat with handles' for lamb chops, as opposed to 'meat') and is found to be a functional process for bilingual children who often produce substitutes for specific verbs they do not know (van der Heijden, 1997).

Adjectives

Adjectives emerge later than nouns and verbs, are scarce in early CDS and increase in frequency after 2;6, as in other languages (Aksu-Koç *et al.*, 2008; Caselli *et al.*, 1995; Ravid & Levie, under review; Sofu, 1995). Simple adjectives precede derived adjectives. In Sofu's data, the overall order of emergence for structurally different adjectives is as follows: lexical (*kırmızı* 'red', *güzel* 'pretty') > derived with suffixes *-lI* (*kötü kalp-li* 'bad hearted') and *-Ik* (*kır-Ik* 'broken') > suffix *-En* (*koş-an* 'running') > *-cIk* (*küçü-cük* 'small-DIM') and *-sIz* (*uyku-suz* 'sleepless').[6] Attributive and predicative uses emerge at the same time but predicative use is the more frequent strategy. On the task designed to elicit participial adjectives with *-En* and *–mIş* discussed previously (Aksu-Koç, 1988a), three-year-olds preferred predicative to attributive constructions, confirming the trends observed in English or Hebrew (Ravid & Levie, under review). Sofu (1995) has proposed that predicative use may be simpler because it expresses a focus on a single aspect of the entity: the attribute mentioned in the predicate. Attributive use where the adjectival phrase is embedded in a larger clause, on the other hand, implies focusing on both the attribute expressed by the modifier in the attributive slot and that expressed by the predicate of the clause. Furthermore, predicative use fits the schema of simple SOV sentences.

Demonstrative pronouns

Demonstrative pronouns in Turkish present a tripartite system that rests on social-interactive in addition to spatial contrasts (Özyürek & Kita, 2000): *bu* 'this' and *o* 'that' are used, respectively, in referring to a proximal or distal object when the participants share attention on it, whereas *şu* is used when joint attention on objects has not been achieved. Küntay and Özyürek (2006: 345) explored the use of these demonstratives by four- and six-year-olds and adults and found that children prefer *bu*, whereas adults use *şu* more frequently. Both children and adults use *bu* for objects close to speakers, and *şu* for all spaces. Adults use *şu* for control and *bu* for ideational utterances, whereas children do neither. Even six-year-olds do not display adult-like use for *şu*, which is used for 'conversational management of joint attention' by adults. These findings, which illustrate another case of protracted development, are surprising given the early sensitivity of infants to contexts of joint attention for communication (Tomasello,

2003); the authors explain them by noting that children may have difficulty in integrating nonverbal pragmatic factors with verbal expression.

Later Grammatical Competence: Complex Sentences

During the third year, children start producing complex syntactic constructions that serve information packaging (Berman & Slobin, 1994; Diessel, 2004). They learn how to balance their communicative goals with the needs of the listener, how to present new information while keeping the shared in the background, what to express in a main versus subordinate clause, and what type of clause structure to use for different types of contingency relations (Yumrutaş, 2008). Thus, in trying to become effective discourse participants and narrators, children put to use their syntactic, semantic and pragmatic knowledge as well as their cognitive resources. In the following sections, I summarize research on the acquisition of clausal structures for syntactic packaging providing evidence from conversational and narrative discourses.[7]

In English complex sentences, the two clauses preserve their canonical form and subordination is realized by the use of conjunctions in adverbial clauses and the pronoun *that* in complement and relative clauses. The acquisition of these constructions is mostly completed by age 3. Turkish subordinate clauses, on the other hand, undergo a number of syntactic operations such that the surface form does not reflect underlying meaning in a transparent fashion as in simple structures. Furthermore, the type of complementizer changes with the properties of the matrix verb and subject and object relatives require different relativizers. Hence, complex sentences pose problems and need the scaffolding adults provide in discourse. Conversational data show that dependent clauses are produced first in response to adult questions that contain the matrix clause, and only afterwards occur in self-initiated independent child utterances (Aksu, 1978; Aparici *et al.*, 2003; Bloom *et al.*, 1976; Clancy *et al.*, 1976; Hoff, 2006; Tomasello & Brooks, 1999, among others).

Coordination

Coordination involves joining two functionally equivalent independent clauses with conjunctions in order to link or contrast events. Conversational data from 29 children between 1;9 and 4;6 (Aksu, 1978) and narrative data from three-, five-, seven- and nine-year-olds and adults (Aksu-Koç, 1994; Topbaş & Özcan, 1995) show that coordination is the earliest means of connectivity observed up to 2;6. First observed are the particle *işte* 'there' used to affirm what has gone before in discourse, and the emphatic particle *dA* used to present one event as equivalent to (e.g. *çocuk uyuyor, hav hav da uyuyor* 'the boy is sleeping, the dog is sleeping too' (3;0)) or contingent on another event (e.g. *üşümüşler de örtüyorum* 'they are cold so I am covering them' (3;0)). The conjunction *ve* 'and' is not observed at all and very few instances of the adversative *ama/fakat* 'but' are observed before age 7. Most frequent are the temporal connectives *sonra* 'then' and *ondan sonra* 'after that', which function to sequence utterances in discourse as well as events in narrative.

Around 2;6–3;0, children either juxtapose sentences in the cause–effect order without any connective or use *ondan* 'from that' and *onun için* 'that's why' that point anaphorically to the previous clause as causal. They use the effect–cause order to justify an intended action with *çünkü* 'because' or without explicit connectives. They sometimes come up with wrong ordering of clauses, as in Example (11), showing how conceptual organization of notions may cause problems independent of syntax.

(11) MOT: *Niçin aradın?*
Why did you call?
CHI: *Onun için ara-dı-m, siz-e gel-ecek-ti-m.* (2;4)
that-GEN for call-PAST-1S, you:2S-dat come-FUT-PAST-1S
I called for that reason, I was going to come to you
(Correct order= *size gelecektim, onun için aradım*)

Coordinating conjunctions that relate chunks of utterances describing events temporally or causally connected (e.g. *bu sırada/o sırada* 'at this/that time', *öte yandan* 'on the other hand', *ve* 'and') are observed in the narratives of older children and adults. However, their complexity is more a function of the type of discourse than of the syntax or the semantics of the form.

Subordination with adverbial clauses

Adverbial clauses are formed by appending to the verb of the subordinate clause either (1) a suffix that results in a nonfinite form transforming it to a *converb* or (2) a nominalizer marked for possession and case and followed by a postposition. Converbs most frequent in early CS between 2;6 and 3;6 are *V+IncA* 'when/cause' expressing sequence/contingency (e.g. *Bu bas-ınca çalış-ır değil mi?* this push-CONV work-AOR, doesn't it? 'This works when you push it doesn't it?' (2;8)) and *V+Arken* 'while' expressing simultaneity (e.g. *Bu-nu ben gid-erken giy-iyor-um.* this-ACC I go-CONV wear PROG-1S 'I wear this when I am going.' (3;4)). These constructions set reference time, and there is no coreferentiality restriction on the subjects of the two clauses. *V+Ip* 'having V+ed' and *V+ArAk* 'by V+ing' appear around 3;6–4;0 in spontaneous conversations. *V+Ip* expresses a tight sequential relation between the actions denoted by the main and subordinate verbs, and *V+ArAk* expresses a temporal/causal/instrumental relation or manner of action. The conjoined events are interpreted in terms of background–foreground relations within a single complex event since the subjects of the two clauses are coreferential (Aksu-Koç, 1988b, 1994; Slobin, 1993).

While *-IncA*, *-Arken* and *-Ip* are absent from the narratives of three-year-olds, there are few examples in the narratives of five- and seven-year-olds (Aksu-Koç, 1994; Slobin, 1993; Topbaş & Özcan, 1995) as in Example (12). However, *-ArAk* is scarce because children have trouble in choosing which aspect of the situation to foreground and which aspect to background with *-ArAk*, as illustrated in Example (13).

(12) *Sonra camdan bak-**arken**, bir kavanozu al-**ıp** da köpek başına geçirmiş* (5;2)
Then while looking [V+Arken] out the window, taking [V+Ip] the jar, the dog put it on its head.

(13) **Çocuk ağaca çık-**arak** kurbağanın bir deliğe saklanmış olduğunu sandı.* (9;1)
The boy, climbing [V+ArAk] the tree, thought that the frog had hidden in a hole.
(Correct order: *Çocuk kurbağanın bir deliğe saklanmış olduğunu san-**arak** ağaca çık-tı.*
The boy, thinking the frog had hidden in a hole, climbed the tree.)

Slobin (1993) suggests that errors as in Example (13) arise due to the complex requirement of managing attention flow to the temporal–causal organization of events in narrative in addition to the ability to mark two actions as constituent parts of a complex event. Such examples again show how discourse genre makes a difference to the mental load of using a given structure.

Adverbial clauses formed by nominalized forms of the verb (*V+mA/-mAk/-DIK/-(y)AcAK*) and followed by a postposition (e.g. *için* 'for', *zaman* 'time', *sonra* 'after') are also observed around 3;6–4;0 in conversational discourse. The causal adverbial *-DIğI için* 'because of V+ing' and the semantically more general temporal adverbial V+*DIkta* 'at time of V+ing' are observed earlier than the more specific *V+DIKtan sonra* 'after V+ing' and *V+mAdAn önce* 'before V+ing', both in spontaneous speech and in narratives (Aksu-Koç, 1994; Topbaş & Özcan, 1995). Example (14) is produced in response to an adult why-question, and Example (15) is from the narrative of a five-year-old.

(14)	*Oyuncak*	*ol-duğ-u*	*için*	*uç-ma-z*	(3;8)
	Toy	be-NOM-POSS:3S	for	fly-NEG-AOR	

It does not fly because it is a toy.

(15)	*kurbağayı*	*orada*	*gör-e-me-**dik-leri***	***zaman***	*her yere*	*bakıyorlar.*	(5;0)
	frog-ACC	there	see-POT-NEG-NOM-POSS:3P	POST	everywhere	look-PROG-3P	

They look everywhere when they cannot see the frog there

In these adverbial structures where the verb has lost its canonical surface shape, the two clauses are syntactically integrated, but the distance between surface form and underlying meaning is increased (Aksu-Koç & Slobin, 1985).

Complement clauses

In Turkish complement structures, the subject of the embedded clause receives the genitive, the nominalized verb is marked by the possessive for agreement, and the whole clause is marked for case. Complementizers *-DIK* and *–(y)ACAK* express factivity, while *-mAk* and *-mA* express nonfactive notions such as wish, manner and appreciation (Özsoy, 1988). The semantics of the complementizers have to be compatible with that of the matrix verbs (Taylan, 1998), which may be volitional (e.g. *want, like*), aspectual (e.g. *start, try*), perceptual (e.g. *see, hear*), causative (e.g. *make, have*), and communicative verbs (e.g. *tell, ask*) (Diessel, 2004; Givon, 1989). The conjunctions *ki* and *diye*[8] and the verbs: *zannet-/san-* 'assume/think', *bil-* 'know' and *tahmin et-* 'guess' take sentential complements where the complement verb maintains its finite form (Taylan, 1998). Infinitival complements with (*-mAk*) are simpler since the subjects of the two clauses are co-referential and the matrix subject appears in the nominative just like the subjects of simplex sentences.

Complement constructions have been traced in our data by Altan (2005) who observed that they are infrequent in the input, either because mothers simplify their speech by using sentential complements or because there are not many occasions to use them. They are also very scarce in children's speech; the only examples before 2;6 are infinitival complements with *-mAk* with aspectual/modal verbs *başla-* 'begin', *çalış-* 'try' and the desire verb *iste-* 'want'.

(16)	CHI:	sen de	***ye-me***	***itte-e mi-sin***	***makana***?	(Azra 2;1,29)
		you too	eat-NOM	want-AOR QUE-2S	spaghetti?	
		Do you want to eat spaghetti too?				

Subject and object complements with *-mA* (Examples (17) and (18), respectively) are observed around 2;8–3;0.

(17)	CHI:	bak	bu-nu	***bul-ma-n***	***la:zım.***	(Mine 2;8,10)
		look	this-ACC	find-NOM-2S	necessary.	
		Look you have to find this.				

(18)	CHI:	*bu-nun*	***kız***	***ol-ma-sı-nı***	***isti-yor-um.***	(Azra 2;9)
		this-GEN	girl	be-NOM-POSS-ACC	want-PROG-1S	
		I want this to be a girl				

-DIK and *-AcAK* complements are observed after 3;0 but pose problems with the irregular verb *ol-* 'be' that is required as an auxiliary in the embedding of sentences with nonverbal predicates. In Example (19), instead of the nominalizer *-DIK*, Azra adds *-DI past* to the complement verb *ol-* and produces two finite clauses that do not form a grammatical unit.

(19) CHI: *Aslı ben-im *ol-ma-dı* *bil-me-den* Edis-e ver-di. (Azra 3;3)
Aslı I-POSS be-NEG-PAST know-NEG-ABL Edis-DAT give-PAST
Aslı gave it to Edis not knowing that it is mine.

The fact that she can produce the *-mA* complement with *ol- 'be'* in Example (27) at 2;9 suggests that the ungrammatical construction in Example (28) results from the interaction of semantic (meaning of the main verb *bil-* 'know'), morphosyntactic (nominalizing the auxiliary *ol-* 'be' with *-DIK*), and processing (an adverbial and a complement clause embedded in a main clause) factors.

A similar sequence is observed in the conversations of 36 children between 2;0 and 4;8 of the Berkeley Crosslinguistic Acquisition Project (Altan, 2005) and in the Frog narratives of 30 children between 3;0 and 9;0 (Aksu-Koç, 1994). Two-to-three-year-olds use *-mAk* complements with *iste-* 'want' and *lazım* 'necessary' as predicates. Three-to-four-year-olds prefer sentential complements to *-DIK* complements (e.g. *Büyük hayvan nereye tırmandı biliyor musun?* Big animal where climb-PAST know-PROG QUE-2S 'Do you know where the big animal climbed?' (3;8)) and use *-mA* complements in coreferential 'know how' constructions (e.g. *Ev yap-ma-sı-nı bil-iyor-um.* house make-NOM POSS-ACC know-PROG-1S. 'I know how to make a house.' (4;0)). *-DIK* complements are scarce both in conversational (e.g. *gör-üyor-sun işte nasıl ol-duğ-u-nu* 'You see how it is' (4;4)), and in narrative data. Boeschoten (1990) also reports a preference for *-mAK* and an avoidance of *-mA* complements in picture descriptions of Turkish–Dutch bilingual 5–8-year-olds and their monolingual peers.

The sequence of acquisition can be summarized as follows: *-mAk* object complements > *-mA* subject complements with modal predicates > *-mA* object complements, and sentential complements with *diye* > *-DIK* and *-(y) AcAK* complements with verbs of saying and cognition. *-MAk* complements with coreferential main and embedded subjects are syntactically simpler like the infinitival constructions in English or Korean (Bloom *et al.*, 1984; Limber, 1973; Kim, 1989). Although *-mA* and *-DIK* are equally complex syntactically, *-mA* is earlier because it is selected by the highly accessible desire verb *iste-* 'want' and by the modal predicates *gerek/lazım* 'need/necessary' used frequently by adults to impose normative behavior to children. Sentential complements with *san-* 'suppose/think' and *bil-* 'know' pose complexity due to the semantics of these cognitive verbs acquired around age 4 with developments in 'theory of mind' (Astington & Byrd, 2005; Bartsch & Wellman, 1995; de Villiers & de Villiers, 2000; among others). The late emergence of *-DIK* and *-(y)AcAK* selected by these cognitive verbs can therefore be explained by semantic as well as syntactic complexity plus the fact that they figure in adverbial and relative clauses violating the 'one form–one function' principle. Complements with verbs of saying are scarce because in many contexts the reportative morpheme *-ImIş* appended to a simplex sentence can serve the same function as they do.

In short, the late acquisition of complement structures is a function of the complex syntax of nominalization, the semantic–pragmatic function of the matrix verb, the semantic and the syntactic requirements of the complementizer, the knowledge of what complementizer goes with what verb, and low frequency of occurrence in CDS.

Relative clauses

Relative clauses in Turkish, like complements, are nontransparent, noncanonical structures posing difficulties for comprehension and production (Aksu-Koç & Slobin, 1985; Slobin, 1986). The relativizer is formed with a participial verb form: *–An* marks subject relatives, *-DIK*, *-(y)AcAK*, *-mIş*, and *–Ir* mark nonsubject relatives where the relativized element may be the direct or oblique object. In nonsubject relatives, the subject of the relative clause takes the genitive and the verb carries the possessive for agreement. In subject relatives, there is no genitive and, hence, no agreement. The *-DAki* structure, which does not have a verb form, functions as a simpler means of relativization.

Early examples are in the form of adjectival or postpositional phrases rather than full embedded clauses, as illustrated with the *pronominalizer+ki* construction in Example (20), *–En* in Example (21), *-DIK* in Example (22) and *-(y)AcAK* in Example (23). These examples lend support to Diessel's (2004) proposal that relative clauses emerge from simple sentences that are gradually expanded to multiple-clause structures.

(20)	CHI:	*ben-im-ki-ti*	*bit-ti.*	(Deniz, 1;10)
		I-GEN-*ki*-POSS&3S	finish-PAST	
		Mine is finished.		

(21)	CHI:	*ağlay-**an***	*bebek*	(2;3, Ekmekçi, 1986)
		cry- run-SREL	baby	
		crying baby		

(22)	CHI:	*pazarda*	*abi-nin*	*ye-**diğ**-in-den*	(2;6, Sofu, 1995)
		market-LOC	brother-GEN	eat-NSREL-POSS-ABL	
		Same as what the brother was eating at the marketplace.			

(23)	CHI:	*karıştır-**acak***	*şey*	(2;7, Sofu, 1995)
		stir-FUTURE.PART	thing	
		Thing to stir with (=spoon)		

Early errors show that children have difficulty in defining the set of relativizers but choose from the numerous nonfinite verb forms for clause conjoining as in **yat-arak kedi* (sleep-*CONVERB cat) instead of *yat-an kedi* (sleep-SREL kedi 'sleeping cat' (3;0)). Evidence from experimental studies confirms this picture of complexity and late acquisition.

In an acting out study testing the comprehension of different types of relative clauses such as Example (24a and b), Slobin (1986: 283) observed that even 4–5-year-olds ignored the relative clause (*italicized*) and just acted out the main clause (CAPITALIZED) that corresponds to a canonical SOV simplex sentence. He explained the findings in terms of difficulties in identifying 'these nonfinite participial forms as verbs with their appropriate valences and participants in complex sentences'.

(24a)	*Kuş-un*	*düşür-**düğü***	*İNEK*	ZEBRA-YI	OKŞA-SIN.
	bird-GEN	knock:down-NSREL	cow	zebra-ACC	pat-OPT

'The cow that the bird knocks down should pat the zebra.'

(24b)	KUŞ	*zebra-yı*	*okşa-**yan***	*İNEĞ-İ*	DÜŞÜR-SÜN.
	bird	zebra-ACC	pat-SREL	cow-ACC	knock:down-OPT

The bird should knock:down-OPT the cow that patted the zebra.

A second problem Slobin (1986: 277) noted is that Turkish 'relative clauses are not constructed in a uniform way across different types of relativization'. Children have to figure out the grammatical role the relativized noun plays in the subordinate clause from the relativizer used (subject if *–An*, or *-DAki*, and nonsubject if *-DIK*) and the grammatical role it plays in the matrix sentence from the case marking (subject if nominative as in SS and SO sentences, and object if accusative as in OS and OO sentences [where the first letter designates the role of the relativized element in the matrix clause and the second letter its role in the subordinate clause]). Since both *–An* and *-DIK* relatives can modify either the matrix subject or the object, there is no 1:1 mapping between the relativizer and the syntactic role in the matrix sentence.

Research on relative clauses has benefited from the predictions of a number of hypotheses. Keenan and Comrie (1977) state that subject relatives are easier than object relatives ({SS, OS} > {SO, OO}) due to the universal order of grammatical functions on the accessibility hierarchy (AH). This hypothesis predicts *–An* relatives to be easier than *-DIK* relatives (see 24b above). Sheldon's (1974) parallel function (PF) hypothesis makes the opposite prediction that processing will be easier if the head of the relative clause has the same grammatical role in the relative as in the matrix clause than if the grammatical roles are different ({SS, OO} > {SO and OS}). This hypothesis predicts an equal distribution of *–An* and *-DIK* relatives.

Children's errors that show that *–An* relatives are favored and often substituted for *-DIK* relatives (Aksu-Koç, 1988a) support the AH but not the PF hypothesis on structural grounds. However, this could also be because *–An* is functionally restricted to subject relativization and thus serves as a salient surface cue, whereas *-DIK* structures that relativize different nonsubject roles and figure in complement and adverbial clauses are multifunctional. Research results are informative about the role of underlying structural factors versus attention to local surface cues.

In conversational data from matched Turkish and English child samples between 1;0 and 4;8 and their mothers, Slobin (1986) found an almost equal distribution of nonsubject and subject relatives in English where the canonical form of simple sentences are preserved, but there is a preference for subject (88%) over object relatives (12%) in Turkish. These differences show that when the language presents equivalent means for relativization on different roles, as does English, subject relatives are not necessarily more accessible than object relatives (Slobin, 1986) contrary to the prediction of the AH. The preference for subject relatives in Turkish then may be due to the properties of *–An* as a surface cue, and the low percentage of nonsubject relatives to the complexity of the *-DIK* construction that results in a deformation of the sentence away from the canonical form.

Özcan's (2000: 312) study with five–nine-year-olds provides support in this regard. In a production experiment, correct responses averaged around 40–50% for subject relatives {SS and OS} with *–An*, but between 2% and 8% for object relatives {SO and OO} with *-DIK*. Özcan concluded by stressing the importance of 'the morphological marking of the relativized constituent', that is, the salience of *–An* as a surface cue that satisfies the *one form–one function principle*. Ketrez (2007) found a higher proportion of subject than object relatives in adult narratives, but a preference for PF structures (SS and OO sentences with an equal distribution of *–An* and *-DIK* relatives) in the stories of five- and nine-year-olds. Both Özcan's child data and Ketrez's adult data support the AH as well as the surface cue hypothesis. Children's narrative data, which support the PF hypothesis that favors the same subject relatives, on the other hand, can be explained by their tendency to maintain the same protagonist as the topic across utterances (Aksu-Koç & Tekdemir, 2004),[9] whereas adults who can easily shift from the perspective of one actor to another are not so constrained and use different subject OS relatives more freely. In fact, in another set of adult narratives, we found that *-DIK* constructions, which can relativize on any nonsubject role, outnumber *-(y)En* relatives (Taylan & Aksu-Koç, 1998), indicating that with mature subjects what determines frequency of use is functionality in a given discourse genre rather than complexity of structure.

Other surface cues investigated in relation to processing of relative clauses are prototypical N-V-N schemas developed for simplex sentences in English (de Villiers *et al.*, 1979) and inflectional marking in Japanese and Korean (Clancy *et al.*, 1986). In Turkish, nominal inflections rather than word order have cue value. Case marking in simplex sentences matches that in center-embedded relatives where the first noun that is the subject of the matrix clause remains unmarked for the nominative (see 24b). In left-branching relatives (24a), on the other hand, the first noun that is the subject of the relative clause is marked for genitive, deviating from the canonical schema. Slobin (1986) reports experimental evidence that shows that adults prefer relatives beginning with unmarked nouns despite center embedding in addition to preferring *–An* over *-DIK* relatives. For speakers of Turkish, then, inflectional cues play a more significant role than interruptions in the unity of the clause, particularly once they have developed strategies for holding units of information in memory before closure. Considering all five factors together (subject versus object role in the relative clause (AH), same versus different grammatical role in the relative and matrix clauses (PF), left branching versus center embeddedness, canonical versus different case marking of first noun, unifunctionality versus multifunctionality of relativizer), we get Table 4.3. The structures that are easiest and acquired earliest satisfy four out of five determining criteria, whereas those that are the hardest satisfy only one. It is observed that *-An* relatives in Turkish are favored both on structural and processing grounds.

To conclude this section on complex sentences, let me summarize a study where we tested five- and six-year-olds on different complex morphosyntactic structures, using the technique of elicited imitation (Taylan & Aksu-Koç, 2003). The results revealed the following order of complexity for the structures tested, from the least to the most difficult: adversative conjunction *ama* > converb *-IncA, conditional -sA* > converbs *-ArAk* and *-Ip*, adverbial *-DIĞI zaman > adverbial -mAdAn önce,* comparative *daha* > relativizer *–An* > complementizers *-mA* and *-DIK*, relativizer *-DIK*, adverbials *-DIĞI için, -DIKTAn sonra.* Children who could not repeat a sentence verbatim simplified it by deleting the complex constituents such as relative clauses, coordinated NPs, complex verbal or nominal

Table 4.3 Distribution of the subject versus object relative clauses in terms of the parameters they satisfy

	SS –An	*OS –An*	*OO -DIK*	*SO -DIK*
Accessibility hierarchy	+	+	–	–
Parallel function	+	–	+	–
Left versus center embedding	+	–	–	+
Uni-versus multifunctional	+	+	–	–
Canonical first N	–	+	+	–

morphology (modal *-mAlI*, causative and passive suffixes; the genitive marker of the subject of a complement clause). They also tended to delete nonobligatory constituents such as subject pronouns (*ben* 'I'), adverbial phrases (*biraz önce* 'a while ago'), and conjunctions (*ve* 'and', *ama* 'but') in accordance with the typological characteristics of the language. They replaced nonfinite verb forms with finite ones and specific terms with general terms (e.g. *her sabah* 'every morning' with *her zaman* 'always'; *-(y) AcAK* adverbials with *-DIK* adverbials). This order of difficulty and the simplification operations identified reflect very closely the order and the processing strategies observed in the acquisition of complex sentences discussed above.

Concluding Remarks: Implications for Speech and Language Pathologists (SLPs) Working with Turkish Clients

In this overview of the acquisition of Turkish, I focused on the early phase where the basic morphosyntax of the language is established and the later phase when complex constructions tend to be part of the grammar. We saw that acquisition is an active learning process and its timing is a function of the interaction among the complexity of the structures of the specific language being acquired, the functionality of a given structure at a given time and the social, cognitive and processing capacities of the child. Let me now briefly consider some implications of the patterns observed for SLPs working with language delayed or deviant populations acquiring Turkish.

(1) *Language deviance or delay may be caused by problems related to the social, cognitive and perceptual capacities necessary for attending to and analyzing linguistic input.* These range from attention, auditory perception, phonological memory, working memory and other executive functions, to capacities for abstraction, generalization, symbolic-representation and social interaction (Chiat, 2001; Johnston, 1993, 2004; Paul, 2001). For example, O'Hara and Johnston (1997) observed that in assigning thematic roles to objects on the basis of two-argument versus three-argument verbs, SLI children omitted arguments in sentence-initial or -medial positions more often than in final position, and more often in cases of three-argument than two-argument verbs. Such errors reveal the importance of recency and length effects and indicate problems with processing load due to memory limitations. Therefore the first step for the SLP is to take these capacities into primary consideration and check whether they are developing and functioning normally.

(2) *Order of acquisition of the linguistic structures in normal development is informative about what may be vulnerable to deviance or delay in that*

language. Knowledge of what aspects of the system are acquired at roughly what time informs the SLP about what is easy versus complex in the language and gives a baseline for expectations, a standard for comparison and guidelines for intervention. For example, we saw that inflectional morphology is acquired early and with few errors due to the regularity and transparency of the paradigms and saliency of individual morphemes that are word final and stressed. This pattern suggests that noun and verb inflections in Turkish will not pose problems for children showing SLI symptoms, whereas they do in English where the inflections are phonologically weak forms and the inflectional system is neither regular nor rich (O'Hara & Johnston, 1997). Complex clausal constructions, on the other hand, are acquired late in Turkish because subordinate clauses lose their canonical sentential forms and existing strategies need to be modified to accommodate the new structures. Children showing SLI symptoms are likely to experience difficulties with this part of the system. In designing intervention schedules, the SLPs can plan on reinforcing simple morphosyntactic structures before moving on to complex clauses.

We also noted that in interpreting sentences Turkish children rely on morphological cues and knowledge of specific verbs rather than syntactic frames (Göksun *et al.*, 2008), whereas children acquiring English are sensitive to syntactic frames for transitive or intransitive verbs (Naigles, 1990). O'Hara and Johnston (1997) have experimentally shown that SLI children who have problems with temporal morphology can make successful inferences from syntactic frames in making thematic role assignments for nonsense verbs. This suggests that the SLPs working with Turkish clients will be more successful if they focus on morphological cues (case and agreement marking) rather than syntactic frames in teaching how to interpret sentences.

(3) *Acquisition involves complex interactions among the phonological, semantic, syntactic and pragmatic components leading to reorganizations within each component and within subdomains*. It was observed, for example, that generalization of productive inflectional schemas is closely tied to an increase in the number of verbs, the semantic properties of which have a bearing on the development of case and of t-a-m marking. Similarly, the emergence of voice morphology is observed to result in a reorganization of existing schemas whereby the semantic roles of agent and theme and syntactic roles of subject and object decouple and become more flexibly aligned. An example for a problem arising from the interface is the inability of one of our subjects to produce the first person agreement marker due to difficulties she had

pronouncing the /m/ sound in word-final position. In short, the SLP must be aware of the possibility that delayed or deviant patterns of learning in any one component may have effects on the rate and quality of developments in the other components.

(4) *Input should represent the different structures of the ambient language in a stage appropriate, meaningful way*. We saw that early in development, there is a close correspondence in terms of frequency and complexity between the structures modeled by the mother and those acquired by the child. Mothers display a rich variety of morphosyntactic constructions in their speech, but they modulate its level of complexity according to the level of competence of the child. The SLP should similarly be sensitive to the existing level of knowledge of the language delayed child. We saw that different types of cues may be functional at different stages for figuring out the meaning of words and functions of forms. The SLP, therefore, needs to set appropriate teaching goals, using cues available to the learner and building on what she already knows.

(5) *The modes of social interaction whereby input is presented are culturally specific*. In our discussion of complex sentences, we emphasized the role of adult–child discourse as a social-interactional framework within which children develop preferred strategies to 'learn about the structure of the language, the semantics of words and constructions and conversational pragmatics' (Küntay & Slobin, 2002: 12). However, the literature on the cultural and social dimensions of adult–child interaction shows that there are differences that have consequences on aspects of children's language development. Word knowledge, definitional skills, and narrative production abilities are particularly vulnerable to the effects of socio-educational standing of parents (Aksu-Koç *et al.*, 1999; Aksu-Koç, 2004; Hart & Risley, 1995; Johnston & Wong, 2001; Küntay & Ahtam, 2004; Sofu, 1995). These findings indicate that language delayed or deviant children will benefit from conscious intensification of normal interaction patterns; it is therefore important for SLPs to educate parents in this regard, but it is also important to do so in culturally consistent ways (Johnston, 2004).

To conclude, let me share our experience of preparing a short-term language intervention program for 5–6-year-old mono- and bilingual children of disadvantaged families (Bekman *et al.*, under review) and illustrate three principles that Johnston (1985) has proposed for SLPs to follow in therapy: *FIT, FOCUS* and *FUNCTIONALITY*. The program was designed for the socially interactive contexts of kindergarten classrooms, with a highly structured daily routine that allows for predictable language–context matching. In devising the syntactic component, our guide for determining where to start and what structures to include was the order of acquisition displayed by normally developing children and elicited imitation data obtained from the target population revealing the structures produced with most errors (Aksu-Koç *et al.*, 2002). The curriculum was thus devised to FIT the particular needs of the target population; the starting point was the highest level of competence displayed by most of the target children. For the target level of linguistic competence to be reached at the end of the intervention, we relied on developmental profiles obtained from normal, monolingual middle-class children of the same age. This way we tried to ensure FUNCTIONALITY of the constructions taught for the learner. During the 20 min language training period in the daily routine of what could be called a language immersion curriculum, structured exercises, games and stories were used to teach the particular linguistic constructions targeted for the day. This highly structured approach was chosen to help children FOCUS on the semantic–pragmatic functions of the linguistic forms by supporting them with the visual experiential context. I hope that this example, albeit at the community rather than the individual level, illustrates how knowledge of normal language development can be used for intervention purposes.

Notes

1. Abbreviations (adapted from MacWhinney, 2000): ABL: ablative, ACC: accusative, AOR: aorist, CAUS: causative, CHI: child, COM: comitative, CONV: converb, DAT: dative, DIM: diminutive, EVID: evidential, FUT: future, FUTURE.PART: future participle, GEN: genitive, IMP: imperative, INS: instrumental, INDEF: indefinite, LOC: locative, MOT: mother, NEG: negation, NOM: nominalization marker, NSREL: nonsubject relative, OPT: optative, PAST: past tense, PAST:PART: past participle, PASS: passive, PRES.PART: present participle, PROG: progressive, POSS: possessive, POSS.PRO: possessive pronoun, POT: potential, PL: plural, 1/2/3P: 1/2/3 person plural, 1/2/3S: 1/2/3 person singular, QUE: question particle, SREL: subject relative, V: verb, N: noun, PRO: pronoun, (&) morphological fusion, (+) compound marker, (–) morpheme boundary, (0): omission of the following morpheme, (*0): ungrammatical omission, (&): undecipherable form.
2. These data were collected and analyzed as part of three consecutive projects supported by grants from the Boğaziçi University Research Fund to A. Aksu-Koç. (1) 'A Longitudinal Study of the Acquisition of Turkish: The First Phase' (Project No. 94S007) (2) 'A Longitudinal Study of the Acquisition of Turkish: The Second Phase' (Project No. 96S0017); (3) 'A Longitudinal Study of the Acquisition of Turkish: The Third Phase' (Project No. 98 HB 702). Data from the 'frog-story' narratives come from the project 'The development of temporality in narratives: Evidence from Turkish', funded by Boğaziçi University Research Fund, Project No. 86 B 0724.
3. The children are Azra (1;1–3;3), Deniz (1;3–2;0), Mine (1;6–2;10) and Tuna (1;3–1;7). Monthly recordings were made at home by one of the parents. The data were transcribed, coded morphologically and entered into a computer by following the CHAT conventions of the CHILDES project (MacWhinney, 2000) and analyzed quantitatively using the CLAN program.

4. The highest and lowest MLUs in the first and the last recordings calculated in morphemes are as follows: Azra's (MLU = $0.00_{\text{at }1;1}$–$5.13_{\text{at }2;11}$); Deniz (MLU = $1.26_{\text{at }1;3}$–$4.32_{\text{at }2;0}$), mine (MLU = $1.49_{\text{at }1;6}$–$5.75_{\text{at }2;7}$) and Tuna (MLU = $1.13_{\text{at }1;3}$–$1.33_{\text{at }1;7}$).
5. The accusative and the third person singular possessive have the same phonological shape (*-I*) on nouns ending in consonants. The word *bebeğ-i* means either baby-ACC (the baby) or baby-POSS&3S (somebody's baby).
6. Sofu's data are from Adana in the eastern Mediterranean region of Turkey where there are dialectal differences, which is probably why no adjectives derived with the –mIş participle are observed.
7. The conversational data comes from Slobin's Berkeley Crosslinguistic Acquisition Project, and the narrative data comes from Aksu-Koç's frog story data based on the book *Frog Where Are You?* by Mercer Mayer, 1969.
8. For example, *Sen git-ti-n san-dı-m.* (I you go-past-2nd person think-past-1st person) 'I thought you have left.' (Taylan, 1998). Or they are constructed *with ki and diye* (e.g. *Sen gel-ecek-sin diye kek yap-tı-m.* (You come-future-2nd person comp cake make-past-1st person) 'I made cake since you are coming', and *Süt-ün-ü iç ki çabuk büyü-ye-sin.* (milk-2nd poss-acc drink comp quickly grow-optative-2nd person) 'Drink your milk so that you grow very fast.').
9. Ketrez offers to reconcile the conflicting pieces of evidence by using the two hierarchies together: The high frequency of SS relatives is supported by all types of data – except the frog stories of children – and the low frequency of SO relatives is supported by all types of data, findings that are predicted by both hierarchies. OO relatives, which are easier than SO relatives both in experimental and narrative data, fit the PF hypothesis. The high frequency of OS relatives as reflected in errors where *–An* replaces *-DIK* is predicted by the AH hypothesis and the principle of one form–one function, which Ketrez seems to equate with the one function–one role requirement of the PF hypothesis, and suggests that when faced with complexity introduced by multifunctional forms, children may be introducing the PF strategy together with AH. I find this claim arguable since the unifunctionality of the *–An* suffix is a surface rather than an underlying structural feature, and in OS relatives *-En* marks the subject of the relative clause, which is, however, coreferential with the object of the matrix clause. I suggest instead that structural and processing factors should be considered together rather than reducing one to the other.

Chapter 5

Mean Length of Utterance as a Tool for Morphological Assessment in Turkish Children

PINAR EGE

Introduction

In the process of acquiring the language(s) they are exposed to, children learn separate, but in many aspects interrelated, sets of rules in the five components of language: syntax, morphology, phonology, semantics and pragmatics. Since both normally developing children and children with language impairments display varying levels of performance in these components, each component is assessed individually to provide an accurate picture of the child's language.

In a descriptive–developmental approach to assessment, the goal is to decide if the child has a significant deficit in any of the components of language, and if a deficit is identified, to describe that deficit as accurately as possible to eventually determine therapy goals. There are four basic methods used in language assessment: standardized tests, developmental scales, non-standardized or criterion referenced procedures and behavioral observations, each with its advantages and limitations (Paul, 2001), and each contributing a different type of information at a different level within the assessment process.

One way grammatical development is assessed is by computing *mean length of utterance* (MLU) in morphemes. The concept of 'utterance length' has been around for over 50 years (Nice, 1925). In 1973, Brown claimed that MLU determined by morpheme count is a much more accurate tool in quantitatively predicting expressive language in preschool children than is age. According to Brown, children show variation in achieving syntactic skills when age is considered a criterion. Much less variation is observed if MLU stages are used as a descriptive measure. MLU has since been regarded as a reliable general measure of syntactic and morphological complexity for children learning Standard American English. It has been applied to British English (Wells, 1985), Finnish (Bowerman, 1973) and Spanish (Linares, 1983); however, there have been problems in extending the concept to other languages, especially those with wide use of inflections, such as Russian or Hebrew (Dromi & Berman, 1982).

Being an agglutinative language and having relaxed rules regarding word order, Turkish is a highly inflected language and relies on suffixes attached to mostly verbs and nouns to convey information about tense, aspect, negation, person, question, dative, accusative, ablative as well as reflexive, passive, etc. Contrary to the flexibility in word order, the order in which these suffixes are used is unchangeable. In Turkish, it is common to have sentences with just one word and words can be of considerable length, containing as many as 12 morphemes, one free and the others bound. Verbs with 4–5 morphemes are widely encountered in any sentence.

As explained in the previous chapters, although children learning Turkish adhere to many universals of language acquisition, language-specific differences in the acquisition of grammatical structures are observed. For example, as opposed to children learning English, Turkish children do not seem to go through a distinct period during which only two-word combinations with no bound morphemes are used to express various semantic relations. Instead, early morphemes such as the past tense *-di* attached to verbs or the accusative *-i* or dative *–e* attached to nouns (Özcan, 1996; Author, unpublished manuscript) are observed simultaneously with two-word combinations as soon as children reach the two-morpheme stage. Therefore, 'morphemes' rather than 'words' seem to be more critical in determining syntactic complexity in Turkish. It follows that MLU should turn out to be a useful tool in assessing syntactic development in Turkish.

MLU as a Measure for Assessing Syntax

The three normally developing children known as Adam, Eve and Sarah, that Roger Brown followed, showed variability in their development of grammatical structures, as do all children. For example, the structures that Adam and Sarah expressed between the ages of 2;2 and 3;6 were observed in Eve between 1;7 and 2;3. Therefore, Brown concluded that MLU was a better predictor of syntactic/morphological development than age. He and his colleagues divided the MLU continuum around the midpoint values of 1.75, 2.25, 2.75, 3.5 and 4.0, known as Brown's stages I–V, and described the structural achievements of each stage. Regardless of age, the three children Brown studied seemed to demonstrate similar grammatical structures at each MLU stage. Although these stages are rather arbitrary and are not claimed to be discrete, they are associated with qualitatively different levels of development in children's language. Brown's stages are characterized as follows:

Stage I	MLU 1.0–2.0	12–26 months	Semantic relations
Stage II	MLU 2.0–2.5	27–30 months	Grammatical morphemes
Stage III	MLU 2.5–3.25	31–34 months	Sentence modalities
Stage IV	MLU 3.25–3.75	35–40 months	Embedding
Stage V	MLU 3.75–4.25	41–46 months	Sentence coordination

Brown's observations were confirmed later using a much larger sample of children (de Villiers & de Villiers, 1973). De Villiers and de Villiers have also modified Brown's stages to smaller increments of 0.5 morphemes which proved useful in capturing rapid development at early MLU ranges.

Based on data from 123 children between the ages of 17 and 59 months, Miller and Chapman (1981) have shown that there is a linear relationship between age and MLU. MLU increased, on the average, by 1.24 morphemes every year. The Pearson correlation between age and MLU was found to be 0.88. These results were confirmed to a large extent by studies that followed (Rondal *et al.*, 1987; Scarborough *et al.*, 1986). Arguing that the socio-economic status of the children in the Miller and Chapman study was too high, Klee *et al.* (1989) repeated the study with 24 children with a lower socio-economic status and found the correlation between age and MLU to be 0.75.

Miller and Chapman also found the average age at which their subjects displayed MLUs and age ranges for their eight stages based on ±1SD from the average. Two linear regression equations were derived: one predicting age from MLU and the other MLU from age. Klee and Paul (1981) state that when one wishes to determine whether a child's MLU is within normal limits of development for a certain age, a measure of variability is necessary.

Taking the language sample

MLU is a measure based on a free language sample obtained from the child in a natural setting. For the MLU measurements to be valid, obtaining a reliable sample is of utmost importance. Samples can be obtained anywhere such as home, school, a clinical setting, etc. as long as the child is comfortable with the clinician, materials are used properly as facilitators of conversation and the clinician adapts to the cognitive level, interests and other aspects of functioning of the child. In addition, Miller (1981) cautions against the following characteristics of the sample which might affect the reliability of the obtained MLU:

(1) high rate of imitation of the previous speaker;
(2) frequent self-repetitions within a speech turn;

(3) high proportion of questions and answers in the child's speech;
(4) frequent routines, such as counting, nursery rhymes, songs, jingles, etc.; and
(5) high proportion of utterances in which clauses are joined by coordinating conjunctions such as *and, and then* and the like.

The language sample should also be long enough to be representative of the child's speech. Miller (1981) indicates that 30 min of interaction usually produces from 100 to 200 utterances in children 24 months of age or older. Younger children produce about half the number of utterances within the same time period. Generally, 50–100 utterances are considered sufficient for a representative sample if the sample is reliable. The sample is then transcribed. It is also common to exclude the first page of the transcript to allow for the warming-up period between the child and the clinician.

Calculating MLU

To calculate MLU, the transcript is divided into utterances. An utterance is a physically identifiable stretch of speech lacking any grammatical definition. It may be a sentence or a shorter unit separated from other utterances by a pause, a drop in intonation or other physical cues. The utterances are then analyzed into their morphemes. The total number of morphemes in the speech sample is counted and this number is then divided by the total number of utterances.

$$\text{MLU} = \frac{\text{Total number of morphemes}}{\text{Total number of utterances}}.$$

Decisions need to be made as to what should be considered a morpheme. Although Brown has listed the counting rules, one often needs to exercise judgment about whether certain structures should be considered separate morphemes or undivided wholes. Quite often the evidence is available in the language sample itself. The productive use of a morpheme by the child indicates that it should be regarded as separate.

MLU as a Measure in Turkish Samples

It has been mentioned before that MLU as a measure of syntactic development has been shown to be problematic for inflected languages, and adaptations have been necessary. Ege *et al.* (1998) set out to test the applicability of the measure to Turkish, a highly inflected language. The purpose was to investigate the relationship of MLU to age in Turkish and, if a relationship existed, to make the necessary adaptations to be able to employ the concept as a measure of expressive language development in Turkish.

The sample

A total of 95 children between the ages of 17 and 59 months participated in this study. None of the children had any observable disabilities based on parent and teacher reports and observations by the authors. All the children attended age-appropriate classrooms. The half-hour language samples from the children were obtained by experienced clinicians in environments that the children were familiar with, such as home or school. Books, dolls, toy animals and cars were used to facilitate conversation. The conversations were recorded on audio tape.

The samples were transcribed and separated into utterances by the consensus of the three authors. The generally accepted rules for selecting utterances to include in the computations were followed: Unintelligible or partially unintelligible utterances were excluded from the count, but transcriptions marked doubtful were included. The first 50 utterances after the warm-up period were included in the study. However, some very young children could not produce 50 utterances in half an hour. Therefore, for a few children with limited language development in the youngest age group, a 25-utterance sample was set as the limit. Children with fewer than 25 utterances were not included in the study. A 50-utterance language sample rather than the more traditional 100 was chosen to reduce the gap between children with high and low levels of language production.

Calculation of MLU

Brown (1973), Lund and Duchan (1993) and Miller (1981) with slight modifications have clearly set the rules for counting morphemes in each utterance in English; however, owing to differences in the structures of the Turkish language considerable adaptations had to be made to arrive at rules for identifying phonemes. All known information for acquisition of grammatical structures in Turkish was considered. The appendix lists the rules for separating utterances into phonemes in Turkish according to Ege *et al.* (1998).

Predicting MLU from age

The results of this study were obtained following the methodology used by Miller and Chapman (1981). The sample was grouped by age into three-month intervals. The midpoint age was assigned to subjects within each group. For example, 17-, 18- and 19-month-old subjects were placed in one group and 18 months was the label of the group. This kind of grouping increases the number of subjects in each group and allows for comparisons among groups. A high Pearson correlation of 0.83 ($p < 0.01$) was obtained between age and MLU. Figure 5.1 depicts this relationship and

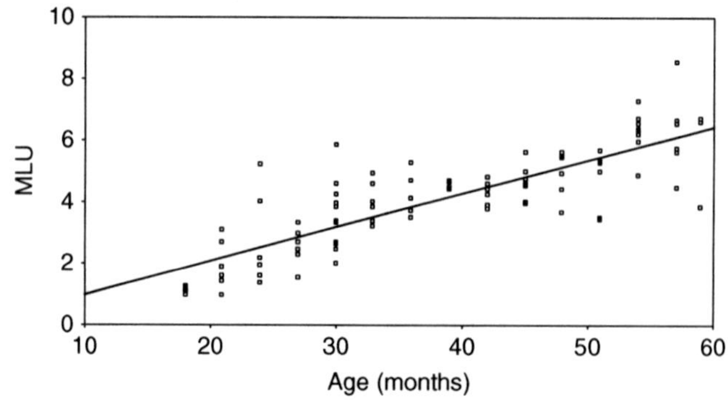

Figure 5.1 The relationship between MLU and age

the regression line. A regression equation was obtained that predicted MLU from age (months):

$$\text{MLU} = 0.110 \times (\text{age}) - 0.008. \quad (5.1)$$

Table 5.1 includes age groups, the number of subjects in each group, obtained and predicted MLUs and the standard deviation (SD) of actual MLUs from the predicted MLUs. The sign of the difference shows the direction of the prediction in relation to the actual data. No significant deviation from the regression line is observed in any age group. When the SDs of obtained MLUs from the predicted MLUs are calculated as a function of age group, it is observed that SD increases with age. The regression equation obtained is used to calculate predicted SDs for each age group:

$$\text{SD MLU} = 0.008 \times \text{age} + 0.551. \quad (5.2)$$

Then, MLU ranges were obtained by adding and subtracting the predicted SD from the predicted mean MLU for each age group. The results are shown in Table 5.2.

Predicting age from MLU

It is also possible to predict the age value of an obtained MLU. Following the Miller and Chapman study (1981) and based on de Villiers and de Villiers' modification of Brown, the subjects were grouped into 0.5 morpheme ranges and the midpoint value of each group (1.25, 1.75, 2.25 morphemes, etc.) represented each group. The upper value of 6.99 morphemes for the group with the midpoint value of 6.75 was set as the

Table 5.1 MLU prediction for age groups based on the equation

Age±1 month	*Number of subjects*	*MLU*	*Predicted MLU*	*Difference MLU and predicted MLU*	*Difference squared*	*SD of MLU from predicted MLU*
18	5	1.17	1.89	–0.72	0.518	0.724
21	6	1.97	2.22	–0.25	0.063	0.772
24	6	2.77	2.55	0.22	0.048	1.118
27	6	2.59	2.88	–0.29	0.084	0.626
30	11	3.57	3.21	0.36	0.130	1.121
33	6	4.03	3.54	0.49	0.240	0.779
36	5	4.30	3.87	0.43	0.185	0.788
39	5	4.56	4.20	0.36	0.130	0.381
42	8	4.22	4.53	–0.31	0.096	0.480
45	7	4.68	4.86	–0.18	0.032	0.561
48	6	4.97	5.19	–0.22	0.048	0.741
51	7	4.84	5.52	–0.68	0.462	1.087
54	8	6.33	5.85	0.48	0.230	0.800
57	6	6.32	6.18	0.14	0.020	1.260
59	3	5.77	6.40	–0.63	0.397	1.465

MLU = 0.110 (age) – 0.008.

limit. Two subjects with MLUs above that value who would need to form another group were left out ($N = 93$). A linear regression equation was obtained using the midpoint MLU value:

$$\text{Age} = 6.351 \times (\text{MLU}) + 12.236. \tag{5.3}$$

Listed in Table 5.3 are the MLU groups, the number of subjects in each group, actual and predicted ages, the difference between the two, the square of the difference and the SD of the actual ages from the predicted age for each group. According to Table 5.3, the group with the midpoint value of 3.75 shows the largest variation. Table 5.4 depicts the predicted age when the MLU value is known. This table provides the MLU values in 0.10 morpheme increments, the average predicted age for the MLU value and the age range ±1SD around the predicted age, based on Equation 5.3.

Table 5.2 Predicted MLU ranges for groups within ±1SD of the predicted mean

Age (months)	*Predicted MLU*[a]	*Predicted SD*[b]	*Predicted MLU±1SD*
18	1.89	0.695	1.20–2.59
21	2.22	0.719	1.50–2.94
24	2.55	0.743	1.81–3.29
27	2.88	0.767	2.11–3.65
30	3.21	0.791	2.42–4.00
33	3.54	0.815	2.73–4.36
36	3.87	0.839	3.03–4.71
39	4.20	0.863	3.34–5.06
42	4.53	0.887	3.64–5.42
45	4.86	0.911	3.95–5.77
48	5.19	0.935	4.26–6.13
51	5.52	0.959	4.56–6.48
54	5.85	0.983	4.87–6.83
57	6.18	1.007	5.17–7.19
59	6.40	1.023	5.38–7.42

[a]From the equation MLU = 0.110 (age) − 0.088.
[b]From the equation SD = 0.008 (age) + 0.551.

Discussion and Conclusion

MLU is a general indicator of syntactic and morphological development that includes the use of both free and bound morphemes. Because it provides too general a picture, it does not help in identifying targets for intervention. It may also be a time-consuming endeavor since it requires transcription and analysis of recorded language samples. However, it is a quantitative measure that allows the clinician to chart the changes in the child over the course of time. It has now been demonstrated that such a measure can be reliably used for a highly inflected language such as Turkish, which relies on bound morphemes for expression of syntactic relationships and conveying meaning. The relationship between MLU and age ($r = 0.81$) was found to be very high and quite comparable to the MLU–age relationship in English. Furthermore, when Brown's stages of language development are compared with the MLU values for Turkish in Table 5.4, it can be observed that Brown's stage I, which includes the

Table 5.3 Prediction of age based on MLU

MLU	*Number of subjects*	*Predicted age*[a]	*Obtained age*	*Difference between predicted age and obtained age*	*Difference squared*	*SD of actual age from the predicted age*
1.25	8	20.17	19.00	1.17	1.37	2.94
1.75	4	23.35	22.50	0.85	0.72	3.00
2.25	4	26.53	25.50	1.03	1.06	2.51
2.75	6	29.70	27.33	2.37	5.62	4.06
3.25	7	32.88	29.00	3.88	15.05	5.62
3.75	12	36.05	42.50	−6.45	41.60	10.30
4.25	12	39.23	37.83	1.40	1.96	7.12
4.75	15	42.40	42.00	0.40	1.16	7.32
5.25	7	45.58	43.71	1.87	3.50	9.88
5.75	8	48.75	48.38	0.37	0.14	8.21
6.25	4	51.93	54.00	−2.07	4.28	2.30
6.75	6	55.11	56.50	−1.39	1.93	2.74

[a]From the equation age = 6.351 × MLU + 12.236.

single-word stage and expression of semantic relations using two words without the use of bound morphemes, ends at around 26 months. In Table 5.4, the predicted average age for Turkish children with an average MLU of 2.00 is 25–26 months. In both languages, children move to the two-morpheme stage at about the same time. The similarity also holds for Brown's stage III.

MLU as a tool for syntactic assessment in Turkish has been used for the last 10 years. It has proven to be a useful tool in determining the child's language level based on a natural language sample, in the absence of standardized language tests in Turkish to be employed for the same purpose. In addition to determining the child's syntactic level, MLU can be used to compare other areas of the child's language development to his/her syntactic and morphological development. Paul (2001) also suggests that knowing the child's MLU can guide the clinician about how to proceed next. For example, if the MLU is less than 3, it would perhaps be wise to consider doing a semantic analysis such as Lahey's (1988) semantic–syntactic analysis procedure. If the MLU is greater than 4.5, complex sentence development might be the focus of attention. For MLU values in between,

Table 5.4 MLU, average predicted age and age range (in months)

MLU	*Predicted age*[a]	*Predicted age±SD*[b]
1.00	18.59	15.65–21.53
1.10	19.22	16.28–22.16
1.20	19.86	16.92–22.80
1.30	20.49	17.55–23.43
1.40	21.13	18.19–24.07
1.50	21.76	18.76–24.76
1.60	22.40	19.40–25.40
1.70	23.03	20.03–26.03
1.80	23.67	20.67–26.67
1.90	24.30	21.30–27.30
2.00	24.94	22.43–27.45
2.10	25.57	23.06–28.08
2.20	26.21	23.70–28.72
2.30	26.84	24.33–29.35
2.40	27.48	24.97–29.99
2.50	28.11	24.05–32.17
2.60	28.75	24.69–32.81
2.70	29.38	25.32–33.40
2.80	30.02	25.96–34.08
2.90	30.65	26.59–34.71
3.00	31.29	25.67–36.91
3.10	31.92	26.30–37.54
3.20	32.56	26.94–38.18
3.30	33.19	27.57–38.81
3.40	33.83	28.21–39.45
3.50	34.46	24.16–44.74
3.60	35.10	24.80–45.40
3.70	35.73	25.43–46.03
3.80	36.37	26.07–46.67

(Continued)

Table 5.4 *Continued*

MLU	*Predicted age*[a]	*Predicted age±SD*[b]
3.90	37.00	26.70–47.03
4.00	37.64	30.52–44.76
4.10	38.27	31.16–45.40
4.20	38.91	31.79–46.03
4.30	39.55	32.43–46.67
4.40	40.18	33.06–47.30
4.50	40.82	33.50–48.14
4.60	41.45	34.13–48.77
4.70	42.09	34.77–49.41
4.80	42.72	35.40–50.04
4.90	43.36	36.04–50.68
5.00	43.99	34.11–53.87
5.10	44.63	34.75–54.51
5.20	45.26	35.38–55.14
5.30	45.90	36.02–55.78
5.40	46.53	36.65–56.41
5.50	47.17	38.96–55.38
5.60	47.80	39.59–56.01
5.70	48.44	40.23–56.65
5.80	49.07	40.86–57.28
5.90	49.71	41.50–57.92
6.00	50.34	42.13–58.55

[a]From the equation age = 6.351 × MLU + 12.236.
[b]Based on SDs in Table 5.3.

an examination of basic morphological and syntactic development in simple sentences would be the appropriate choice since children's development of grammatical morphemes falls within that stage.

In addition to being too global, another criticism of MLU has been with regard to its validity and reliability, particularly with individuals at the higher MLU levels. Brown (1973) cautioned against its use as a measure of development beyond MLU 5.0. Subsequent studies have argued that MLUs beyond 3 are less valid indicators of syntactic maturity than lower values (Lahey *et al.*, 1992; Rondal *et al.*, 1987). Scarborough *et al.* (1991) have demonstrated that MLU above 3 overestimated the grammatical complexity of individuals with delayed language, Down's syndrome, Fragile X syndrome and autism, even more than normal preschoolers. It is recommended that other measures of grammatical complexity be also used beyond MLU 3.

MLU provides quantitative information; however, a qualitative analysis of the child's bound morphemes appears to be of crucial importance in assessment, especially for Turkish children. Work is in progress to see if MLU phases and stages can be characterized by syntactic and morphological developments in Turkish as in Brown's work, and to determine what those developments would be at each stage. There is evidence that Turkish children acquire most of the grammatical morphemes at relatively early ages. The accusative *–i*, the directive *–e* and the possessive *–m* noun suffixes are observed by 15 months (Topbaş *et al.*, 1997). Locative *–de*, ablative *–den* and instrumental *–le* follow by one-month intervals. The past tense *–di* and present tense *-iyor* verbal suffixes are observed at around the same time (Aksu-Koç & Slobin, 1985). Even generally late-occurring suffixes for passive (*-il*), reciprocal (*-iş*) and reflexive (*-n*) were reported to be observed in two-year-old Turkish children's language (Maviş & Ege, 2002).

Last but not least, it should be noted that grammatical morpheme development may not be congruent with what MLU might suggest. For example, according to Leonard (1998), in children with specific language impairments, grammatical morpheme development is usually more delayed relative to MLU than are other components of language. In a recent study of Turkish mentally impaired children, Ege and Erdem (2008) showed that although mentally retarded children had lower MLUs than mental age-matched normally developing children, the difference was insignificant. There was a significant difference, however, between the type-token ratios (TTRs) of the two groups: TTR for the mentally retarded group was higher. Further investigation suggested that the mentally retarded children relied on using a higher number of different words relative to their number of total words to raise their MLU to their capacity and to make up for their delayed use of grammatical morphemes. As long as one is aware of its advantages and limitations, MLU has been shown to be a useful tool for the assessment of language development in Turkish-speaking children.

Appendix: Rules for Counting Morphemes in Utterances in Turkish Utterances (The underlined sections are counted)

1. Repetitions of words or syllables are not counted. A word is counted in the most complete form produced. (**Ex**: Bu bu <u>bu kitabı ver</u>. [This this <u>this book give</u>].)

2. Incomplete utterances or incomplete sentences when the child decides to change topic are not counted. (**Ex**: Haydi seninle- annem bunu dün getirdi. [Come on with you – Mom brought this yesterday].)
3. Partially or completely unintelligible utterances are not included.
4. Utterances by rote, such as poems, songs or jingles are not counted.
5. Fillers such as *Ahh, oh, şey* ([*Well*]) and *yani* ([*I mean*]) that do not have a syntactic function in the sentence are not counted.
6. Counting out loud or listing of words is not included; however, if the list occupies syntactic space in the sentence, only one is counted. (**Exs**: Ben mavi, yeşil, sarı renkleri severim. [I blue, green yellow colors like]; Dayım beni, abimi sinemaya götürdü. [My uncle me, my brother to the movies took].)
7. If any of the listed items are separated by a conjunction, items on either side of the conjunction are counted. (**Ex**: Dayım annemi, beni ve abimi sinemaya götürdü. [My uncle my mother, me and my brother to the movies took].)
8. The child's self-repetitions are not counted. (**Ex**: C: Bunu oynayalım. [Let's play this]). A: Ne ([What])? C: Bunu oynayalım ([This play lets].)
9. All uninflected words are counted as one morpheme. (**Exs**: koş [run], iç [drink], kalem [pencil], ilaç[drug], güzel [pretty], duygu [feeling].)
10. Proper names are counted as one morpheme even if they consist of two or more free morphemes. (**Exs**: Dalmaçyalı [The Dalmatian] = 1 morpheme; Pamuk Prenses [Snow White] = 1 morpheme.)
11. The shortened form of the tag question *değil mi* [isn't it] *'di mi'* at the ends of utterances is counted as one morpheme because there is no evidence that the child is aware of the question suffix *-mi* in that form.
12. Ritualized forms such as *Hoşça kal [good bye]* and *güle güle [good bye]* are counted as one morpheme.
13. Nouns derived from other nouns by suffixes but have different referents than the nouns they were derived from are counted as one morpheme. (**Exs**: gözlük [eye + nominal suffix *-lük* = glasses] and dişçi [tooth + nominal suffix *-çi* = dentist].)
14. Nouns that refer to animate or inanimate objects that are derived from verbs by suffixes are counted as one morpheme. (**Exs**: yargıç [judge (verb) + nominal suffix -ç] = judge (noun); dalgıç [dive + nominal suffix -ç] = diver.)
15. In adverbs that are repeated, the repeated word is not counted a second time. However, if one of the adverbs includes a suffix, the suffix is counted. (**Exs**: yavaş yavaş/ gel [slow slow /come] = 2 morphemes; koşa koş/ a /git/ti [running runn/ing /go/ + past tense -di] = 4 morphemes.)
16. Suffixes for time, person, question and negation added to verbs and dative, accusative, locative and ablative suffixes added to nouns are each counted as a separate morpheme. (**Exs**: git/ti/m [go + past tense

-di + first person singular *-m*] = 3 morphemes; Yer/e /otur/acak /mı? [Floor + locative *-e* // sit + future tense *-acak* + question *-mi*] = 5 morphemes.)

17. Adjectives derived from nouns with suffixes are counted as two morphemes if there is evidence that the child is using the suffix generatively. (**Ex:** Çiçek/li /elbise [flower + suffix *-li* (meaning *with*)// dress] = 3 morphemes.)
18. In adjectives, gerunds, infinitives, nouns, adverbs or causative, reflexive or passive verbs derived from a verb root, all suffixes are counted separately. (**Exs:** kır/ık [break + adjectival suffix *-ık* = broken] = 2 morphemes; yüz/me [swim + nominal suffix *–me* = swimming] = 2 morphemes; koş/unca [run + adverbial deverbative *-unca* = when running] = 2 morphemes; yap/ tığ/ım [do + nominal suffix *-ık* + first person singular *-m* = that I did] = 3 morphemes; ölç/mek [break + infinitive suffix *-mek*] = 2 morphemes; sık/ıl/dı/m [squeeze + passive suffix *-ıl* + past tense *-dı* + first person *-m* = I am bored] = 4 morphemes; del/in/miş [make-a-hole + passive suffix *-n* + reported past tense suffix *-miş* = has a hole] = 3 morphemes; koş/up [run + conjunctive suffix *–up* = running] = 2 morphemes.)

Chapter 6

Turkish SALT: Computer-Assisted Language Sample Analysis

FUNDA ACARLAR and JUDITH JOHNSTON

Introduction: Formal and Informal Approaches to Language Assessment

Assessment of a child's language is a multilayered and complex process that utilizes a wide range of procedures and instruments. In general terms, however, there have been two basic approaches; *formal* language assessment, making use of standardized tests, and *informal* language assessment, making use of criterion-referenced measures. The relative efficacy and adequacy of the two approaches depend in part on the purposes of the assessment, that is, on whether the goal is to judge the age appropriateness of a child's language, to describe current language knowledge and behavior or to measure progress in a language intervention program (Kennedy, 2007; Owens, 1999). In this chapter, we will first outline the strengths and weaknesses of formal and informal assessment relative to these goals; then we will describe a new hybrid approach, namely computer-assisted language profiling, and illustrate its clinical use with children who are learning Turkish as their first language.

Norm-referenced tests

Norm-referenced tests provide a standardized set of language tasks and a scoring scheme that allow us to compare a given child's language performance to that of typically developing age peers. Assuming the test is psychometrically sound, any observed differences in language behavior can be taken as evidence of differences in language proficiency rather than as differences in contexts of language use. Tests thus play an essential role when the purpose of the assessment is to determine the normalcy of a child's language learning.

Use of test data for intervention planning is more problematic. In many cases, the sample of verbal behavior that is elicited by a test is not representative of the child's everyday language use. Young children in particular may produce more complex language when they are motivated by their own communicative intents. Older children, on the other hand, may be more error-prone when they are faced with the demands of real-life discourse. In both cases, an analysis of the language elicited by tests fails to capture the child's strengths or weaknesses and hence provides a poor basis for intervention planning (McCauley & Swisher, 1984; Nelson, 1998; Owens, 1999; Paul, 2001).

The utility of tests for program planning is further limited by their content. Few are designed to compare different aspects of language ability, and even fewer examine conversational skills or other context-sensitive aspects of language use (Lund & Duchan, 1993; Paul, 2001). Test content and norms are also frequently culture biased – a limitation of importance in our increasingly multicultural societies (Ball & Lewis, 2004; Campbell *et al.*, 1997; Crago & Westernoff, 2002; Huang *et al.*, 1997).

The normative comparisons provided by tests are a critical component of developmental diagnosis, but are less important in intervention planning. Instead, individualized educational programs require detailed descriptive data about a child's actual use of language in daily-life situations (Johnston, 2006). The noncommunicative and decontextualized language produced in the test situation does not reliably provide this information.

Criterion-referenced procedures

Like tests, criterion-referenced language assessments measure the child's level of achievement in prescribed areas of structure and use. However, rather than asking whether a child's language meets age expectations, this approach asks only whether a child gives evidence of knowing a given language form or of being able to accomplish a given language task (McCauley, 1996). The set of criteria used can be comprehensive, systematic and detailed, and will reflect the examiner's particular theories about the nature of language and language learning (Duchan, 1982). Such criteria-referenced assessment yields a descriptive account of a specific child's language that can be used to determine baseline function, identify intervention targets and measure progress (Johnston, 1993; Paul, 2001). This individualization is particularly important given evidence that children with equivalent degrees of overall language delay, or even identical test scores, may nevertheless show quite different profiles of language ability (Colozzo *et al.*, 2006; Johnston & Kamhi, 1984).

Criteria-referenced language assessment may make use of structured probe tasks, particularly for forms that naturally occur at low frequencies.

More typically, however, criteria-referenced assessment uses observations of language behavior in minimally structured situations such as interactive play with peers or with the examiner. Following the lead of Roger Brown and his students in the early 1960s, research scientists and clinicians now commonly record children's conversation or storytelling and use transcripts of these samples of verbal behavior as the basis for criterion-based description within one of a number of taxonomies that have been developed for this purpose (e.g. Johnston, 2006; Miller, 1981). This set of procedures, that is, the recording, transcription and use of criterion-referenced measures to guide descriptive analysis, is generically known as 'language sample analysis' (LSA) (Klee, 1985).

The Evolution of LSA

LSA has been used for mainstream educational planning in North America since at least the early 1970s when the Los Angeles County classroom program for children with specific language impairments began to accept language sample data in support of program placement. A monograph reviewing clinical research on, and use of, LSA was published in 1978 and indicates the growing interest in this approach (Barrie-Blackley *et al.*, 1978). By 1997, surveys of North American speech language pathologists (SLPs) showed that some 85–90% of them were using LSA for assessment purposes (Eisenberg *et al.*, 2001; Kemp & Klee, 1997). A number of studies have provided evidence that measures derived from language samples are both sensitive to developmental change and valid clinically in identifying children with language disorders (Condouris *et al.*, 2003; Dunn *et al.*, 1996; Klee, 1992; Klee *et al.*, 2004; Miller, 1981, 1991; Watkins *et al.*, 1995). The clinical literature further attests to its value in determining goals for intervention and for describing the extent and nature of language disorders (Johnston, 2006; Paul, 2001).

LSA as it has been practiced over the last 40 years has had certain limitations that have hindered its full use. The fluidity and flexibility that are the strength of LSA have made it difficult to determine standard errors of measurement, thereby compromising investigations of program efficacy. For individual practitioners, the more immediate difficulty has been the level of language expertise, and the time, required to elicit and descriptively analyze a child's language (Barrie-Blackley *et al.*, 1978; Kelly & Rice, 1986). Eisenberg *et al.* (2001) for example report that while 90% of the SLPs in their survey used LSA, most of them only calculated mean length of utterance (MLU), and did so over a relatively short sample.

Traditional forms of LSA are evolving in response to these challenges, in at least three directions. First, there are attempts to standardize the language task without losing its communicative, real-world character. Narrative samples, preset conversational topics and interview protocols have been used to reduce the variance in contexts of use and thus improve the psychometric characteristics of LSA data (e.g. Evans & Craig, 1992; Miller, 1981, 2004; Schneider *et al.*, 2006). Recent reports suggest that with such changes, LSA can yield assessment measures with acceptable levels of reliability, at least for general indices of development such as MLU (Acarlar, 2005; Heilmann *et al.*, 2006; Miller *et al.*, 2006).

Secondly, computer programs are increasingly available to assist in LSA. Some, such as the CLAN program at Carnegie Melon University (MacWhinney, 1996), were designed primarily for researchers and require use of elaborate coding systems. Others such as Linquest (Mordecai & Palin, 1982) require coding schemes that are simpler, but also less flexible. Still others, such as Computerized Profiling (Long *et al.*, 2000) and Systematic Analysis of Language Transcripts (SALT) (Miller & Chapman, 1984–2000; Miller & Iglesias, 2003–2007), offer a mixture of user coding and automatized analysis. Computer programs can increase the accuracy of LSA as well as reduce the time and expertise required (Miller, 1992). These changes in traditional LSA practice, although not entirely eliminating the measurement and practical costs noted earlier, have at least reduced them.

The third direction of change, rather than solving old problems, introduces new possibilities. The normative potential of LSA is now being realized through the use of reference databases. Clinicians were always prone to viewing criterion-based descriptions of language competence through a quasi-normative lens. Based on their general knowledge of the child language literature, they might, for example, inform a family that their child's language achievements were comparable to those of a two-year-old child. Now, detailed scoring systems in conjunction with criterion-based taxonomies and reference databases can yield standard scores. Developmental Sentence Scoring (DSS; Lee, 1974), the Index of Productive Syntax (IPSyn; Scarborough, 1990) and SALT (Miller & Chapman, 1984–2000; Miller & Iglesias, 2003–2006; TSALT, Acarlar *et al.*, 2006) are three such systems. The standard scores they generate can be used to identify the presence and extent of language delay and can also, in the case of SALT/TSALT, indicate a child's relative competence in a wide range of language domains.

Systematic Analysis of Language Transcripts

Overview

SALT is a flexible, user-friendly computer program designed to assist researchers and educators with LSA tasks. It is essentially a set of complex search-and-count algorithms that identifies and measures various characteristics of a transcribed language sample. These 'scores' can be used to describe different aspects of a child's language knowledge and performance, to compare a child's language to that of a peer group (matched by age, gender, sampling context and transcript length), or to compare one sample to a second one from the same, or a different, child. These options can be applied to user-created variables as well as to a standard set. The program can also locate and list all utterances containing particular words or codes – a capability that encourages and supports the systematic investigation of patterns of error or use.

Developed over a 20-year period by Miller and his colleagues at the University of Wisconsin (Miller & Chapman, 1984–2000; Miller & Iglesias, 2003–2006), SALT now includes a number of normative databases for English speakers and also accepts local databases, making it possible to adapt SALT for use with other languages. All coding is optional, but the standard analyses can be greatly enhanced with a few simple tags that separate affixes from roots and note the presence of grammatical errors at the word and/or utterance level. Further coding of grammatical, semantic and discourse features of a child's language can be done using both preprogrammed and self-designed codes.

Development of the Turkish version of SALT (TSALT)

The TSALT was published in 2006, the product of a five-year collaborative project conducted by Acarlar and Johnston with consultative and programming support from Miller and his Madison team. The project was motivated in large part by the limited availability of assessment tools in Turkish that could identify and describe the language of children with atypical development. The development of TSALT thus entailed not only adaptation of the program to fit the grammatical characteristics of Turkish, but also the creation of a reference database (Acarlar & Johnston, 2006). Although there had been a number of studies of language acquisition in Turkish (Aksu-Koç & Ketrez, 2003a; Aksu-Koç & Slobin, 1985; Ege *et al.*, 1998; Ketrez & Aksu-Koç, 2009; Topbaş *et al.*, 1997), very few had provided the sort of quantitative data that are appropriate for normative purposes.

The adaptation process for Turkish included the creation of 15 lists of grammatically pertinent words or inflections. The lists are specified in ways that take vowel harmony into account, disambiguate homonymous forms and require only a small number of transcription codes. With these lists as a guide, TSALT automatically provides normative and descriptive data for question words, negatives, conjunctions, prepositions, pronouns, case markers, plural markers, possessive constructions, tense/aspect/modality markers, verb suffixes for person, voice (passive, transitive, reflexive), infinitives and participles, adverbs of location, yes/no words and filled pause forms. The user can also add whatever lists might assist in answering child-specific assessment questions. An example of a TSALT printout is provided in the appendix. Further details about the Turkish adaptation of SALT can be found in Acarlar and Johnston (2006).

The Turkish reference database

The Turkish reference database consists of language samples collected from 140 children aged 2;6–6;6, 30–40 at each yearly interval, evenly divided between girls and boys. The children were drawn from preschools in Ankara, Turkey, were monolingual speakers of Turkish and were typically developing according to scores on the Denver Developmental Screening Test, teacher opinion and observations of the researcher. Children were predominantly from middle-class families with parents who had completed at least a high school education. Language samples were collected in conversations conducted in a room at their schools or during home visits. At least 150 complete and intelligible utterances were obtained from each child. A standard set of materials (e.g. playdough, books) and topics (e.g. holidays, home activities) was used to structure the interaction with the children.

All samples were transcribed and edited in SALT format by using procedures similar to those recommended in Brown (1973) and Miller (1981) for English. Reliability of the transcription was determined following the consensus transcription protocols developed by Miller and his colleagues (Heilmann *et al.*, 2006). Coded elements in the transcripts include (1) bound morphemes, (2) instances of overlapping speech, (3) unintelligible segments, (4) omissions of words and suffixes, (5) mazes (i.e. false starts, filled pauses, self-repetitions and self-corrections), (6) abandoned or interrupted utterances and (7) nonverbal communication acts and contextual comments. This initial Turkish database does not include timing information.

Language profiles using normalized SALT variables

Acarlar's (2005) analysis of the Turkish reference database (RDB) indicates that MLU in morphemes, number of different words (NDW) and total number of words (TNW) are all strongly correlated with age ($r = 0.74$, 0.76, and 0.72) and thus have good potential as global assessment indices.

As well as these general measures, TSALT allows the user to develop a more differentiated view of a child's language abilities. The relative strength shown in specific verbal domains can be determined by using the database to generate one or more normalized *z*-scores in each area. TSALT offers a wide array of potential measures for such profiling. The following list indicates the seven domains we currently include along with a selection of associated measures. Wherever possible we have chosen measures that have some history but this profile protocol should be considered only illustrative. Further research is needed to identify the best variables to use for this sort of descriptive assessment.

General developmental level (MLU, MLU2)

MLU has been used as a general index of language growth since the 1930s (McCarthy, 1930; Templin, 1957). It correlates with age throughout the preschool and school years, and predicts the presence/absence of specific forms (Brown, 1973; Leadholm & Miller, 1992; Miller & Chapman, 1981). Despite these indications of validity, some critics have questioned the use of MLU, noting in particular the increasing influence of discourse context as language skills mature (e.g. Barrie-Blackley *et al.*, 1978). To meet this concern, TSALT offers the option of calculating MLU only on utterances that are not single-word responses or answers to questions, thereby minimizing the effects of ellipsis (Johnston, 2001; Johnston *et al.*, 1993). The program also provides the option of an MLU based on word counts rather than the traditional morpheme counts. Use of MLU in words allows us to separate measures of length from measures of morphology and in general makes cross-linguistic data more interpretable (Parker & Brorson, 2005; Thordardottir & Weismer, 1998).

Syntax (number of conjunctions, participles, infinitives, converbs)

The fact that SALT is designed to identify words without assigning them to functional categories means that any true syntactic coding must be done by the clinician or scientist. Nevertheless, certain words and morphemes do imply structural complexity and their presence can serve as proxies for syntactic analysis. In Turkish these would include conjunctions, participles, infinitives and converbs. TSALT provides normalized frequency counts for these forms.

Morphology (number of omitted affixes)

Measures of grammatical morphology would seem to be particularly important in an agglutinative language. Initial cross-linguistic studies of Turkish acquisition had suggested that the semantic transparency of Turkish morphology led to unusually early competencies in this domain (Aksu-Koç & Slobin, 1985). Current research presents a more differentiated picture with possessive expressions and case markers in less frequent word orders still not mastered by seven-year-olds in bilingual contexts (de Jong & Çavuş, 2007). In general, however, morphological errors are rarely produced in the normal course of development, making the omissions and substitutions frequently seen in clinical cases even more intriguing (Acarlar & Johnston, 2006).

Lexicon (NDW)

The best candidate for a lexical measure derived from LSA is a measure of lexical diversity, namely NDW per 250 (150, 200, etc.) words. Greater lexical diversity reflects vocabulary growth and also an increased ability to make pragmatically motivated lexical choices. NDW has recently shown promise in identifying children with specific language impairment (Klee, 1992; Watkins *et al.*, 1995) and is being investigated as a phenotypic marker for this condition.

Social discourse (percentage of examiner questions that are answered; number of utterances per turn)

SALT has limited capacities for discourse analysis since it focuses on only one utterance at a time. There are nevertheless two variables of interest in this domain. TSALT indicates the percentage of adult questions that are immediately followed by a child utterance. This turns out to provide a reliable estimate of the child's responsiveness to adult questions (Johnston *et al.*, 1993). TSALT also provides several measures of the child's contribution in each conversational turn, for example the number of utterances per turn. These measures seem to estimate what Fey calls conversational assertiveness (Fey, 1986). Higher values on this variable would indicate a greater degree of social engagement and/or communicative ease, as well as knowledge of the current topic.

Formulation processes (words in mazes/total words; number of utterance-level error codes)

TSALT provides a thorough analysis of 'maze' material, that is, filled pauses, repetitions, revisions and false starts. A high frequency of mazes can indicate word-finding difficulty or problems in coordinating the incremental construction of an utterance. In younger children, maze frequency increases with age and with the complexity of language, both in typically developing children and in SLI children (Leadholm & Miller, 1992; MacLachlan & Chapman, 1988; Rispoli & Hadley, 2001; Thordardottir & Weismer, 2002). The second variable we use in this domain is the number of utterance-level errors. These utterances are often ungrammatical to a degree that makes them uninterpretable, and they are undoubtedly a mixed set, some reflecting a lack of knowledge and others a processing failure to deploy known schemes. In both instances, they reflect a gap between the child's communicative intention and his/her linguistic means.

Intelligibility (number of totally intelligible utterances/total utterances)

SALT/TSALT is not meant to be used with phonetic transcription and cannot support a detailed phonological analysis. It does provide a single index of intelligibility, however, which can flag the need for further investigation.

Advantages of SALT/TSALT Language Profiling

The idea of generating a profile of relative ability and/or knowledge in various language domains is not new. There are a number of standardized tests and criteria-referenced taxonomies that incorporate this feature (e.g. Crystal, 1982; Miller, 1981; Newcomer & Hammill, 1977) They differ, however, in degree of detail, number of domains, requirements for coding or analysis, inclusion of quantitative norms and the fundamental nature of the data they use. Computer-assisted language profiling with SALT or TSALT offers a combination of these characteristics that is both unique and attractive. It allows the user to measure relative ability in a decent number of domains, at a reasonable level of detail, with little or no precoding or analysis and impressive speed. Moreover, it does so using spontaneous speech samples and quantified comparisons with an age-matched group of normal learners. Each of these features carries an advantage that may be shared by other procedures, but to our knowledge only SALT/TSALT offers this particular combination of advantages.

Firstly, SALT-based language profiling eliminates the need to equate units of measurement across different linguistic domains and avoids the comparison of scores drawn from different standardization samples.

Secondly, SALT-based language profiling goes well beyond single summary measures such as verbal IQ and provides a richly differentiated view of language capabilities. Clinical experience indicates that some children may have particular difficulty with the social context of communication, others may have particular difficulty in the analysis and representation of speech sounds, and still others may never fully automatize syntactic frameworks (e.g. Catts *et al.*, 1999; Miller, 1991; Rapin, 1996; Rapin & Allen, 1998). Even for children who are developing normally, levels of achievement and rates of learning for different aspects of language can differ (Klee *et al.*, 2004).

Thirdly, when we use the SALT database to quantify the characteristics of a child's everyday language, we combine some of the best features of formal and informal language assessment. Like criteria-referenced approaches, LSA uses spontaneous rather than elicited language data. Since these data are drawn from communicative and fully contextualized speech, they are more likely than test responses to be representative of the child's everyday language patterns. On the other hand, like norm-referenced language tests, the databases used in conjunction with LSA allow us to make judgments about the age appropriateness of a child's language. Norm-mediated uses of LSA, such as the profiling we have just described, thus become a new assessment hybrid that stands somewhere between the traditional formal and informal approaches.

Using TSALT to Answer Clinical Questions

In this section we will illustrate the use of TSALT to assist in educational and clinical problem-solving. Language sample data were collected from children enrolled in special education centers and preschools in

Ankara, Turkey. Conversations were taped, transcribed, coded and analyzed with TSALT as described above, yielding individual profiles of language ability. The normalized scores (in standard deviation units) that comprise these profiles indicate each child's performance level in specific domains of language relative to each other and to the performance of age peers from the reference database.

Identifying delays and describing strengths and weaknesses

Profile data for the first three cases illustrate how TSALT can help educators answer both diagnostic and descriptive assessment questions. A is a 6;2-year-old boy diagnosed with global developmental delay. His mother works outside the home and his grandparents care for him during the day. His teacher feels that A does not receive sufficient learning support and could be making better progress. K is a 4;8-year-old girl diagnosed with Down's syndrome and global developmental delay. She is a classroom favorite, friendly and attention seeking. Her parents are both university graduates who work outside the home, but are nevertheless viewed by the school as providing good support for their daughter's social and intellectual growth.

A global judgment about the presence or absence of delayed language development is often the first goal of a language assessment. Clinicians ask whether or not a child's language meets age expectations. In the cases of A and K, the TSALT data shown in Table 6.1 and Figure 6.1 provide initial answers to this question. Note first that both children are using sentences that are much shorter than would be expected for their age group, earning z-scores of –4.1 and –4.3. When we look further to determine the reasons for this reduced length, we find high rates of bound morpheme omission and the near absence of complex sentences in the language of both children. A did not use any conjunctions; K used only one type of conjunction {de, da}, albeit 6 times. K did not use any participles or converbs; A used the converb {/ınca, /ince} only once. For both children, these more advanced syntactic forms occurred less frequently (z-scores of –1.9 to –2.9), and bound morphemes were omitted more frequently (z-score > 6) than in the control groups. Interpretation of these facts will depend upon one's theory of language acquisition, but from our cognitive constructivist perspective they point to significant delays in language learning.

Having established the presence of delays in language learning, clinicians and educators can then use TSALT data to describe the relatively strong and weak aspects of a child's verbal communication. As is clear in Figure 6.1, the language profiles for A and K indicate considerable variability from one domain to the next. In contrast to the large developmental delays in syntax and morphology, both A and K show

Table 6.1 Absolute scores (AS) and standard scores (SS in SD units) in seven verbal domains for three children with atypical language development

Children	***A***		***K***		***CT***	
Language measures	***AS***	***SS***	***AS***	***SS***	***AS***	***SS***
General						
MLU2 – words	1.67	–4.3	1.65	–4.1	3.2	1.1
Grammar/form						
Number of conjunctions	0	–2.8	3	–2.9	29	0.1
Number of participles	2	–1.7	0	–1.9	1	–1.2
Morphology						
Number of omitted bound morphemes	12	–16	5	–6.2	1	0.8
Lexicon						
NDW/250	109	–0.5	101	–1.4	77	–2.6
Discourse						
Responsiveness						
% questions answered	95	0.3	90	–0.2	84	–0.2
Initiative						
Number of utterances/ turns	1.5	–2.8	1.6	–2.5	3.9	0.4
Intelligibility	98	0.1	88	–3.1	89	–2.5
Formulation processing						
% words in mazes	1	–1.1	1	–1.4	7	0.5
Utterance-level error	1	1.1	0	–0.9	5	3.2

considerable strength in vocabulary development and in conversational responsiveness. Vocabulary diversity (NDW) is almost at the levels that would be expected for children of this age; both answer virtually all of the examiner's questions. A third 'peak' in the profiles occurs in the area of utterance formulation. Neither child was likely to self-correct, self repeat, or use many filled pauses and neither child produced many uninterpretable utterances. In fact, they showed somewhat less difficulty with utterance formulation than would be expected for their ages, suggesting that this 'strength' may instead be a side effect of using only simple sentences that are well within their production control. Further observation would be needed to choose between these possibilities.

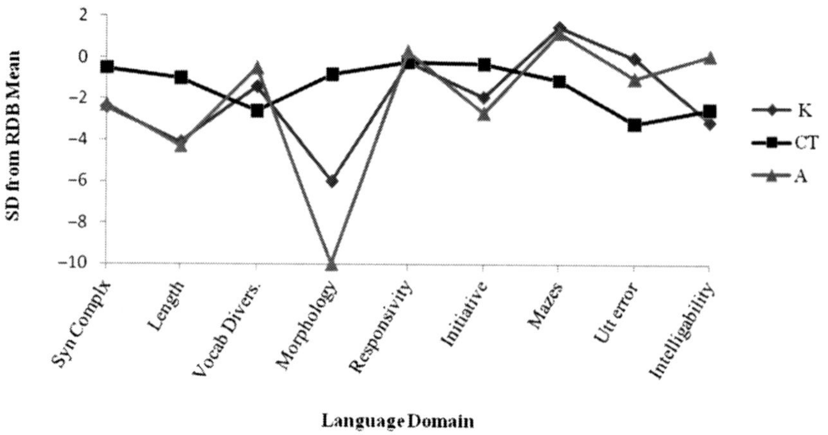

Figure 6.1 Language profiles for A, K and CT. *Note*: The signs have been reversed for variables that measure errors so as to maintain a constant visual direction for the less desirable scores

Apart from some differences in their degree of difficulty with morphology and intelligibility, A and K show remarkably similar patterns of strength and weakness across the various aspects of verbal communication that can be profiled with TSALT. Moreover, the particular profile that they show is one that finds support in the literature on global developmental delay. A number of research studies, for example, report that vocabulary knowledge, especially for words that refer to objects and events rather than conceptual relations, can surpass mental age expectations in children with global delays (Chapman *et al.*, 1998; Fazio *et al.*, 1993). A recent study by Moyle *et al.* (2007) suggests that these findings may even point to a more general dissociation between lexical and grammatical development. These investigators report that grammatical development for 'late talkers' does not predict lexical development to the same extent as is typically seen and speculate that late talkers rely more on lexical bootstrapping and less on syntactic bootstrapping in the learning process. While 'late talkers' are by definition children with normal nonverbal intelligence, this pattern may also be true for children whose late talking is accompanied by global delays.

Other aspects of this profile also resonate with the literature on retardation. One body of research points to a certain lack of inquisitiveness and intellectual energy that can result from slow rates of learning (Inhelder, 1968). This might explain the relatively low conversational assertiveness seen in these children. Also the fact that K shows reduced intelligibility (–3.1 standard deviation, SD) and A does not is consistent with K's diagnosis of Down's syndrome with its associated abnormalities in oral structure and movement (Chapman & Hesketh, 2000; Kumin, 1996; Miller, 1999; Stoel-Gammon, 2001).

These correspondences between the data from A and K and the research literature on retardation serve to validate the LSA profile approach to assessment. The broader literature on atypical development suggests that we might find additional correspondences between particular verbal profiles and other developmental conditions (Rice *et al.*, 2005). Children on the Autism Spectrum, for example, are often unresponsive conversationalists, and many children with language learning disabilities have particular difficulties mastering English grammatical morphology (Johnston & Schery, 1976; Redmond, 2004).

When studied more carefully, however, these associations between profile patterns and diagnostic groups have proven to be imperfect at best. In one large-sample, longitudinal project designed to test the validity of traditional diagnostic categories, North American researchers concluded that although SLI children showed somewhat fewer pragmatic deficits and fewer errors in lexical selection than children in other groups, there was considerable overlap in performance patterns for both verbal and nonverbal variables (Rapin, 1996; Rapin & Allen, 1998). Similar overlapping profiles have been reported by researchers in Great Britain (Hick *et al.*, 2005; Laws & Bishop, 2003; Mawhood *et al.*, 2000; see also Roberts *et al.*, 2004). Such findings suggest that profile patterns are best used for individualized program development rather than for differential diagnosis.

TSALT profiles of the sort portrayed in Figure 6.1 provide evidence to guide the first stage of educational program planning, namely, selection of the general areas of language learning and use that will be targeted for intervention (Fey, 1986). TSALT can also guide the finer details of program development. The profile variables we have discussed are included in the program's initial default analyses, but the capacities of TSALT for investigating language patterns extend well beyond this standard set and include a powerful set of tools for customized searches. To illustrate these follow-up analyses, we used TSALT to search through the A and K transcripts and list all utterances in which a grammatical morpheme had been omitted. Reviewing this list, we found that the majority of the omitted forms were noun affixes, possessive constructions for A and possessive, dative and accusative affixes for K. These forms could be the focus of individualized language learning programs.

The third child in Figure 6.1/Table 6.1 shows a very different language profile. CT is a somewhat overprotected child who prefers the comfort of familiar toys and activities. He has been diagnosed as having a pervasive developmental disorder that, although mild, is reflected in difficulties with topic maintenance and in the occasional inclusion of nonsense words in his speech. In contrast to the first two children, most of the standard scores in CT's profile fall within or nearly within the normal range.

The primary exceptions are in the areas of vocabulary, intelligibility and formulation processes. His *z*-score for lexical diversity is –2.6. Follow-up analyses indicated a frequent reliance on general purpose expressions such as 'doing something', which suggests that the low diversity may reflect word-finding difficulties rather than a limited lexicon.

1 **E:** What did you do at the zoo?
C: At the zoo I >
E: Yes at the zoo~
C: I was doing something at the zoo.
2 **E:** What is he doing to the cat later on?
C: He is doing something to the cat later on.

Further evidence of difficulty with utterance formulation can be seen in the unusually high number of utterance-level errors and abandoned utterances, with *z*-scores of 3.2 SD and 2.0 SD, respectively. The following utterance is typical of this set.

3 Ama biz tavşan da o-nu ol-uyo [EU].
But we rabbit too that-acc. become-ing.
(But we rabbit is becoming that too)

Although CT's sample does not include an unusually high proportion of maze words, the TSALT maze analysis indicates that those that do occur primarily involve syntactic revision, which again is consistent with formulation difficulties.

4 (Ben bıçak el-im-i bıçağ-ım-ı) Ben bıçağ-ım-ı kes-iyor-um.
(I knife hand-poss-acc. knife-poss-acc) I knife-poss-acc cut-ing-1sing
I am cutting my knife

Finally, a listing of the utterances with unintelligible segments suggested that CT's problems in this domain are due to the use of invented words rather than to phonological immaturity, and further, that these apparently meaningless syllables are more likely to occur when CT is having formulation problems. A larger sample would be needed to confirm this possibility.

This brief exploration of CT's language profile illustrates a further advantage of computer-assisted LSA. Transcripts of a session remain available for repeated and in-depth analysis, allowing for the investigation of the same behavior from different perspectives. Prior to the profile analysis, CT's communication problems had been described primarily from a social and pragmatic point of view, that is, failure to maintain a collaborative topic and inappropriate use of nonsense words. However, TSALT profile data indicated good conversational responsiveness and assertiveness, which seemed to be inconsistent with the emphasis on social limitations. Additional TSALT data revealed a high number of abandoned and uninterpretable utterances, which in turn introduced the possibility of significant difficulty with language processing. When we looked at the profile data from this perspective, there was greater coherence. Abandoned and uninterpretable utterances, unintelligibility and low lexical diversity could all be reflections of a fundamental processing deficit that might contribute to coexisting social limitations but would not inherently require them.

Measuring progress

The first three cases illustrated the use of computer-based LSA to assess the presence of language delay and describe a given child's language strengths and weaknesses. The fourth and final case study illustrates the unique advantages of this approach in documenting a child's progress in language learning. T is a shy and serious six-year-old boy who enjoys computerized games and activities. He is high functioning with a diagnosis of pervasive developmental disorder and a history of hyperlexia. He has difficulty initiating his own play, but is cooperative within the structure of the kindergarten program. Language samples were collected from T at three points over an eight-month period. Figure 6.2 portrays the changes that occurred for a selection of TSALT variables during this time.

Note first the accelerating increase in mean length of utterances in words (MLUw). The *z*-score for this variable changes from –4 to –2.5 in the

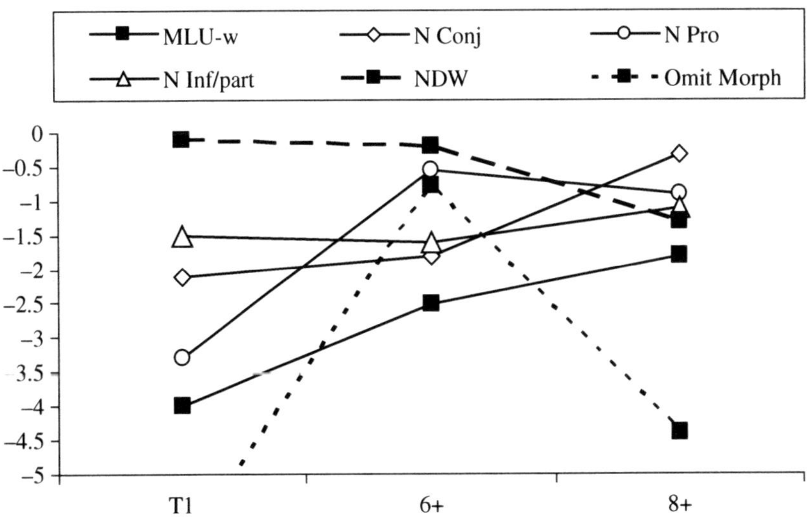

Figure 6.2 Longitudinal changes in standard scores for LSA variables

first six months, with an additional improvement to –1.8 in the next two months. Several lines of argument suggest that these changes represent real and significant language growth. Firstly, the change in T's standard score implies that his MLUw is increasing more rapidly than that of age peers. Although we lack data from children learning Turkish, studies of children learning other languages indicate that MLU continues to increase throughout the school years. It is thus unlikely that this improvement in *z*-scores can be attributed to ceiling effects in the comparison group. Secondly, by analogy to calculations of effect size, we can compare the absolute value of the MLUw gain score with the variance observed in the control group at T1. MLUw increases from 1.7 to 2.8 over the eight months. This gain is 2.8 times as large as the SD for the control group at T1 and can thus be viewed as substantial. Finally, this increase in length is accompanied by clear changes in the syntactic complexity of T's utterances. Gains in both absolute scores and *z*-scores for frequency of conjunctions are nearly equivalent to those for MLUw when similarly evaluated, and frequency of infinitives/participles begins to increase during the last two months. Interestingly, strong gains are also seen in T's use of anaphoric pronouns, suggesting a growing facility for linking linguistic forms across discourse as well as within sentences.

The growth trends seen in the length and complexity of T's language are not seen in all of the TSALT profile variables. The *z*-scores for lexical diversity (NDW) actually decline during the eight-month period. We lack information about T's educational program during this period, but it is possible that the difference between the lexical and syntactic growth curves indicates a need to change the focus of the educational program in the months ahead. New syntactic schemes could be allowed to consolidate, while T's literacy skills were used to support vocabulary learning.

The dramatic ups and downs seen in the data on morphological omissions are a good reminder that error rates for given linguistic forms will rise and fall as they are first attempted and then mastered (Rispoli & Hadley, 2001). Variation of the sort seen in T's longitudinal profile data is to be expected. Follow-up computer searches could identify the particular forms that emerged during this period and were responsible for the observed error spike.

This brief longitudinal analysis serves to illustrate the value of TSALT for documenting progress in language learning. The quantified variables provided by the computer-generated comparisons with reference data permit us to explicitly consider variability and magnitude of change. In this respect, profiling shows characteristics more typically found in standardized tests than in criteria-referenced measures. LSA is, however, more sensitive to change than test scores and can be focused on those aspects of language that have been emphasized in the child's educational program (Fawcett *et al.*, 2001; McCauley & Swisher, 1984). Moreover, there is no question that whatever learning has taken place has been incorporated into the child's everyday repertoire and is not restricted to the tasks practiced in test or therapy activities.

Conclusion

In our experience, detailed examination of the real-life language produced by children with learning difficulties provides insight into the programming needs of individuals and helps us understand the nature of developmental language disorders in general. The potential contributions of computer-based language profiling to this endeavor seem to be very promising. By combining age-based comparisons with the use of relatively spontaneous, communicative language, LSA procedures using SALT/TSALT greatly blur the traditional distinction between normative and criterion-referenced approaches to assessment. Further research will be needed to determine the predictive power and measurement characteristics of this hybrid approach. But as we have attempted to demonstrate in this chapter, this procedure provides a wide and flexible range of comparisons to a single normative database, rapidly and with a minimum of coding. The resulting scores have good face validity and address a variety of assessment questions, both descriptive and diagnostic. There are also tools to facilitate follow-up explorations, in the moment and over time. The availability of TSALT should thus prove valuable to Turkish-speaking educators and early language specialists.

Appendix: Example of SALT Printout

TRANSCRIPT INFORMATION
Speaker: **CHILD T**
Sample Date: 16.4.2007
Current Age: 5;11
Context: Conversation
150 C&I Verbal Utts

DATABASE INFORMATION
Database: Turkish Soh.SDB
Subjects: 20 females, 24 males
Age Range: 5;5 - 6;5
Context: Conversation
150 C&I Verbal Utts

STANDARD MEASURES

	CHILD		DATABASE				
LANGUAGE MEASURE	***Score***	***+/- SD***	***Mean***	***Min***	***Max***	***SD***	***%SD***
Current Age	5.92	-0.24	5.99	5.42	6.42	0.30	5
TRANSCRIPT LENGTH							
Total utterances	162*	1.29	156.59	151	168	4.21	3
# C&I Verbal Utts	150	0.00	150.00	150	150	0.00	0
Number of complete words	260**	-3.19	485.45	341	713	70.64	15
SYNTAX/MORPHOLOGY							
# MLU in words	1.70**	-4.03	3.29	2.40	4.42	0.39	12
# MLU in morphemes	3.47**	-3.73	6.08	4.87	8.45	0.70	12
SEMANTICS							
# TTR	0.48	-0.08	0.48	0.40	0.54	0.03	7
# Number of different word roots	107	-0.91	114.77	97	129	8.57	7
# Total main body words	223*	-1.76	237.89	211	250	8.44	4
DISCOURSE							
% Responses to questions	90%	-0.38	92.08	78	100	5.75	6
Mean turn length (words)	1.47**	-2.62	5.16	2.95	9.54	1.41	27
Utts With overlaps	2	0.28	1.57	0	6	1.55	99
INTELLIGIBILITY							
% Intelligible Utts	99%	0.39	97.88	90	100	2.07	2
MAZES & ABANDONED UTTS							
# Utterances with mazes	20	0.32	16.64	1	40	10.65	64
# Number of mazes	20	0.19	17.73	1	46	11.90	67
# Number of maze words	30	0.12	27.50	1	81	20.74	75
# % Maze words/total words	12%*	1.60	5.57	0	14	3.89	70
Abandoned utterances	4*	1.78	1.25	0	5	1.54	123
OMISSIONS & ERROR CODES							
# Omitted words	0	0.00	0.00	0	0	0.00	0
# Omitted bound morphemes	5**	6.07	0.41	0	3	0.76	185
Word-level error codes	1*	1.20	0.36	0	2	0.53	146
Utt-level error codes	0	-0.72	0.39	0	2	0.54	139

Calculations based on C&I Verbal Utts.
* At least 1 SD (** 2 SD) from the database mean.

Chapter 7

Specific Language Impairment in Turkish: Adapting the Test of Early Language Development (TELD-3) as a First Step in Measuring Language Impairments

SEYHUN TOPBAŞ

Introduction

Communication through language is the central building block for children's social and educational development. Any interfering difficulty may hamper the children's future learning throughout their entire lives. Over the past decades, a variety of labels have been used for childhood or developmental language disorders. The current consensus is to use the label *specific language impairment* (SLI) for those children who exhibit significant deficits in one or all aspects of language development (including grammar, phonology, semantics and pragmatics) with no evidence of concomitant cognitive, sensory, socioemotional or motor deficits (Bishop, 1992; Leonard, 1998; McCauley, 2001). The validity of this label has been called into question by considerable research devoted to defining the nature of the condition and to find its correlates to other developmental disorders over the past 30 years. The results of these studies have shown that SLI is a heterogeneous disorder affecting approximately 7% of children (Leonard, 1998; van der Lely, 2005). Late onset of speech acquisition is shown as the earliest typical characteristic of these children (Bishop, 1997; Conti-Ramsden, 2003), and several studies of children at different ages have shown deficits in grammatical knowledge. Related problems for these children include somewhat increased risk for emotional, behavioral and social difficulties, as well as a greater risk for persistent academic difficulties. Moreover, language impairments can range from mild to severe and may manifest as both receptive and expressive deficits

(Conti-Ramsden & Hesketh, 2003). As Conti-Ramsden and Hesketh (2003) have noted, clinicians draw from their knowledge of normal language development to ascertain whether the children in question behave like younger children developing normally or whether they behave differently in some way as to indicate SLI. However, there are large individual differences among children especially at the early ages, which lead to difficulty in differentiating late talkers from children who will have a persistent impairment. Researchers have placed special emphasis on identifying those children, at an early age, who are at risk of later language difficulties and on describing the nature and severity of their problems so that appropriate interventions can be designed. At present, these children are identified primarily through the use of exclusionary measures (i.e. a discrepancy between nonverbal intelligence and expressive language measures). More recently, researchers have been motivated to identify inclusionary symptoms as possible *clinical markers* or *key aspects* that may be helpful in differentiating late talkers from SLI. However, this is a challenging task in that language symptoms may differ and change with development. Moreover, symptoms of SLI are not the same across languages. For example, cross-linguistic studies have made it clear that children with SLI do not display uniform grammatical profiles across different languages (Bishop, 1996; Gopnik, 1996; Johnston, 2001; Leonard, 1989, 1998, 2000, 2002; Rice & Wexler, 1996; Stokes & Fletcher, 2003; van der Lely, 2005; Marton *et al.*, 2006). Given that languages differ, it is not surprising that different linguistic aspects may be impaired in different languages. To illustrate, some structural characteristics of languages that influence the types of linguistic forms that pose problems for children with SLI may be universal, whereas others may be language specific (Leonard, 2000; Paradis & Crago, 2001). Language-specific differences have been reported in German (Roberts & Leonard, 1997), Swedish (Hansson *et al.*, 2000), Italian (Bortolini *et al.*, 1997), Spanish (Bedore & Leonard, 2001), Hebrew (Dromi *et al.*, 1999), and Arabic (Abdalla & Crago, 2008).

Few investigations of linguistic descriptions of childhood language disorders, pertaining to either SLI or other developmental disorders, have been reported in Turkish. Most of the studies conducted were generally restricted to phonological disorders (an extensive summary can be found in references Topbaş and Yavaş (2006) and Topbaş (2007)). One reason for the focus on phonology was that SLI was not seen as a distinct diagnostic entity until recently. Language disorders were (1) included along with developmental disabilities occurring secondary to hearing impairment, mental retardation (MR), learning disabilities and other organic, neurological or psychiatric disorders or (2) denied altogether. In the latter case, *a wait-and-see approach* was often implemented for many years. The second reason for lack of language focus might have arisen from differences in the descriptions of what language impairment means to medical doctors and other professionals such as special educators, psychologists, researchers and the general public. Thus, the identification of these children who would now be diagnosed with SLI was left to intuition or semi-professional opinion. No doubt that many children were either inappropriately diagnosed or unattended. As discussed in the first chapter, the development of the speech and language pathology (SLP) profession in Turkey, the implementation of a new special education law and the adaptation of the International Classification of Functioning, Disability and Health (ICF) (WHO, 2001) procedures to the Turkish health system have presented new challenges. Among these are the inclusion of the characteristics of communication disorders within the ICF classification and the need for valid and accurate identification of communicatively impaired children. Identification of language impairment and subsequent qualification for services require comparison of a child's performance to a normative group (Merrell & Plante, 1997; Spaulding *et al.*, 2006). McFadden asserted that 'the major utility of norm-referenced testing lies in its contributions to the diagnosis of a language impairment and the assignment of a label for accurate and efficient service delivery' (McFadden, 1996: 3). A logical and timely first step in normative assessment has led to a new trend (i.e. translating and adapting tests from English to Turkish). In this chapter, one of these adaptations will be presented. The ultimate goal of this research is to describe the patterns of language development displayed by normally developing Turkish children in order to provide a basis for a comparison of patterns of impaired and/or delayed development with normal development. Such normative comparisons are particularly necessary in identifying language patterns that may be symptomatic of an uneven course of development.

Background to the Adaptation of the Test of Early Language Development (TELD-3) to Turkish

Although there are sufficient studies that provide a picture of typical language acquisition in Turkish (see Chapter 4 of this book), most of these studies were conducted with small groups of children. In addition, the picture is incomplete because there are no norms available indicating which structures are acquired at which ages. Thus, as a first step, a project began in 2005 to adapt the TELD-3 (Hresko *et al.*, 1999) to Turkish (Topbaş & Güven, 2007; by permission of PRO-ED). The TELD-3 was developed for English children and adapted to Spanish in the United States (Ramos & Ramos, 2007). It was chosen mainly because it is widely used, is easy and short to administer and provides a good picture of a child's language performance.

Translating or adapting a test from one language to another for a new target population is a complex task. First, considering typological differences between English and Turkish, it was necessary to preserve semantic or syntactic information in the test items. Importantly, the Turkish translation (TELD-3: Turkish version, TELD-3:T) is both a *translation* and an *adaptation*. Therefore, performance on the original and the adapted tests cannot be compared directly. Several researchers have cautioned potential users of problems and issues related to developing equivalent forms of language tests (Geisinger, 1994). Although the items may appear similar, there are inherent linguistic differences in vocabulary, sentence structure, morphology, linguistic cues, word order, subject–verb agreement, verb morphology and so on. The standardization populations also cannot be equivalent; each population has different sociocultural and environmental contexts including variables that affect parents or caregivers and their interactions in the home. The actual standardization of TELD-3:T is ongoing; to date, the development of the test has progressed through three pilot studies (Topbaş, 2006; Topbaş & Güven, 2008).

According to Plante and Vance (1994), tests used to identify individuals with impaired language (identification tests) should discriminate with a high degree of accuracy between children with normal language and children with language impairment. With accurate discrimination as a basis, this chapter will report the final pilot field testing that has been carried out with a large-scale sample to measure whether the adaptation of TELD-3:T has the capacity to discriminate between those children who are typically developing and those who have language impairments in Turkish. The chapter is organized into two parts. In Study 1, the pilot field testing will be summarized with a special emphasis on validity, reliability and sensitivity in the identification of SLI. In Study 2, the sentence completion tasks of the test with some qualitative data will be compared between the pilot normative sample and a sample from another group of children who have been suspected as SLI.

Study 1: Pilot Field Testing

Method

The participants

The TELD-3:T pilot sample assessed typically developing and disabled children ($n = 359$), aged 2–7, residing in 14 cities from five geographical regions in Turkey. All of the children speak Turkish as their first language. A total of 335 typically developing children, who were divided into six age groups, were recruited from private and state preschools, elementary schools and university nursery schools by a formal permission from the Ministry of National Education. In all cases, permission was also granted by the parent, guardian, student and school authorities prior to testing. Spaulding *et al.* (2006) and Andersson (2005) proposed that the standardization sample of a test should represent subgroups of children in proportions similar to those found in the population, and these subgroups should be included in the standardization sample. Keeping in mind this criterion, we included 24 children in a disability group, of which 18 had language delay and/or language learning difficulties (hereinafter referred to as SLI), and six had a diagnosis of MR. These subgroups constitute 6.7% of the Turkish sample and 2% of the total population (Andersson, 2005). The characteristics of the pilot sample with regard to geographic region, gender, family income, parents' educational attainment, disability status and age compared, when possible, to proportions in the population are reported in Table 7.1.

The disabled group

Identifying children with SLI has challenging problems because of the lack of detailed normative receptive and expressive language tests at present. Thus, 18 children who were referred for speech and language therapy as presenting language delay and language learning difficulties were chosen for the study after meeting several criteria in the literature. Criteria for inclusion in the study consisted of (1) expressive language performance that was markedly below the developmental milestones expected for typically developing children as well as (2) meeting the following criteria:

- Normal hearing: Any speech and language difficulties could not be attributed to hearing loss; thus, each child was required to pass a hearing screening bilaterally at 20 dB for 1000 and 2000 Hz and at 25 dB for 550 and 4000 Hz.
- Normal range on a measure of nonverbal cognitive ability: with IQ, Leiter and Wechsler intelligence scale for children (WISC-R) test, (Savaşır & Şahin, 1995) performance scores higher than their verbal scores.
- No report of other special education categories: no congenital problems, no diagnosis of autism and MR; no major/specific neurological and motor problems or any evidence of abnormal social behavior could be present as reported by a formal report from medical teams.
- The SLI participants were tested first, Peabody picture vocabulary test: Turkish version (PPVT) (Dunn & Dunn, 1997) (the M age = 5;7 for province).

The six mentally retarded children were recruited from special education schools where the SLPs who were responsible for data collection worked. The children were diagnosed as educable mentally retarded according to school files. Two children had Down's syndrome. All background information about the children's development was taken from their schools.

Procedure

The TELD-3:T was administered by SLPs who were graduates of DİLKOM and were trained to administer the TELD-3:T during their education, as well as by SLP students in master's and doctoral degree programs.

Table 7.1 Demographic characteristics of the TELD-3:T sample in pilot field testing (N = 359)

Characteristics	*n (number)*	*Percentage of sample*	*Percentage of total population in Turkey*
Gender[a]			
Male	198	55.2	50.6
Female	161	44.8	49.4
Residence[a]			
Urban	307	85.5	64.9
Rural	52	14.5	35.1
Family income[b]			
Below 1000 YTL	61	17.0	NA[c]
1000–2500 YTL	158	44.0	NA
2500 and above	140	39.0	NA
Educational attainment of parents			
Illiterate	4	1.1	21.5
Primary school	42	11.7	37.0
Secondary school	36	10.0	10.1
High school	131	36.5	13.4
University graduate	146	40.7	3.2
Kindergarten[a]			
Enrolled	117	32.6	28.5
Not enrolled	242	67.4	71.5
Disability status[a]			
No disability	335	93.3	98.2
Disabled	18	5.0	1.8
Speech–language disorder			
MR	6	1.7	
Ages			
2 (N = 29)			
3 (N = 71)			
4 (N = 88)			
5 (N = 74)			
6 (N = 61)			
7 (N = 36)			

[a]Based on total population data in the Current Population Survey and data reported in The Statistical Abstract of the Turkish Statistical Institute (2008).
[b]Based on Income, Poverty Information in Turkey: 2008 (Kamu-Sen).
[c]Information not available.

The SLP graduates who agreed to participate were sent materials to test students in their area. Examiners followed a standard administration protocol throughout the pilot testing period. Both alternate forms (Form A and Form B) of the subtests were administered to all children.

Results of reliability measures

Content sampling, time sampling and scorer differences were computed for investigators to examine reliability. For each of these sources of error variance, the degree of reliability is reported in terms of correlation coefficients.

Content sampling

Two methods were used to investigate the TELD-3:T's content sample reliability: internal consistency (coefficient α and its associated standard error of measurement) and alternate forms (immediate administration).

The internal consistency of the pilot test was measured by computing Cronbach's α for each subtest at six age intervals using the entire sample. The coefficients were averaged using the *z*-transformation technique and are shown in Table 7.2. Averages are listed in a column on the right side of the table. The coefficients along with the standard errors of measurement for both Forms A and B of the subtests indicate that the test has high internal consistency in that all comparisons exceeded or rounded to 0.90.

The adapted test should also be equally reliable for every subgroup within that population. The coefficients for selected subgroups within the pilot sample are reported in Table 7.3. The αs, shown in Table 7.3, range from 0.91 to 0.96 and demonstrate that the TELD-3:T was about equally reliable for all the subgroups investigated and support the idea that the test contained little or no bias relative to the subgroups.

Alternate forms of the subtests, which were given during one testing session, show the correlation between the two forms as a reliability index that can be used to estimate content sampling error. The means and standard deviations for Forms A and B of the subtests and the correlation

Table 7.2 Reliability coefficient αs (and standard errors of measurement) for the TELD-3:T at six ages

TELD-3:T		*Age*						
Subtests	*Form*	2	3	4	5	6	7	*Average*
Receptive language	A	0.90 (5)	0.90 (5)	0.86 (6)	0.93 (4)	0.92 (4)	0.98 (2)	0.93
	B	0.86 (6)	0.88 (5)	0.88 (5)	0.91 (5)	0.93 (4)	0.98 (2)	0.92
Expressive language	A	0.87 (5)	0.91 (5)	0.91 (5)	0.96 (3)	0.94 (4)	0.98 (2)	0.94
	B	0.86 (6)	0.92 (4)	0.87 (5)	0.92 (4)	0.92 (5)	0.98 (2)	0.92

Table 7.3 Coefficient αs for selected subgroups of the TELD-3:T sample

	TELD-3 scores			
	Receptive language		*Expressive language*	
Subgroups	*A*	*B*	*A*	*B*
Males (*N* = 198)	0.96	0.95	0.95	0.95
Females (*N* = 161)	0.95	0.94	0.95	0.93
Enrolled in school (*N* = 242)	0.95	0.94	0.95	0.93
Not enrolled in school (*N* = 117)	0.95	0.94	0.95	0.94
Language delay/ disorder (*N* = 18)	0.92	0.91	0.94	0.94
Urban (*N* = 307)	0.95	0.95	0.95	0.94
Rural (*N* = 52)	0.95	0.95	0.95	0.94

between the two forms at six ages are found in Table 7.4. The two forms of the TELD-3:T seem equivalent at this piloting stage. The means and standard deviations for Forms A and B are quite similar at every age interval. The correlation coefficients depicting the relationship between Forms A and B show a moderate-to-high reliability, ranging from 0.60 to 0.97 at different ages. This might be due to the low number of children in some age groups. Nevertheless, it should be kept in mind that a revision was made after the pilot field testing due to the results of item analyses before the actual standardization.

Table 7.4 Alternate forms (immediate administration) reliability for TELD-3:T scores: Means (and standard deviations) for Forms A and B and correlations between forms

	TELD-3:T scores					
	Receptive language			*Expressive language*		
Age	*A*	*B*	r_{A+B}	*A*	*B*	r_{A+B}
2	11 (5)	12 (5)	0.70	14 (4)	15 (4)	0.60
3	18 (5)	18 (5)	0.64	20 (5)	21 (5)	0.72
4	24 (5)	24 (5)	0.69	26 (5)	26 (4)	0.82
5	29 (6)	28 (5)	0.68	31 (6)	29 (4)	0.80
6	32 (5)	31 (4)	0.81	34 (5)	32 (5)	0.76
7	33 (8)	32 (8)	0.96	35 (7)	34 (8)	0.97

Table 7.5 Test–retest reliability for Forms A and B of the TELD-3:T (ages 5, 6 and 7) (n = 20; 12 male + 8 female)

	First testing			*Second testing*			
TELD-3:T	*Forms*	*M*	*SD*	*M*	*SD*	*r*	r_{A+B}
Receptive language	A	33	(5)	33	(5)	0.96	0.95
	B	33	(6)	33	(6)	0.93	
Expressive language	A	35	(6)	36	(5)	0.89	0.86
	B	33	(6)	34	(6)	0.83	

Time sampling (test–retest)

A test–retest correlation method was used to study the adapted test's time sampling error with 20 children, aged 5–7. Both forms of the test were administered twice, and the intervening time was approximately two weeks. The means and standard deviations for the first and second testing and the correlation between the two testing periods can be found in Table 7.5 for Forms A and B. The correlation coefficients were corrected for a restricted range of the sample where appropriate. The resulting coefficients were consistently high and significant, indicating that the TELD-3:T has significant acceptable test–retest reliability in this pilot study.

Interscorer reliability

Two master's degree students in SLP at Anadolu University independently scored a set of 20 completed protocols, which were drawn randomly from the sample. The results of the interscorer reliability were 0.98 and 0.99 for receptive and expressive subtests of Form A and 0.99 and 0.99 for receptive and expressive subtests of Form B, respectively. These coefficients provided initial evidence supporting the TELD-3:T's interscorer reliability.

Results of validity measures

Content, construct and convergent validity were computed as indicators of the validity of the adapted test.

Content validity

The format of the original TELD-3 was followed to construct TELD-3:T subtest items. During adaptation of the items, adherence to accepted standards for translating and adapting tests was used as a guide (Andersson, 2005; Geisinger, 1994). Research studies of Turkish language acquisition as well as instructional materials used in early childhood, kindergarten and first-grade curricula were reviewed before items were selected. The critiques of TELD and its editions by several authors (Andersson, 2004, 2005; Dale & Henderson, 1987; Plante & Vance, 1994; Spaulding *et al.*, 2006) were also considered to strengthen the validity of the TELD-3:T. For example, special problems exist in comparing measures of normal development in languages like Turkish where measures are typically translations of English versions. As a result, these adapted measures may not reflect the structural characteristics of a richly inflected, subject–object–verb language. Thus, items such as sentence repetition (SR) tasks were not direct translations; rather, they were expanded and selected to reflect the grammatical structure of Turkish.

As a next step, *expert review* from 10 practicing SLPs, assistant professors and special education teachers was used to determine the appropriateness of the items, the vocabulary and the instructions used in the adapted TELD-3:T. After the completion of these procedures, two trial administrations of the adapted tests were carried out to learn any further potential problems. The first one was conducted with 13 typically developing children and 15 learning-disabled children who were potentially language impaired (i.e. referred for speech therapy with unknown diagnoses). Based on results of the first administration, the test was revised and a second pilot study was carried out with an expanded sample of 90 normal and 20 learning-disabled children. After the second administration, some items were changed and additional SR items were added to the existing SR tasks.

The validity of the items should be supported by the results of conventional item analysis (i.e. differential item functioning analysis) before the actual standardization. Thus, the third pilot field testing discussed in this chapter was conducted with a large sample of children. To demonstrate that the item characteristics were satisfactory for the TELD-3:T, we performed an item analysis using all of the third pilot sample. The resulting median item discrimination coefficients and item difficulties indicate that the test items satisfy the requirements and provide evidence of content-description validity.

Construct-identification validity

Since this was a pilot study, only the basic constructs that appear to underlie the TELD-3:T were computed.

Age differentiation: Language is developmental in nature; therefore, performance on the TELD-3:T should be strongly correlated with age. The means and standard deviations for the TELD-3:T subtests at six age levels between 2 and 7 can be found in Table 7.6. An inspection of the table illustrates that the means became progressively larger between ages 2 and 7. Recall that this was pilot sampling, and the sample was low at each age; thus, as expected, the coefficients showing the relationship of age to performance were considered moderately high.

Table 7.6 Construct validity: Age differentiation for receptive and expressive subtests, Forms A and B of the TELD-3:T and correlations to age

	TELD-3:T scores			
	Receptive language		*Expressive language*	
	Form A	*Form B*	*Form A*	*Form B*
Age	*M (SD)*	*M (SD)*	*M (SD)*	*M (SD)*
2	11 (5)	12 (5)	14 (4)	15 (4)
3	18 (5)	18 (5)	20 (5)	21 (5)
4	24 (5)	24 (5)	26 (5)	26 (4)
5	29 (6)	28 (5)	31 (6)	29 (4)
6	32 (5)	31 (4)	34 (5)	32 (5)
7	33 (8)	32 (8)	35 (7)	34 (8)
Correlations to age	**0.78**	**0.76**	**0.77**	**0.76**

Group differentiation: Because the TELD-3:T measures language, its subtests should differentiate between children with normally developing language and children who have disabilities that include language impairments or who have disabilities that affect language acquisition (i.e. children with MR). A test whose results do not differentiate between such groups would have limited clinical or diagnostic value; therefore, it would be lacking in construct validity (Hresko *et al.*, 1999). At this stage, a series of analyses have been done regarding the construct validity of the test. First, a group differentiation was made by a *t*-test following the TELD-3 original manual (Hresko *et al.*, 1999) as shown in Table 7.7 (the MR children were not included in this analysis since the number of children was very low). The result of the *t*-test was significant in that TELD-3:T was able to distinguish between groups of children with differing language abilities in this piloting sample.

Convergent validity

As Merrell and Plante (1997) have suggested, tests in use should aid in answering the question of whether or not there is a language impairment. Thus, the test should be *sensitive* and *specific* enough for a clinician to use with confidence in diagnosing children of unknown language status. In order to do so, a discriminant analysis was run to assess TELD-3:T's strength in discriminating between children from the pilot sample and children with impaired language. This analysis can also be evaluated as evidence for the convergent validity of the test.

For this measure, 30 new SLI children were matched with 30 normally developing age-matched (NDAM) children from the pilot sample. Matching

Table 7.7 Group differentiation, *t*-test scores for the selected subgroups

TELD-3:T subtests	*Disability status*	*Form A*		*t*	*p*	*Form B*	*t*	*p*
Receptive language	Normal	*M*	25.66	2.14	0.033	25.16	2.42	0.016
		SD	8.43			7.89		
	SLI	*M*	21.33			20.61		
		SD	7.00			5.47		
	MR	*M*	10.83	4.30	0.000	10.83	4.44	0.000
		SD	2.14			2.40		
Expressive language	Normal	*M*	27.90	3.20	0.002	27.13	2.90	0.004
		SD	8.11			6.95		
	SLI	*M*	21.67			22.28		
		SD	6.86			5.95		
	MR	*M*	12.33	4.68	0.000	13.00	4.97	0.000
		SD	4.18			2.83		

was one-to-one on age in months (*M* = 62.5, SD = 13.2), on gender (5 girls, 25 boys), on family income levels (high: 33%; middle: 46%; low: 6%) and on educational attainment of parents (primary: 6.7%; middle school: 16.7%; high school: 43.3%; university graduates: 33.3%). The SLI children were administered the TELD-3:T at DİLKOM by a qualified research assistant who participated in the adaptation project. All testing took place in a video-circuited therapy room and recorded using digital recorders and a microphone. Children's utterances were transcribed simultaneously by a second assistant to verify the scoring.

Discriminant analysis provides information concerning a test's sensitivity and specificity. The measure of a test's *sensitivity* is the accuracy with which the test identifies children with language impairment as language impaired. The measure of a test's *specificity* is the accuracy with which the test identifies children with normally developing language as having normally developing language. The percent of error in sensitivity and specificity provides evidence of the number of false positives and false negatives a clinician might encounter in using the test to identify children with language impairment. Low sensitivity would indicate a higher false-negative rate (i.e. under-identification); low specificity would indicate a higher false-positive rate (i.e. over-identification) (McCauley, 2001; Plante & Vance, 1995). Plante and Vance (1995) recommended that a higher standard be met for sensitivity than for specificity. Specifically, they recommended that sensitivity should be at 90% or above, whereas for specificity, they accepted levels of 80% as 'good' and 70% as 'fair'.

Discriminant analysis consists of two steps. The first stage evaluates whether the variance in test scores among subjects can be accounted for by group membership (NDAM versus SLI). This is accomplished through a regression formula in which the predictor variable is the test and the criterion variable is the group categorization. The second stage involves the use of the regression information to categorize children as normally developing or language impaired and to check the accuracy of the statistical categorization against the children's true categorization. Statistical significance only indicates that the amount of variance in test scores that is associated with group categorization (NDAM versus SLI) is above chance levels. A significant analysis does not indicate in and of itself that categorization based on this analysis would be clinically useful. A second step for evaluating categorization accuracy is needed. This is known as the test's sensitivity. This analysis also shows the frequency with which the test identified NDAM children. This is known as the test's specificity. The raw scores for each subject were converted to *z*-scores. The *z*-scores represent the difference between a child's score and the normative sample mean, divided by the standard deviation of the normative sample. Therefore, each *z*-score maintains its tie to the normative sample of the test. All remaining statistical analyses were calculated using *z*-scores (Plante & Vance, 1995, 1994).

Considering these guidelines, both of the receptive and expressive subtests including the alternate forms of TELD-3:T were subjected to discriminant analysis and cross-validation (SPSS, 1997). The analysis used the test scores to place each child into either SLI or NDAM group (NDAM $M = 1.53$, SD = 0.80; SLI group $M = -1.53$, SD = 1.17). The results of the discriminant analyses indicated a statistically significant group classification on both receptive (Receptive Form A $F = 75.23$, $p < 0.000$; Form B $F = 48.81, p < 0.000$) and expressive (Expressive Form A $F = 97.30, p < 0.000$; Form B $F = 129.20$, $p < 0.000$) subtests. This indicated that group membership accounted for a significant proportion of the variance in test scores. The first discriminant function explained 100% of the variance where the canonic correlation coefficient was 0.85, and overall Wilks's λ was significant, $\Lambda = 0.27$, $\chi^2(2, N = 30) = 72.43$, $p < 0.000$. Thus, this function successfully differentiated between the two groups. However, as Plante and Vance (1994) noted, significance alone does not guarantee that a test is a clinically accurate identifier of impaired skills. Therefore, sensitivity and specificity analyses had to be undertaken. The percentage and actual number of cases that were correctly classified in the cross-validation analysis are summarized in Table 7.8 (Plante & Vance, 1994).

As illustrated in Table 7.8, the receptive subtest classified 93.3% of the NDAM children and 83.3% of the SLI children. The expressive subtest

Table 7.8 Percentage and total number of children correctly classified in the TELD-3:T subtest scores, cross-validation analysis of SLI and NDAM children

	SLI	*NDAM*
Receptive subtest	93.3% (28/30)	83.3% (25/30)
Expressive subtest	100% (30/30)	86.7% (26/30

classified 100% of the NDAM children (specificity) and 86.7% of the SLI children (sensitivity). Using the total scores, 100% of the NDAM children and 86.7% of the SLI children were classified accurately. Using the total scores, all the NDAM children were classified highly accurately, whereas 4 children out of 30 with SLI were misclassified in this investigation. The findings of this pilot study seem particularly noteworthy because the TELD-3:T has a significant potential to correctly identify children with impairments.

Study 2: Comparison of Performance on SR Tasks of the TELD-3:T

Over the past decade, elicited sentence imitation or SR tasks have been shown as a reliable and powerful method for assessing grammatical knowledge (Crain & Thornton, 1998; Lust *et al.*, 1996; Thornton, 1995). Many test batteries including the Clinical Evaluation of Language Fundamentals, fourth edition (CELF-4) (Semel *et al.*, 1989), the TELD-3 (Hresko *et al.*, 1999) and the test of Early Language Development-4: Primary (TOLD-4:P) (Newcomer & Hammill, 2008) include SR tasks to assess children's language and processing abilities. Although there is still controversy over whether the SR tasks may underestimate or overestimate children's linguistic competence, some authors observed that the child could reorganize the model sentence presented in a way that more closely reflects standard word order, but may omit, introduce or substitute a new morpheme, keeping the sense of the sentence and showing that he/she understood it (Kuczaj & Maratsos, 1975; Slobin & Welsh, 1973). According to Blake (2000), sentence imitation involves related words and knowledge of syntax, at least for correct repetition of longer sentences. Some authors observed that normal children can easily imitate the same language forms that they use spontaneously while rarely repeating sentences that have never previously occurred in their spontaneous speech (Bloom *et al.*, 1975; Kuczaj & Maratsos, 1975; Menyuk, 1963). Similarly, Bates *et al.* (1988) suggested that the ability to imitate sentences may be an individual difference variable. Some children imitate in advance of their spontaneous language abilities, while others imitate very little, and when they do imitate, they restrict their repetitions to structures that they already produce and understand.

Nevertheless, more recent studies have suggested that SR skills are potential key markers for language impairments, and for SLI specifically, they are important in measuring syntactic and/or morphosyntactic abilities of children (Conti-Ramsden *et al.*, 2001). SR measures are easy to administer and permit the assessment of specific target structures in controlled situations (Devescovi & Caselli, 2007). SR as a clinical marker has also been investigated in identifying children with normal development and children with different developmental disorders (Botting & Conti-Ramsden, 2003; Eadie *et al.*, 2002) as well as children with SLI-speaking languages such as Cantonese (Stokes & Fletcher, 2003), Italian (Vicari *et al.*, 2002; Volterra *et al.*, 2003; Bortolini *et al.*, 2006) and Dutch (Rispens, 2004). Importantly, special SR tests have been developed for this purpose in Italian (Devescovi & Caselli, 2007), English (Gardner *et al.*, 2006; van der Lely, 1997) and Dutch (Rispens, 2004). An SR task was also used in determining the language abilities of ND Turkish children during a project on the educational needs of 5–8-year-old children (preschool, primary first and second graders) living in the eastern part of Turkey (Aksu-Koç *et al.*, 2002).

Since the TELD-3:T includes SR tasks, it would be valuable to evaluate the utility of SR in identifying ND children from SLI by focusing on key grammatical structures in Turkish. Thus, in Study 2, leaving detailed qualitative analyses for future studies, we aimed to focus on quantitative analyses of SR items before the actual standardization of the test. It is assumed that if SR tasks are able to identify the differences between ND and SLI children's capacity in repeating sentences of syntactic complexity (simple versus complex sentences and errors), then the construct validity of the TELD-3:T would be strengthened.

Method

Participants and procedure

For this part of the study, we used data from the previously described children (30 SLI and 30 NDAM in Study 1) whose performance was evaluated for discriminant analysis. To evaluate the differences, the children were grouped according to five age groups: 3;0 ($n = 5$), 4;0 ($n = 5$), 5;0 ($n = 9$) and 6;0–7;0 ($n = 11$). The 6;0–7;0-year-olds were combined because there were only two children with SLI at age 7;0 for whom matching was possible.

Analysis of the SR tasks of TELD-3:T

The TELD-3:T requires a criterion tick response for correct repetition of various questions for each test item. For example, out of six sentences on one SR test item, the child must repeat at least five sentences correctly to receive 1 point, depending on the child's age. However, during this pilot study, all the sentences in each item had to be repeated correctly to receive a point.

In this study, all sentences were modeled in a play situation wherein the child was given the role of a *parrot* that listens carefully and imitates exactly what he hears. One repeat was permitted for the trial items if the child's response was incorrect; however, no test items were modeled again. The number of sentences differed for each age level. Twenty-two sentences were included as follows: 3–4-year-olds repeated 10, 5 -year-olds repeated 17 and 6–7-year-olds repeated 12 of them. All the sentences were scored separately and a total corpus of 385 sentences was ereanalyzed.

The coding during the testing time was carried out as follows: (1) incorrect or error parts of the sentences were highlighted by a colored marker pen, and the child's repetition was written down on the response form, and (2) a second examiner wrote down the child's responses to verify the scoring as well. The sessions at DİLKOM with the SLI group were recorded by digital video and audio recorders, whereas the normative group's sessions were audio recorded only and transcribed later. For this analysis, we followed a procedure similar to that reported by Volterra *et al.* (2003) and Aksu-Koç *et al.* (2002). The scoring of the number and type of errors in each sentence was as follows:

(1) The numbers of complete repetitions (CRs), incomplete repetitions (InCRs) and nonrepetitions (NoRs) were compared to the target sentences (Volterra *et al.*, 2003):
   (a) *CR* was defined as a repetition that reproduced all the content words and function words with the inclusion of all sentence elements of the target sentence. Children were not penalized on this measure if they altered or substituted words in their repetitions without a change semantically.
   (b) InCR was defined as any attempt of repetition that omits or alternates one or more of the content or function words, phrases, subordinate clauses or simplifications of the target sentence.
   (c) NoRs were defined as failures to repeat any part of the target sentence (including silence or irrelevant comments).
(2) Specific error types in each incomplete SR were subjected to further analyses of omission, addition of new elements, word-order (WO) inversion, errors of bound morphology and lexical substitutions. In this step, we counted
   (a) each element omitted (specifying also the number of omissions in obligatory contexts such as omitting the subordinate clause);
   (b) each element substituted (the child repeated the target sentence, substituting one or more elements such as noun, verb, etc.);
   (c) each morphological modification of a word (the child used in the repeated sentence a different morphological form of the same word – a singular form instead of a plural one, tense, voice, negation, case modifications, subordinating morphology, etc.); and
   (d) each repetition with word order (WO) inversion (a different order of one or more elements in the sentence repeated).

(3) The target sentences were grouped as simple and complex sentence types, and we identified whether or not the errors differed between the NDAM and SLI with respect to sentence types. Then, the specific error types were further analyzed qualitatively in simple and complex sentences (adverbial clause, relative clause, noun clause or coordinate clauses).

Results

Table 7.9 presents the means and standard deviations for each age group in the SR task for CR, InCR and NoR measures. As can be seen, the differences between the SLI and NDAM children in CR were evident at each age level for the two groups. All the NDAM children attempted to repeat the sentences, whereas three of the SLI children did not make any attempt to repeat the sentences.

The total percentages of CR, InCR and NoR sentences are illustrated in Figure 7.1, which also shows the difference between the two groups.

One-way analysis of variances (ANOVAs) were used for each age group to determine the statistical significance for the three measures. The mean difference for the NoR measure was high and statistically significant, $F(1, 20) = 28{,}832$, $p = 0.00$, which may mean that the SLI children were not able to repeat most of the sentences. Thus, group differences at different ages were computed for CR and InCR measures only. At age 3, there was a significant group difference on the CR measure ($F(1, 8) = 22{,}563$, $p < 0.001$); however, no significant group difference was observed for the InCR measure ($F(1, 8) = 3500$, $p = 0.098$). At age 4, there was a significant group difference both on CR ($F(1, 8) = 41{,}806$, $p < 0.000$) and InCR measures ($F(1, 8) = 39{,}200$, $p < 0.000$). At age 5, although there was a significant group difference on CR measure ($F(1, 16) = 6411$, $p < 0.022$), no difference was found between children with SLI and NDAM in InCR measure ($F(1, 16) = 3792$, $p = 0.069$). At ages 6–7, group differences were significant

Table 7.9 Means and standard deviations for each age group in SR tasks for CR, InCR and NoR measures by NDAM and SLI children

	NDAM						*SLI*					
	CR		*InCR*		*NoR*		*CR*		*InCR*		*NoR*	
Age group	*M*	*SD*	*M*	*SD*	*M*	*SD*	*M*	*SD*	*M*	*SD*	*M*	*SD*
3	5	1.58	2	1.58	3	2.74	1.20	0.84	3.40	0.54	5.40	0.89
4	9.20	0.84	0.80	0.84	0	0	2	2.35	3.60	0.55	4.40	2.70
5	9.11	5.62	2.89	2.32	5	5.57	3.33	3.91	5.78	3.80	7.89	5.49
6–7	9.18	2.36	1.72	1.95	1.10	2.43	0.36	0.92	4	3.16	7.64	3.23

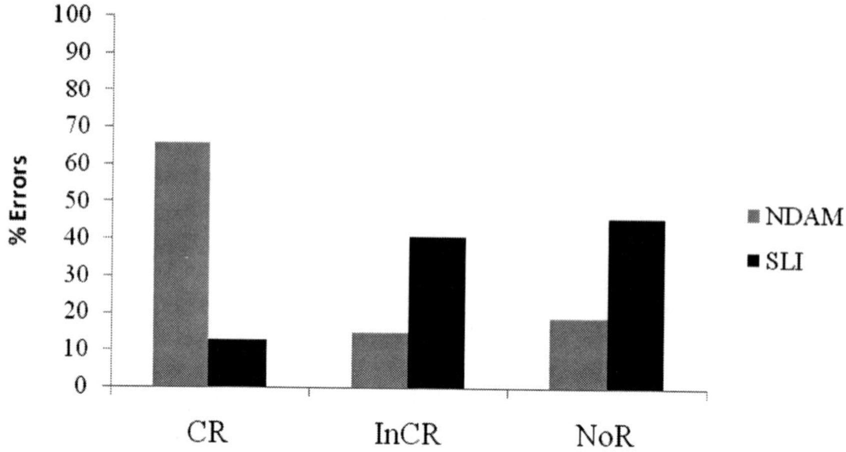

Figure 7.1 Total percentages of CR, InCR and NoR in NDAM and SLI children

both in the CR measure ($F(1, 20) = 133{,}272$, $p < 0.000$) and in the InCR measure ($F(1, 20) = 4112$, $p = 0.05$). In this age group, only two children scored a few sentences on CR, while eight children's attempts were InCRs.

The second task was to analyze the specific error types produced in InCR sentences. We calculated the total number of errors produced by children in each InCR, and a proportional calculation was done to see which of the error types were more significant in the two groups. Figure 7.2 presents the proportion of the different types of errors

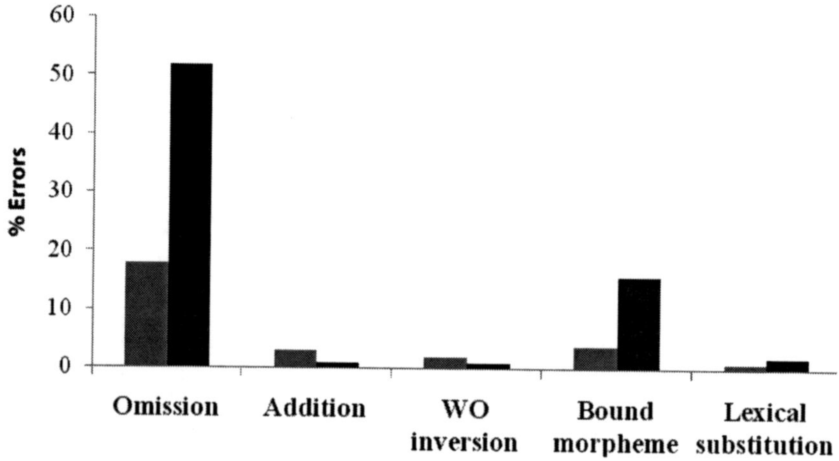

Figure 7.2 Proportion of specific error types in InCR by NDAM and SLI children

produced by the two groups of children in terms of omission, addition of new elements, WO inversion, errors of bound morphology and lexical substitution.

In the 385 sentences, a total of 59 InCRs occurred for NDAM and 159 for SLI children, or about three times as many. Among these, omission errors were proportionally the most frequent type produced by both groups of children; yet, the percentage of omissions was lower (18%) for NDAM than that of the children with SLI (52%). Errors in bound morphology were present in both groups but were much lower in the NDAM group (4%) than in the SLI group (16%). Additions of new elements were rare but were higher in NDAM (3%) versus SLI participants (2%). WO inversions were very slightly higher in NDAM (2%) than in SLI (1%). There was a very slight difference in lexical substitutions between the two groups: NDAM (1%) and SLI (2%). In general, children with SLI performed worse than their age-matched peers with the majority of the errors observed being of the omission type and bound morphology type.

The next analysis considered the errors in simple versus complex sentences constructed by the two groups. Initially, we searched for sentence types that resulted in the most errors. Overall, the NDAM group had 23 errors in simple sentences and 36 errors in complex sentences. These are comparable to analogous totals of 58 and 101 errors in the SLI group. Table 7.10 presents the proportion of error types in relation to simple and complex sentences across the two groups. As can be seen, the NDAM children were quite able to repeat sentences of different complexity, either simple or complex. Fewer errors occurred in simple sentences compared to complex sentences, and most of these were made at younger ages. Although the NDAM children made omission errors in simple and complex sentences, their proportions of such errors were lower than the SLI children's omissions. A relational analysis showed a significant correlation

Table 7.10 Proportion of error types in simple and complex sentences repeated by NDAM and SLI children

	NDAM		*SLI*	
Error types	***Simple%***	***Complex%***	***Simple%***	***Complex%***
Omission	8	9	20	33
Addition	2	2	0	0
WO inversion	0	2	0	0
Bound morpheme	0	3	7	11
Lexical substitution	0	1	0	2
Total proportion	10	17	27	46

between the errors in simple and complex sentences produced by NDAM children ($r = 0.568$, $p < 0.01$); however, this relation was negatively correlated in SLI children ($r = -0.353$, $p = 0.05$), implying that SLI children were relatively prone to make errors in complex sentences. To evaluate the group differences in simple and complex sentences, the Mann--Whitney nonparametric test was conducted. Error scores in repeating simple sentences were not significantly different between NDAM and SLI children ($U = 302.00$, $p = 0.022$), whereas there was a significant difference between the two groups in the repetition of complex sentences ($U = 288.00$, $p = 0.013$).

Next, the complex sentences were analyzed in relation to their structure (adverbial clause, relative clause, noun clause and coordinate clause). The number of sentences with relative clauses, noun clauses and coordinate clauses was lower than that of the sentences with adverbial clauses as targets. Thus, it was not possible to carry out a statistical comparison. Nevertheless, a qualitative analysis was undertaken to provide insights into difficulties experienced by the children in their InCR.

The analysis of complex sentences yields differences between NDAM and SLI children with the SLI group producing an appreciably higher percentage of errors in complex sentences, primarily by omitting important elements of the sentence. This was particularly notable in adverbial clauses where the NDAM group's errors totaled 14% and the SLI group's errors totaled 30%. Both groups committed errors in relative clause sentences by omitting the subordinate clause. The NDAM group did not make any errors in the production of noun clauses, but the SLI group did (7%). Bound morphological errors were evident in both simple and complex SRs of SLI children, while NDAM children had errors in only 3% of their complex sentences.

Since syntactic relations are marked by noun and verb inflections in Turkish, major difficulties arose in attempts to repeat sentences of increasing complexity and length in which morphosyntactic errors were more common. Consider the following examples[1]:

(1) Task:	*Pijama-lar-ın-ı*	*kendi-si*	*katla-dı.*
	Pyjamas-P-POSS-ACC	him+GEN	fold-PAST-3S
	IP[NP[Pro] I′ [VP]V[V′[NP[himself] V [fold] I [PAST]		
CHI-SLI (F, 5;1):	*Pijama*-(0)-(0)-(0)	*kendi*-(0)	*katla-dı.*
	Pyjama	him(self)	fold-PAST-3S
	(He folded his pyjamas by himself.)		

(2) Task:	*Zeynep*	*arkadaş-lar-ın-a*	*hediye*	*ver-di.*
	Zeynep	friend-P-POSS-DAT	gift	give-PAST-3S
	IP[NP*Zeynep*][I′[VP[NP*to her friends*][V′ [N*gift*] [V*give*] [IPAST-3S]]]			
CHI-SLI (M, 4;4):	*Zeynep*	*a:kadaş*-(0)-(0)-*a*	*hediye*	*ve:-di.*
	Zeynep	friend-DAT-3S	gift	give- PAST-3S
	(Zeynep gave a gift to her friends.)			

(3) Task: *Barış tek başına çalışma-y-ı sev-me-z.*
Barış alone study-BL-ACC like-NEG-3S
CHI-SLI (M, 4;4): *Barış kendi çalış-ma-z iste-me-z*
Barış himself study-NEG-3S want- NEG-3S
CHI-SLI (M, 4;6): *Barış tek başına* (0) *sev-me-z*
Barış alone like-NEG-3S
(Barış doesn't like studying by himself.)

(4) Task: *Çocuk-lar [cam-ı kır-ıp] kaç-tı-lar.*
Child-P [window-ACC break-GER(V+*Ip*)] run away-PAST-3P
IP[NP*children*][I'[VP[V'[NP*window*][V*break*]]CP[IP[NP*Pro*][I'[VP*escape*][IPAST-3P]]]
CHI-SLI (M, 4;4): *Çocuk-lar cam-ı kıy-ınca kaç-tı*-(0)
Child-P window-ACC break-GER(V+*Inca*) run away- PAST-3S
(Having broken the window, the children run away.)

(5) Task: *[Yeni giysi-m-i kirlet-ir-se-m] çok üzül-ür-üm.*
new cloth-1POSS-ACC dirty-AOR-CON-1S very get sad- AOR-1S
IP[NP[N'[AP*new*][N*cloth*]]I'[VP*dirty*][IAO-CON-1S]]CP[IP[NP[N-PRO][Deg*very*][I' [VP*get sad*] [I AOR 1S]]]
CHI-SLI (M, 4;4): *[Yeni giysi-m-i kirlet-ince]* (0) *üzül-ür-üm.*
[new cloth-1POSS-ACC dirty-GER(V+*Inca*)] get sad-AOR-1S
(If I get my new clothes dirty, I get very upset)

In Examples (1) and (2) the case markings are all absent whereas in (3) the case markings, as well as the tense inflections are observable but a different inflectional morpheme have been used instead of the original one which changed the semantic meaning of the sentence. In Examples (4) and (5), the substitution of the earliest acquired *V+Ince* (*when/cause*) for *V+Ip* (having V+ed) and *V+sA* (conditional) has been observed.

(6) Task: *[Ağac-a tırman-an kedi] köpek-ten kaç- ı -yor- du.*
[Tree-DAT climb-GER cat] dog-ABL escape-ACC-PAST-CONT
IP[NP[AP*climbing to tree*][N*cat*]][I'[VP[V'[NP*from dog*][V*escape*][IPAST-CONT]]]
CHI-SLI (M, 4;4): *Kedi köpek-ten kaç-ı-yor-du,* (0) *ağac-a çık-tı.*
cat dog- ABL escape-ACC-PASTCONT tree-DAT climb-PAST-3S
(The cat that climbed the tree was running away from the dog.)

(7) Task: *Anahtar-ı anne-m-e ver-diğ-i-mi unut-muş-um.*
Key-ACC mother-GEN-POS-DAT give-GER-ACC-1S-POSS fotget-PERF-ASP-1S
CHI-SLI (M, 6;8): *Anahtar*-(0) (0) *ver- diğ-i* (*0) *unut-tu-m*
Key give-GER-ACC forget-PAST-1S
CHI-SLI (M, 4;10): *Anahtar-ı ver-miş anne-m-e unut-tu*-(*0)
Key-ACC give-PERF-ASP mother-POS-DAT forget-PAST-3S
(I forgot that I gave the key to my mother.)

(8) Task: *Ece anne-si-nin al-dığ-ı oyuncağ-ı kaybet-ti.*
Ece mother-3S-GEN buy-GER-ACC toy-ACC loose-PAST-3S
CHI-SLI (M, 5;8): *Ece anne-si* (*0) (0) *oyuncağ-ı kaybet-ti.*
Ece mother-3S toy-ACC loose-PAST-3S
CHI-SLI (M, 7;11): *Ece anne-si-nin oyuncak al-dığ-ı-nı kaybet-ti.*
Ece mother-3S-GEN toy buy-GER-3S loose-PAST-3S
(Ece lost the toy her mother bought.)

In Example (6) the passive construction of the sentence is changed by the child preserving the meaning.

(9) Task:	*Anne-m*	*film-i*	*sev-di*	*çünkü*	*komik-ti.*
	Mother-1POSS	film-ACC	like-PAST-3S	because	funny-PAST
IP[NP*mother*][I′[VP[V″[NP*film*][V′[V*like*][IPAST]]CP[C*because*][IP[NP[N[Ø]]I′[VP[V′*funny*][IPAST]]					
CHI-SLI (F, 5;0):	*Anne-m*	*film-i*	*sev-di.*	(0)	*Çok komik-*(0).
	Mother-1S-POSS	film-ACC	like-PAST-3S		Very funny.
CHI-SLI (M, 4;0):	*Film-i*	*komik-ti* (*0)			
	Film-ACC	comic-PAST.			
	(My mother liked the film because it was very funny.)				

(10) Task:	*Ayşe-nin*	*arkadaş-ı-nın*	*bebeğ-i-nin*	*elbise-si*	*mavi-y-di*
	Ayşe-GEN	friend-ACC-GEN	baby-ACC-GEN	cloth-3S	blue-BL-PAST
CHI-SLI (M, 5;8):	*Ayşe-nin*	(0)	*bebeğ-i-nin*	(0)	*mavi-y-di*
	Ayşe-GEN		baby-ACC-GEN		blue-BL-PAST
CHI-SLI (M, 6;0):	*Arkadaş-ı-nın*	*anne-si-nin*	(0)	*elbise-si*	*mavi-y-di*
	Friend-ACC-GEN	mother-3S-GEN		cloth-3S	blue-BL-PAST
	(Ayşe's friend's doll's dress was blue.)				

An inspection of the 8, 9 and 10 examples showed that NDAM and SLI children although were able to repeat many of the case markings, they made many errors. However, when the sentences required more processing, either omission or substitutions occurred (i.e. Examples (7) and (8)). In general, children preferred to change the structure of the complex sentence to a simpler construction (NDAM 19, SLI group 49) (see Examples (6), (7), (8) and (10)), either by omitting the whole subordinate clause (NDAM 7, SLI group 27) or by deleting the non-obligatory constituents such as adverbial phrases, whereas some children's repetitions were ungrammatical (NDAM 2, SLI group 26).

General Conclusions

In summary, Study 2 revealed that derivational morphology, which is necessary for verb argument structures, poses problems for SLI children in SR tasks. This may be due to the requirement of knowledge about the semantics of the suffixes. Furthermore, sentences with a subordinate clause undergo a number of syntactic operations and therefore are not as transparent as simple structures. Thus, with increasing sentence length, the morphological structure becomes more complex in Turkish. As an evaluation of potential clinical markers for SLI, we tried to highlight some key aspects of grammatical limitations that may be central to identifying children with language impairments. However, many aspects of typical and atypical language development have yet to be investigated in depth in Turkish children before conclusions can be drawn.

The information presented in Study 1 indicates that the TELD-3:T is a valid measure of language achievement and that examiners will be able to use this test with confidence once the actual standardization and research are completed. Plante and Vance (1994) pointed out that sensitivity is more important for screening measures than specificity because the under-referrals associated with poorer sensitivity may have greater negative effects on children than over-referrals associated with poorer specificity. With this in mind, necessary revisions were made pertaining to the test's usefulness by the data gathered from Study 1 and Study 2 so that the TELD-3:T will be available with relevant information for SLI clients after the actual standardization has been completed.

Acknowledgment

I am grateful to Selçuk O. Güven, who is a research assistant at the Center for Speech and Language Pathology (DILKOM) at Anadolu University. He is the co-author of TELD-3:T and contributed a great deal during the standardization process of TELD-3. I would also like to express my gratitudes to Prof Dr St. Louis for his proofreading.

Note

1. Abbreviations: ABL: ablative, AOR: aorist, ACC: accusative, AOR: aorist, CAUS: causative, COM: comitative, CONV: converb, DAT: dative, DIM: diminutive, EVID: evidential, FUT: future, FUT.PART: future participle, GEN: genitive, IMP: imperative, INS: instrumental, INDEF: indefinite, LOC: locative, NEG: negation, NOM: nominalization marker, NSREL: nonsubject relative, OPT: optative, PAST: past tense, PAST:PART: past participle, GER: gerund, PASS: passive, PRES.PART: present participle, PROG: progressive, POSS: possessive, POSS.PRO: possessive pronoun, POT: potential, P: plural, 1/2/3P: 1/2/3 person plural, 1/2/3S: 1/2/3 person singular, QUE: question particle, SREL: subject relative, V: verb, N: noun, PRO: pronoun, (&) morphological fusion, (+) compound marker, (–) morpheme boundary, (0): omission of the following morpheme, (*0): ungrammatical omission, IP: inflectional phrase, NP: noun phrase, VP: verb phrase, CP: complementary phrase, BL: blending letter, CHI-SLI: child with SLI, M: Male, F: Female.

Chapter 8

Speech Characteristics of Hearing Impaired Turkish Children

UMRAN TÜFEKÇİOĞLU

Introduction

The acquisition of speech and language is a unique human capability that brings about the ability to communicate with oneself, beyond oneself and beyond the boundaries of time and place. However, because the human linguistic system is such that early input develops speech and language skills, hearing impairment with early onset will most probably be responsible for difficulties in speech perception, and delays and disorders in speech production and language acquisition. The more severe losses will be responsible for more severe problems (Ross & Giolas, 1978). 'The phonological system, which includes all the functional intonation and rhythmic patterns as well as the inventory of phonemes, is established in the first place through the reception and recognition of speech' (Fry, 1978: 29). Many researchers point out that hearing impaired children must learn a communication system before they start formal schooling or else they risk struggling with communication proficiency (Easterbrooks & Baker, 2002; Tüfekçioğlu, 2000, 1992) and literacy well into their education (Girgin, 1997; Girgin & Karasu, 2007). In fact, the learning gap found between these hearing impaired children and their hearing peers often increases with the years as a consequence of their limited speech and linguistic skills. Furthermore, unidentified or unmanaged deafness may also have adverse effects on several developmental areas, such as academic achievement and social–emotional development (Joint Committee on Infant Hearing, 2007).

Terms for deafness

Individuals who suffer from hearing loss are most often referred to with the terms deaf, hard-of-hearing, partially hearing or hearing impaired. As a basic classification system, hearing impairment can be defined in terms of degree of loss, time of onset and type of loss. Those with milder forms of hearing loss are called hard-of-hearing (in the USA) and partially hearing (in the United Kingdom). Those with extensive hearing loss who cannot use hearing alone, even with amplification, for speech understanding and language acquisition are called deaf. With regard to speech development, some authors distinguish between hard-of-hearing (mild through severe) and profound as two significant hearing loss categories (Yoshinaga-Itano, 2001). Blamey (2003) reports that Davis and Silverman (1978) placed the boundary between deaf and hard-of-hearing adults at 92 dB HL (this is based on aided speech perception results). For the purpose of spoken language development, Blamey *et al.* (2006) define *hard-of-hearing* as having a pure-tone threshold between 25 and 90 dB HL, and *deaf* as having a pure-tone threshold higher than 90 dB HL. However, as Blamey (2003: 235) reports, 'the situation is more complex, with many congenitally hard-of-hearing children scoring low on speech perception tests even though their unaided hearing thresholds may be much lower than 90 dB HL. Many of these low scores are the result of language abilities that are insufficient to perform the test rather than (or as well as) insufficient hearing levels'. Blamey also reports that the multichannel cochlear implant (CI) has the potential to move a child from the 'deaf' side of this critical level of hearing to the 'hard-of-hearing' side. Nevertheless, this distinction is based on auditory speech perception performance and, as Blamey has also expressed, is not a clear guide for spoken language performance. And besides, additional and confounding variables come into play, resulting at times in low correlations between the level of hearing and spoken language performance or academic achievement. This lack of a direct relationship has led to the wide use of the term *hearing impairment*, which refers to the quantifiable aspect of deafness (Davies, 1993), signifying the presence of a hearing loss, but not necessarily its severity. The severity of the hearing loss is labeled with the terms mild, moderate, severe or profound loss, a classification based on the average pure-tone threshold of the better ear as expressed in dB HL. So for the practical purposes of this chapter, the terms *hearing impairment* or *hearing loss* will be used interchangeably, with the exception of those terms in direct or indirect quotations taken from an outside source. Also, hereafter, all terms relating to deafness, hearing loss and hearing impairment will only refer to the sensorineural type.

The Role of Audition in Speech and Language Acquisition

Audibility of acoustic cues for speech perception

The reception and production of speech require as a prerequisite an intact auditory system that is sensitive to the frequency range where most speech sounds occur (500–4000 Hz). The most obvious effect of sensorineural deafness is a loss in the audibility and analysis of the acoustic cues which are time, frequency and intensity cues (Fry, 1978). Boothroyd *et al.* (1991) have shown that the ability to perceive significant contrasts among acoustic speech patterns decreases with increasing hearing loss. This leads to the loss of the ability to perceive significant contrasts among acoustic speech patterns, which is essential for the identification of the acoustic speech stimuli. 'Examples of significant contrasts are those between front and back vowels, between voiced and voiceless consonants, between stops and continuants, and between rising and falling intonation contours' (Boothroyd *et al.*, 1991: 81).

The majority of children with severe and profound sensorineural hearing loss show audiogram configurations with downward slopes in higher frequencies. Several researchers have established the critical contribution of these higher frequencies to speech understanding. It has been shown that sensorineural hearing losses are likely to be worse in the higher frequencies; moreover, it is consonants that are the major source of intelligibility in the English language (and the Turkish language), having most of their acoustic energy in the higher frequencies. In addition, the acoustic properties of consonants depend on the vowels with which they co-occur, and the vowels with relatively high-frequency second formants are also sensitive to elevated high-frequency thresholds (Bamford & Saunders, 1991). To add to the difficulty of discrimination, consonants with high-frequency formants tend to be spoken at lower intensities than vowels, and the frequency spectrum of speech shows a decrease of intensity in the higher-frequency consonants. Bamford and Saunders (1991: 50–51) explain the crucial importance of high-frequency information for the perception of speech signals: 'The second formant transitions are important cues to the perception of place of articulation of stops, fricatives and affricates; and, particularly for the brief articulations, the frequency of the noise conveys information on place'. Also, the presence of background noise increases difficulties much more for hearing impaired than for normally hearing listeners.

Audition, sensory deprivation and plasticity

Another long-term effect of sensorineural deafness is sensory deprivation. Researchers such as Grimault *et al.* (2000: 191) claim that 'any significant reduction of sensory input to the developing auditory system, such as a hearing loss, will induce both an anatomic and a physiologic alteration of the auditory pathways', which manifests in the slower-than-normal rate of speech and language acquisition in late-identified hearing impaired children. Here the alteration occurs as a result of deprivation; but as a result of later sensory input, reorganization can also take place, referred to as 'acclimatization'. As an example of this type of alteration, Grimault *et al.*

discuss an experiment by Poon and Chen (1992), in which a constant frequency tone was presented to a group of young rats within the first three weeks of their lives. As a result of this, the rats developed a higher number of neurons in response to this particular frequency. This example illustrates an alteration in the physiological properties of neurons in the peripheral and central auditory systems, as described by the term *plasticity* (Grimault *et al.*, 2000). Researchers of brain development claim that during infancy and childhood, neural pathways grow at an explosive rate in children who are able to receive sensory information and that the 'auditory cortex explodes with new connections after birth and maintains this activity until age twelve' (Easterbrooks, 2002: 41).

Fortunately, with today's amplification technology or electrical stimulation technology, together with early and effective intervention, auditory access and development of the brain can as closely as possible resemble the normal developmental stages. However, to enable this development, an aggressive audiological management for maximizing audibility of acoustic cues and linguistic management for maximizing uptake of information should be the core of early intervention. Easterbrooks (2002) draws our attention to *input* versus *uptake*, where uptake signifies what, among all the input in his or her environment, a child takes up as comprehensible units. Early interventionists need to take this into consideration when planning and working with the child in order to maximize the child's learning through interaction with the therapist and parents as part of their implementation of the Auditory–Oral or Auditory–Verbal Approach they practice. Proper audiological management following the principles of the chosen auditory approach to communication is a prerequisite to auditory-based learning. Only then, speech and spoken language acquisition by hearing impaired children can be a realistic expectation.

Auditory Approaches Facilitating Speech and Language Acquisition

'Early intervention' is a broadly used term for a set of early educational management processes that combine to produce the most favorable conditions for the development of hearing impaired children. Since the emphasis of this chapter is on speech and spoken language acquisition, only Auditory–Oral or Auditory–Verbal approaches will be mentioned here. In the implementation of these approaches, the activation of the auditory pathways is what is most important. The guiding principles of both approaches include the early diagnosis of hearing loss, the immediate provision, the proper maintenance and management of amplifying equipment or CIs, and guidance services for the families of these children. 'The whole is an integrated system of early management and each part makes an essential contribution to the prognosis for linguistic development for each child' (Harrison, 1981). However, speech and language acquisition is a continuous process, even more so for hearing impaired children, extending into and beyond the school years. Therefore quality education and the provision of support services during the school years need to follow early intervention services to enable continuous development of the child.

The Auditory–Oral Approach was introduced to Turkey as Anadolu University set out to establish İÇEM, the Education and Research Center for Hearing Impaired Children, and through the pioneering and sustained efforts of overseas advisors, but most specifically of Morag Clark, who is a worldwide recognized proponent of the approach. The results of the interactionist 'Natural Auditory–Oral Approach' is widely known as of today in Turkey, through the pioneering efforts of Clark (1989) and through its implementation at İÇEM. 'The author's (Clark's) recent experience in Turkey substantiates the claim that it is possible to implement this interactionist auditory oral approach in a completely different culture. The program at Anadolu University, Eskişehir, is a completely new one and its growth has been very rapid because it has not been hampered in any way by traditional thinking in relation to hearing-impaired children' (Clark, 1989: 86).

For those who feel that it is more beneficial to use a rather more structured, diagnostic-oriented and completely unisensory auditory approach, which places the responsibility of training the child on the parents, there is the Auditory–Verbal Therapy option. Currently, this approach is being pioneered by Estabrooks (2006a), who has consistently emphasized the exclusive focus on listening and restricting a child's access to lip-reading during therapy sessions. Estabrooks has also emphasized coaching the parents in order for them to develop a similar technique to use in home training.

Both approaches are guided by the principles of early identification of the hearing loss (during the first year of life), followed by the best possible binaural amplification (or when indicated, cochlear implantation), the best use of assistive technology (such as frequency modulated (FM) aids), an effective and 'aggressive' audiological and device management, an active parent/family involvement, a normal natural communicative input of meaningful speech and the development of speech, language and communication skills based on interactive teaching as well as incidental learning at all times through the activation of parents and other family members.

Services available for hearing impaired children in Turkey

The Turkish Ministry of Education is responsible for providing children in Turkey with a free education through the Turkish National Educational System. According to the most recent census figures, Turkey has a population of about 71 million people. According to data from the 2002 Disability

Survey released by the Turkish Statistical Institute and Administration for Disabled People, a projection study of people who are between the ages of 0 and 19 shows that the number of people in the hearing disabled population can be expected to be around 60,910.[1] The number of hearing impaired children who are registered and are receiving an education in schools for the deaf (for the year 2007–2008) is reported by the Turkish Ministry of Education to be around 6270. As roughly estimated by this author, the number of hearing impaired children who are in the mainstream may be around 9000. Alternative forms of educational placement for hearing impaired children who are in formal schooling include: placements in a traditional residential school for the deaf starting at age 6; self-contained class in the mainstream starting at age 6; mainstream starting at age 6; a special school (İÇEM) on the Anadolu University Campus starting at the age of diagnosis and providing education up to university entrance. Only very few enjoy the provision of intervention at an early age; most hearing impaired children start their education at age 6, and in most cases parent guidance is not offered. Such conditions are not conducive to the acquisition of spoken language or for the implementation of a Natural Auditory–Oral or an Auditory–Verbal Approach. This was noticed by interested professionals and the dissatisfaction expressed with the following comment: 'Conditions in these schools make it difficult for new teachers (those specifically trained to teach hearing impaired children) to implement an auditory-oral approach, but it is heartening to meet graduates from time to time who remain dissatisfied with the "status quo" in those schools. Only from such dissatisfaction will progress come out' (Clark & Tüfekçioğlu, 1994).

The development of an auditory–oral program in Turkey

It was due to this dissatisfaction that a truly auditory–oral program was established by Anadolu University in 1979 (Tüfekçioğlu, 1988). Known as İÇEM, the Education and Research Center for Hearing Impaired Children started as a small nursery school program and developed into a fully comprehensive service encompassing early diagnosis, hearing aid (HA) fitting and maintenance, parent guidance (including integration at preschool and a special school for ages 3–18) and a CI program. In addition, there is also now a well-established four-year teacher training program for teachers of hearing impaired children (Clark & Tüfekçioğlu, 1994).

İÇEM is a non-profit university institution, recognized in the country for its exemplary practice in services provided. In addition to providing education to 139 hearing impaired and 41 normally hearing, regularly attending day students,[2] the services provided by the center include a parent guidance program for regular students as well as for families coming from various parts of the country. The philosophy at İÇEM has been to adopt the Natural Auditory–Oral Approach from the very beginning. With CI users or those with good speech reception through modern amplification, an Auditory–Verbal Approach has also been adopted in one-to-one conversation sessions and listening training. A unique feature of the educational program is the implementation of progressive educational practices in teaching children, as opposed to the traditional practices observed in the public system. An HA-maintenance and ear-mold-making laboratory, a graphics studio in which teaching materials are produced and a psychological guidance and counseling unit, all add to raising the quality of education and services provided.

Speech Characteristics of Hearing Impaired Children

One of the major considerations in the habilitation of hearing impaired children has been to improve speech skills and enhance their intelligibility. Documented research provides descriptions of the major problems present in the speech of children with hearing impairments. Detailed studies of speech production characteristics of children using HAs are mostly found in early studies (Abraham, 1989; Gold, 1980; Hudgins & Numbers, 1942; John & Howarth, 1965; Markides, 1970, 1983; Smith, 1975). However, studies of children using CIs are relatively recent (Blamey *et al.*, 2001, 2006; Chin, 2002, 2003; Chin *et al.*, 2001; Chin & Pisoni, 2000; Peng *et al.*, 2004).

The majority of early articles written on the speech production of hearing impaired children focused their attention on prosodic aspects (the first objective studies appearing in the mid-1930s). In later years, research has also focused on segmental aspects (Ling, 1976). The typical speech errors of this group will be very briefly reviewed below. The interested reader may refer to the cited references and other publications in this field for further information.

Detailed characteristics

Suprasegmental characteristics

In relation to respiration, phonation and rate, a general lack of coordination between the articulators (tongue, lips and jaw) and the breath–voice system has been indicated (Ling, 1976). Rhythm (rate, stress, juncture, breath-grouping, pauses) and intonation contribute to intelligibility (Ling, 1976), as shown by several researchers (John & Howarth, 1965).

Vowel production

Defects in vowel production among hearing impaired children have been shown to follow certain patterns (Ling, 1976). The most frequent errors in vowel production are found to be vowel substitution, vowel neutralization, vowel prolongation, vowel diphthongization, diphthong errors (Markides, 1970) and vowel nasalization (Hudgins & Numbers, 1942), 'one vowel tending to sound very much like any other, a finding that indicated very restricted and stereotyped tongue movement' (Ling, 1976: 15). Other vowel errors include tense for lax (and lax for tense) substitutions, especially the front vowels [i] and [ɪ] (Bauman-Waengler, 2004).

Consonant production

Markides (1983, 1970), among others, reported consonant production in hearing impaired children to be generally characterized by omissions, substitutions and distortions. Frequently occurring substitutions included the confusion of voiced and voiceless cognates, the substitution of stops for fricatives and liquids and the confusion between oral and nasal consonants (Ling, 1976). Among deaf students, omission errors were more numerous, followed first by substitutions and finally by distortions. Among the partially hearing, substitution errors were more numerous, followed first by omissions and finally by distortions (Markides, 1983, 1970). Abraham (1989) has also reported omissions to be greater for deaf subjects.

The most frequently misarticulated consonants reported by Markides (1970) were the fricatives /s, ʃ, z/ and the nasal /ŋ/. Bauman-Waengler, reviewing studies of hard-of-hearing children, reported that the consonants produced with the blade of the tongue ([t, d, s, z, ʃ, ʒ, t͡ʃ, d͡ʒ]) are the most likely to be involved in the production of errors. 'The affricates are ranked as most difficult for both profoundly hearing impaired children and the hard of hearing' (Bauman-Waengler, 2004: 325–326). As the place of consonant articulation moves further back in the mouth, correct production decreases. Abraham (1989) reported that the consonants with the lowest percentages of accuracy included [z] and [ð] in word-initial and word-final positions. As a result of all of these processes, overall intelligibility of speech is reduced, even though Law and So (2006) reported that CI users have a significantly higher percentage of correct scores for consonant production than HA users. Other studies have reported intelligibility of speech output to be low, approximately 20% (Brannon, 1964; Dowson *et al.*, 1995; Geers & Tobey, 1992: pre-implant; John & Howarth, 1965; Markides, 1983, 1970; Smith, 1975).

Markides (1983) has observed an order of difficulty in the production of consonants by manner of articulation: the most difficulty was observed in affricates, followed first by the fricatives, then by the nasals and finally by the plosives. Abraham (1989) also reported correct production of sound classes to be in the order of nasals, stops, liquids, fricatives and affricates. The visibility of phonemes proved to be an important factor affecting the articulatory skills of both deaf and partially hearing children. Markides (1983) listed the order of difficulty for place of articulation: Bilabials and labiodentals were produced more correctly than palatals and palato-alveolars, and glottals.

Research has demonstrated that speech perception and/or production of children with profound deafness improves after cochlear implantation (Blamey *et al.*, 2001; Chin & Kaiser, 2000; Dowson *et al.*, 1995; Grogan *et al.*, 1995; Miyamoto *et al.*, 1995; Osberger *et al.*, 1991; Peng *et al.*, 2004; Tobey *et al.*, 1991, 1994; Tobey & Hasenstab, 1991). Acoustic studies contrasting formant frequencies in words when an implant is turned either off or on provide further support for better segmental production with the auditory feedback from a multichannel CI (Tobey & Hasenstab, 1991). Better segmental production was associated with better intelligibility. Tobey and Hasenstab (1991: 54) report observing an improvement in the abilities to imitate segmental aspects associated with consonant and vowel production during the first two years of implant use. However, 'only minimal changes in speech intelligibility or mean length of utterance are evident' within that period. In general, speech perception scores improve more readily, speech production skills improve in time and progress in spoken language is seen much later (Boothroyd *et al.*, 1991).

Several researchers have investigated the relative effects of child and intervention variables on speech and spoken language outcomes. The effects of age of implantation and the duration of implant use are reported to be the most significant factors (Nicholas & Geers, 2007). Several researchers have recently come to identify age of implantation as the most significant predictive factor for successful outcomes. For example, Connor *et al.* (2006) concluded that substantial benefits for both speech and vocabulary outcomes are seen in children who receive their implant before the age of 2.5 years. Nicholas and Geers (2007: 1048), too, concluded that children who received a CI before a substantial delay in spoken language development (between 12 and 16 months of age) were more likely to achieve age-appropriate spoken language skills. Thus, they announced, 'these results favor cochlear implantation before 24 months of age, especially for children with aided pure-tone average thresholds greater than 65 dB prior to surgery'. With age-appropriate language skills now becoming an expectation, the question arises whether these children will be able to catch up with their normally hearing peers. In answer to this question, Nicholas and Geers (2007: 1048) report that 'implantation younger than 16 months of age and enrollment in a good auditory-oral or auditory-verbal program' is promising; however, considerable variability among subjects is consistently reported.

Speech characteristics of hearing impaired Turkish children

The development of speech and language in hearing impaired Turkish children, and their education through the spoken medium, has been a primary concern of educators working in Turkey (specifically at Anadolu University) for the last three decades. The establishment and development of the Center for Hearing Impaired Children (İÇEM) at Anadolu University have been the driving force behind this interest. However, this comprehensive educational program utilizing an Auditory–Oral Approach was the first of its kind in Turkey and started initially with no trained staff and without an existing teacher training program for the hearing impaired (Clark & Tüfekçioğlu, 1994). Therefore, all the efforts of the limited number of staff members and overseas advisors were focused on staff training and on developing educational programs, resulting in a relatively small number of research projects. The review of research, presented in this section, on the speech characteristics of hearing impaired Turkish children will be therefore covering only a limited amount of research work.

In a comparative study, Tüfekçioğlu (1989) examined speech intelligibility (among other language variables) in the spoken language samples of 80 hearing impaired Turkish children enrolled in two different educational programs in Eskişehir. Intelligible and unintelligible utterances were videotaped, transcribed and counted. The number of intelligible utterances of the students attending an auditory–oral educational program was found to be significantly higher than the intelligible utterances of students from a school for the deaf. The subjects were matched in age and hearing loss. In fact, only hearing losses of 90 dB HL or greater were included in the study to control as much as possible for factors causing variability. To check whether there were any differences between the matched groups on hearing levels, *t*-tests were performed, resulting in no difference. Therefore, no significant relationships were found between hearing loss and intelligibility, as expected, proving that this was not to be considered as a factor in this comparison study. The speech intelligibility of children who were fitted with HAs in the third year of life and who had attended an auditory–oral program was significantly superior to the speech intelligibility of children who attended a residential school for the deaf where a different communication methodology was used and where amplification and intervention were provided only after the children had started school.

A very limited number of studies have examined prosodic characteristics in the speech of hearing impaired Turkish children. Girgin (1999, 2000) analyzed the speech samples of 35 secondary school and high school Turkish students with severe to profound hearing losses for prosodic characteristics and intelligibility. The students were enrolled in an auditory–oral program, and all used HAs. Significant differences were found between the hearing impaired group and the similar aged control group in terms of prosodic characteristics and intelligibility. The hearing impaired subjects demonstrated longer sentence and pause duration, more junctures, narrower pitch width and higher pitch when compared with the normal hearing group. Another study (Çeliker & Ege, 2005) also investigated speech intelligibility of hearing impaired Turkish students with severe to profound hearing losses and its relationship to the degree of hearing loss, speech rate, stress and articulation skills. The study group consisted of 9–14-year-old students with losses between 75 and 118 dB who were HA users and attended a special school in Ankara. The students made omission errors, substitution errors and distortion errors; the distribution among the types of errors was not reported. Intelligibility was reported to be low and the strongest relationship was found between intelligibility and articulation skills. A relationship between hearing loss and intelligibility was also reported.

In another study, Girgin and Özsoy (2008) investigated the relationships among formant frequency, duration of vowels and speech intelligibility in 20 hearing impaired Turkish children, all of whom were enrolled in a special program in İstanbul, and all used HAs. The vowel duration of hearing impaired children was significantly longer than that of the control group, and a significant relationship was found between vowel duration and speech intelligibility. The level of hearing loss was also found to be a significant variable that affected speech intelligibility.

Speech Production of Hearing Impaired Turkish Children in an Auditory–Oral Program

Research on the speech production abilities of Turkish children with hearing loss that focuses on segmental analysis has not been a topic of interest until recently. For the purpose of analyzing the speech production skills of hearing impaired Turkish children, Tüfekçioğlu (2008a) examined the speech outputs of eight hearing impaired Turkish children from an auditory–oral program (İÇEM) located in Eskişehir. The study covers their consonant inventory and an analysis of their speech errors. The questions addressed in the study were as follows: (1) What is the size of the consonant repertoire of children using HAs and CIs? (2) What types of consonants are produced by children using HAs and CIs? (3) Is there a developmental trend in acquisition in relation to normal hearing Turkish children? (4) Are the consonant repertoires of children using CIs similar to the repertoires of hearing impaired children using HAs? and (5) What types of speech errors are observed in this group of children? The preliminary findings from data collection at baseline and at an interval of one year will be reported here.

Children in the study

The auditory–oral educational program (İÇEM) was described in the earlier section. The children who participated in the study were randomly selected from the students of İÇEM who had prelingual, profound hearing losses (pure-tone thresholds greater than 96 dB HL bilaterally, except Child C, 89 dB in the better ear). All had either congenital or prelingual deafness, as seen in Table 8.1, none had secondary handicaps, and all had normally hearing Turkish-speaking parents. Children were given the

Table 8.1 Background information for the children

Subject	*Age at data collection (years; months)*	*Age at data collection (in months)*	*Hearing loss[a] (L/R)*	*Age at diagnosis (years; months)*	*Age at ampl. (years; months)*	*Age at change to CI (years; months)*	*Age starting parent guidance (years; months)*	*Age starting school (years; months)*
Child A-CI	5;7/6;7	67/79	98/CI	2;0	2;0	4;9	4;3	4;10
Child B-CI	6;4/7;4	76/88	119/CI	0;8	2;6	4;1	–	4;1
Child C-HA	6;11/7;11	83/95	96/89	3;0	3;0	HA	2;0	6;2
Child D-HA	7;3/8;3	87/99	101/100	0;11	1;1	HA	1;1	3;6
Child E-CI	8;0/9;0	96/108	100/CI	0;3	0;9	2;9	2;0	3;3
Child F-CI	11;7/12;7	139/151	CI/127	1;10	1;11	3;10	1;11	3;10
Child G-CI	12;10/13;10	154/166	114/CI	1;2	1;2	4;8	1;2	3;1
Child H-CI	13;5/14;5	161/173	NR/CI	1;10	1;11	6;6	2;0	3;8

[a]Hearing loss expressed as an average of 5 test frequencies (250–4000 Hz) in dBHL.
NR: no response.

codes A–H, starting from the youngest to the oldest, Child A being the youngest. Hearing ages, with HAs and with CIs based on age at first date of data collection, are presented in Table 8.1. Audiological and educational details for individual subjects are presented in Table 8.1 and reproduced in Figures 8.1 and 8.2 for the convenience of the reader. All CI users were

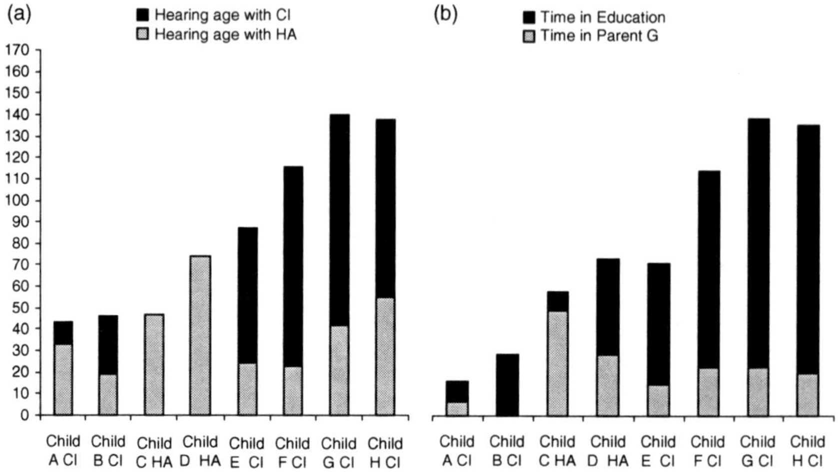

Figure 8.1 (a) Duration of HA and CI use (ages in months). (b) Duration of parent guidance and duration of education in the program (ages in months)

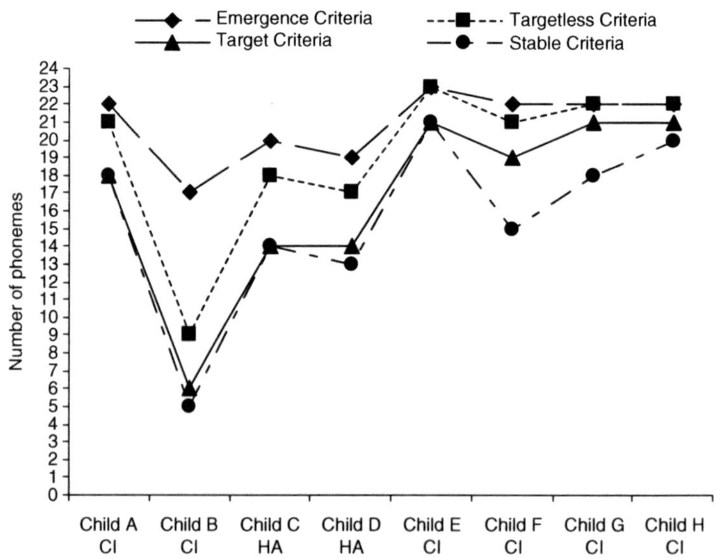

Figure 8.2 Numbers of Turkish consonants reaching the four types of criteria in spontaneous spoken language of eight hearing impaired Turkish children (Year 2007)

fitted with either the advanced combination encoder (ACE) or CIJ speech processing strategy.

The etiologies as recorded in the files are as follows: Child A-infection, Child B-unknown, Child C-hereditary, Child D-unknown, Child E-perinatal asphyxia, Child F-unknown, Child G-hereditary and Child H-unknown.

Speech sampling

Two types of speech sampling procedures were used: (1) *Spontaneous conversational speech samples* and (2) *The subtest of the Turkish Articulation and Phonology Test (SST)*. In (1), each child was videotaped during three sets of continuous spontaneous conversation sessions with his/her teacher. A total of 100 spontaneous utterances were transcribed. Imitations and repetitions were excluded from samples. The resulting samples were examined to determine which sounds a given child pronounced correctly and spontaneously. Correct production required that a target phoneme was the same as a result phoneme according to the broad phonemic transcript, after Blamey *et al.* (2001: 368). The number of correctly produced consonants within the spontaneous language productions was calculated for every sample on four different criteria.

(2) *The Articulation Test*: This subtest, developed for Turkish (Topbaş, 2004/5), contains 93 pictures based on a picture-naming task to examine the child's articulatory competence with speech sounds (Topbaş, 2006b). The production of each consonant, with the two palatal allophones of the velar plosives and the dark-l allophone of the lateral approximant added to the 21 orthographic consonants, totaling 24 consonants, is probed in four different syllable positions in four different target words. The children were expected to say the target word pictured. The test was administered by an MSc graduate trained in speech pathology who also completed narrow phonetic transcriptions, using international phonetic alphabet (IPA) and phonetic representation of disordered speech (PRDS) symbols. The transcriptions were reviewed by this author and a consensus was reached over the entire sample. Only the singleton consonants were used for analysis. All of the eight children were tested for Year 1; however, Child A and Child G were not available for testing in Year 2.

The description of each child's phonological system concentrates on three characteristics: (1) an inventory of correct consonants in conversational speech samples, (2) percentage of consonants correct (PCC) scores on the Articulation Test and (3) error analysis of consonant productions based on the Articulation Test.

Consonant inventories in conversational speech samples

The purpose of this section was to investigate the development of the consonant inventory of the children as 'an emergent system' (Vihman &

Ferguson, 1986). The children's phonemic inventory development was monitored using four different acquisition criteria. Because the aim here was to study the acquisition process itself, a criterion identifying only the endpoint of acquisition (such as the mastery of a particular consonant or a stable one) was not considered appropriate on its own. Of course, some of the hearing impaired children may never reach an acquisition endpoint because of their fundamental limitations in hearing (Serry & Blamey, 1999). Serry and Blamey used 'targetless' and 'target' criteria in their study with children using implants. In the present study, a similar approach was used; however, an 'emergence' criterion and a 'stable' criterion have been added. Each criterion here identifies a different point in the development of individual speech sounds. The study by Tüfekçioğlu (2008a) defined the four different acquisition criteria as follows: The 'emergence' acquisition criterion required at least one correct production of a consonant in a word in a spontaneous conversational speech sample (using a broad transcription). The 'targetless' acquisition criterion required at least two correct productions of a consonant in at least two different words within the same samples, and the 'target' acquisition criterion required at least three correct productions of a consonant in at least three different words within the same samples. The 'stable' acquisition criterion required at least three correct productions of the consonant in three different words in at least two different syllable positions (Topbaş, 2006b), within a spontaneous conversational speech sample. A segment was included in that particular inventory only if it was used according to that criterion.

There are 21 consonants in Turkish, and in the study, the palatal allophones [c, ɟ] and the dark-l allophone [ɫ] of /k, g, l/ were added, after Topbaş (2006b, 2004/5). Hence, there were a total of 24 Turkish consonants in all.

Figure 8.2 presents the number of consonants used in words by each of the children according to the four criteria described.

As seen in Figures 8.2 and 8.3, consonants were acquired steadily, although incompletely, over the one-year period of the study. Based on Serry and Blamey's (1999: 145) description of development, 'The time interval between first attaining the targetless and target criteria, [or between emergence-targetless-target-stable here], is a measure of the rate of development for each sound. The number of new phones attaining the targetless and target criteria in a fixed time interval can also be used as a measure of the overall rate of speech production development'. Year 2 (Figure 8.3), as compared to Year 1, shows steady progressions for all children in consonant acquisitions over the period of the study. It also shows that acquisition is indeed a process in which the children make attempts at using the sounds to form meaningful words. Note that their frequency of use increases as their 'command towards mastery' takes more control. 'Sound features are not just tagged onto knowledge

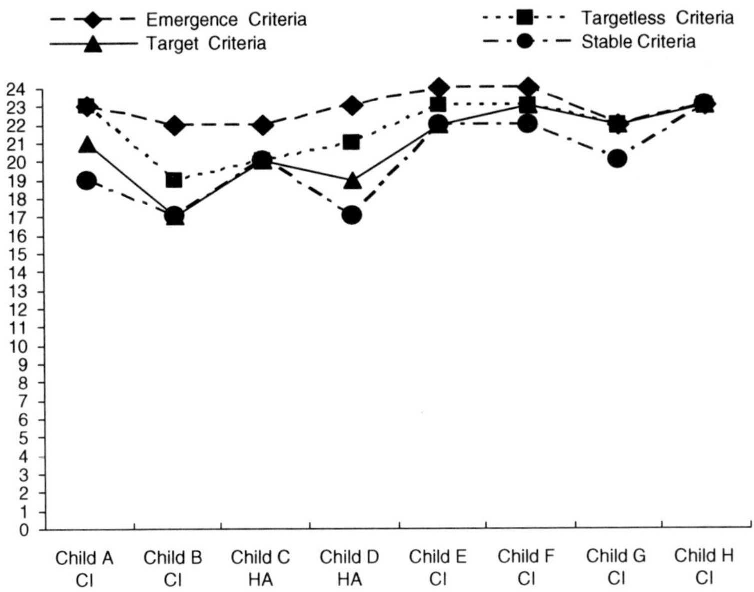

Figure 8.3 Numbers of Turkish consonants reaching the four types of criteria in spontaneous spoken language of eight hearing impaired Turkish children (Year 2008)

structures; they must be integrated into the child's concepts and schemata and become meaningful .... This will also be true for children who have worn hearing aids and subsequently receive cochlear implants' (Laughton & Hasenstab, 2000: 198).

For Year 1, the smallest inventory belongs to Child B, who was a late starter (4;1 years old when admitted to the auditory–oral educational program), followed by the two HA users. Consonants were acquired steadily, although incompletely, over the one-year period, with all children displaying progress without any signs of a plateau effect even though three of them had been using implants for a period of 7–8 years. Although progress is seen in all the children, the youngest ones with the relatively smaller inventories have made the most progress. Blamey *et al.* (2001) also did not see any evidence to suggest a possible plateau in performance for their subjects after six years of implant use. Their finding suggests that these children may in fact keep developing even further.

A discrepancy was evident between the hearing impaired subjects' consonant inventories and their ability to use the sounds from their inventories accurately and appropriately in continuous meaningful speech when listed according to different criteria. With each more stringent criterion, a relatively smaller inventory was profiled. It seemed that the children were producing words containing difficult-to-perceive or difficult-to-perform consonants in less abundance, indicating that their lexicon with these sounds might be more limited when compared to words with more well-established sounds. This may result because of an avoidance strategy known to be used by children who are possibly aware of their difficulties with certain sounds/words and are therefore consciously or unconsciously avoiding their use in spoken language readily. It may also be the result of the impaired auditory capacities limiting the perception of certain sounds so that children need more time to code those sounds with limited acoustic/electrical cues in constructing meaningful linguistic units.

Phoneme acquisition in hearing impaired Turkish children

In Tables 8.2 and 8.3, the Turkish consonants are listed in the upper horizontal column in the order of phoneme acquisition as described by Topbaş (1997) for normally hearing Turkish children ($N = 22$). The list is composed here of the standard 21 phonemes of Turkish plus the palatal allophones for /k, g/ and the velarized allophone of /l/, [c, ɟ, ɫ]. Table 8.2 displays which children in the study are reaching the *emergence* criterion for each consonant at data collection Year 1, and then for Year 2. Each letter corresponds to the phoneme not reaching the *emergence* criterion.

Table 8.2 Hearing impaired Turkish children reaching the emergence criterion for each consonant

		k	c	t	n	j	tʃ	p	ʃ	dʒ	g	ɟ	ɽ	l	s	ʒ	f	z	h	r	ɣ
Child A-CI	07										g					ʒ					
	08										g										
Child B-CI	07			t							g	ɟ				ʒ	f	z	h	r	
	08										g							z			
Child C-HA	07										g	ɟ			s	ʒ					
	08										g	ɟ				ʒ					
Child D-HA	07										g					ʒ		z	h		ɣ
	08										g					ʒ					
Child E-CI	07															ʒ					
	08																				
Child F-CI	07															ʒ				r	
	08																				
Child G-CI	07										g					ʒ					
	08										g					ʒ					
Child H-CI	07		c													ʒ					
	08															ʒ					

Note: Each shaded square corresponds to acquisition by this criterion.

The results indicated a rich inventory of consonants (i.e. the inventory of consonantal sounds that can be combined to form meaningful linguistic units) for all children with implants with the exception of Child B and the HA users. A comparative analysis of correspondences with the inventories of HA and CI users displayed some patterns that are also common in the speech of children with normal hearing. The consonants [b, d, m, n, j, tʃ] were acquired by all in the first two criteria by the second data collection and were among the earliest sounds in Turkish, [tʃ] being in the middle group for Turkish. The consonants [b, d, m, n, j] were also among the earliest, and [tʃ] was in the middle group of sounds in English, as described by Shriberg (1993). The sounds [ʒ, f, z, h, r, ɣ] that are missing from the two children's inventories are also the later acquired ones in Turkish, showing parallels with normal developmental data. However, these show a more widespread absence (Table 8.3), as the next criterion requires more

Table 8.3 Hearing impaired Turkish children reaching the targetless criterion for each consonant

		k	c	t	n	j	tʃ	p	ʃ	dʒ	g	ɟ	ɾ	l	s	ʒ	f	z	h	r	ɣ
Child A-CI	07										g					ʒ					
	08										g					ʒ					
Child B-CI	07	k	c	t				p	ʃ	dʒ	g	ɟ	ɾ	l	s	ʒ	f	z	h	r	
	08										g	ɟ					f	z	h		
Child C-HA	07										g	ɟ			s	ʒ		z	h	r	ɣ
	08										g	ɟ				ʒ		z			
Child D-HA	07										g				s	ʒ		z	h	r	ɣ
	08										g				s	ʒ					
Child E-CI	07															ʒ					
	08																				
Child F-CI	07										g					ʒ				r	
	08															ʒ					
Child G-CI	07										g					ʒ					
	08										g					ʒ					
Child H-CI	07		c													ʒ					
	08															ʒ					

Note: Each shaded square corresponds to acquisition by this criterion.

words to be used. When the consonant inventories at the emergence- and the targetless-criterion point are compared, a decrease is evident in the fricative sound class for HA users (Child C and Child D at first data collection, but also in Child B, an implant user) in addition to a decrease in stop-plosives, affricates and the lateral approximant in Child B's inventory when compared with the emergence criterion.

In the targetless criterion, the sound that is notably missing in the Year 1 inventories of six of the children is [g], and missing in the inventories of eight children is [ʒ], as seen in Table 8.3. In Year 2, only two of the eight children have reached this criterion for [ʒ], and three children have reached this criterion for [g].

Two explanations can be offered for this widespread absence of [g] and [ʒ] consonants from the children's inventories. The words containing the consonant [ʒ] in Standard Turkish have very low frequency of occurrence. Moreover, most of these words are not originally Turkish but have been borrowed from other languages. This consonant was also reported in the Serry and Blamey (1999) study as one of the two consonants missing in the inventories of the children they studied. Serry and Blamey (1999) also reported that this consonant had very low frequency of occurrence in their subjects' samples also and was among the last to be acquired by normally hearing English-speaking children. Those phonemes that have the least frequency of occurrence have less chances of attaining the target and targetless criteria. (Recall that this criterion requires at least two instances in a sample.) As Blamey *et al.* (2001) have pointed out, the low frequency of occurrence for the phonemes may contribute to the slowing down of phonetic inventory development. The consonant [g] also has a low occurrence in Turkish. It is also a back phoneme cited by several researchers as being one of the latest phonemes acquired by hearing impaired English-speaking children (this should also be the case for its allophone [ɟ]). As the place of consonant production moves further back in the mouth, the correct production by hearing impaired children decreases (Markides, 1983).

Abraham (1989) reported that the consonants with the lowest percentages of accuracy included [z] and [ð] in word-initial and word-final positions. The consonants [ʒ], [z], [s] and [h] are fricatives consistently reported by researchers as some of the later acquired phonemes (affricates being acquired the latest) by hearing impaired English-speaking children. The inventory map shows clearly that only the HA users follow this trend with respect to fricatives (with the exception of Child B), and this is expected with known amplification limitations in the higher frequencies and is consistent with previous research findings. Child B is a late starter, without prior attendance at the parent guidance program, who was admitted to the educational program at age 4;1 years (which partly explains her initial difficulties). Her preimplant pure-tone thresholds showed profound to total loss (see Table 8.1 for children's audiological information). Research has shown that the presence of better preimplant thresholds is among the predictive factors for better speech and language outcomes. Her preimplant pure-tone thresholds in combination with a late start to education explain her highly limited initial inventory.

Interestingly, although affricates are the sound class acquired latest by hearing impaired English-speaking children, none of the Turkish children in this study had any unusual difficulties with this sound class, which is consistent with (Topbaş, 1997; Topbaş & Yavaş, 2006) findings for normally hearing Turkish-speaking children. In contrast to normal-hearing English-speaking children, normally hearing Turkish-speaking children were reported to acquire affricates before fricatives.

Percentage of consonants correct

PCC was calculated as described by Shriberg and Kwiatkowski (1982) as a speech production measure. Based on the performance of the target sounds in key words (with four different positions for each sound) in the Articulation Test for Turkish, the PCC scores for Year 2 are as follows: Child A: 71% (Year 1); Child B: 65%; Child C: 69%; Child D: 51%; Child E: 95%; Child F: 68%; Child G: 61% (Year 1); and Child H: 80%. The test required distortions and unexpected allophones to be scored as incorrect and calculations were made following the test procedure. Child A and Child G were not available for Year 2; therefore their scores for Year 1 are given.

Child E has the highest PCC score among all children. Starting to use HAs within the first 6 months of life (Yoshinaga-Itano *et al.*, 1998) or a CI between 12 and 16 months of life (Nicholas & Geers, 2007) is shown to give significant advantages compared to later fittings and is more likely to enable children to achieve age-appropriate spoken language. Connor *et al.* (2006) also concluded that a substantial benefit for both speech and vocabulary outcomes is seen when children receive their implant before the age of 2.5 years. The outstanding PCC score (95%) of Child E, as an indicator of speech intelligibility, and the error type solely consisting of distortions, corroborates these reported findings. Child E had amplification at 9 months and intervention at 24 months (although not within the first 6 months of life). She is the youngest to receive an implant, at age 2;9, and exhibits the positive outcomes of having a relatively early implantation in an auditory–oral program.

Error analysis of consonant productions

Speech errors in consonants as a function of error type

When hearing impaired children's speech errors in consonants are analyzed as a function of error type, the analysis showed (Figures 8.4a and 8.4b) substitutions to be significantly more than omissions, except Child B in Year 1.

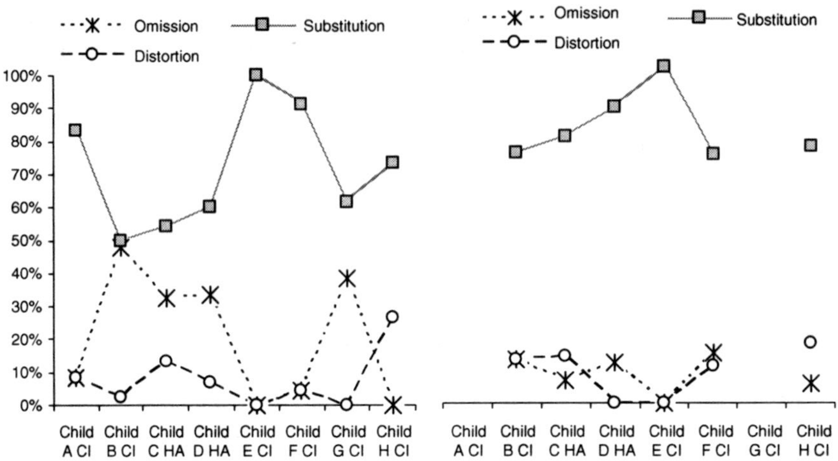

Figure 8.4 (a) Hearing impaired children's speech errors in consonants as a function of error type (Year 2007). (b) Hearing impaired children's speech errors in consonants as a function of error type (Year 2008)

This finding parallels the findings of Markides (1983, 1970), who reported this to be the case for partially hearing children. Omissions of the intended consonant were reported to be the most frequent error type (Markides, 1970; McGarr & Osberger, 1978) for deaf/profoundly impaired children. This is in absolute contrast with the current findings of this study. This changeover in children's error type is regarded by this author as significant improvements, which bring the profoundly impaired children almost to the partially hearing category, just as Blamey (2003) has explained in one of his publications. This finding coincides with what Blamey (2003) stated in relation to speech perception performance of implant users: the multichannel CI has the potential to move a child from the 'deaf' side of this critical level of hearing to the 'hard-of-hearing' side. These findings indicate that in speech production development too, the children exhibit the potential to move to the 'hard-of-hearing' category.

Child B has a similar percentage for omissions and substitutions, which is a reflection of her stage in development. She evidenced the smallest inventory the first year, but progressed significantly, hence the changeover to substitutions in the second year, corroborating the results of present and further analyses. She moved to the 'partially hearing' category by this definition only in the second year of this study, at the end of her third year of implant use. Her second year PCC was 65%, compared to 48% in Year 1, a significant improvement in her score, which confirms her changeover.

Speech errors in consonants as a function of manner of articulation

The analysis according to sound classes as a function of manner of articulation shows that the flap, followed by the lateral approximant,

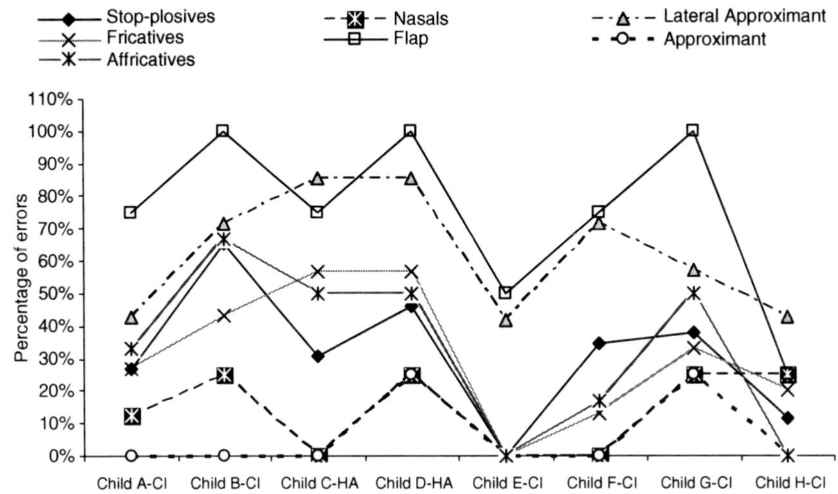

Figure 8.5 Hearing impaired Turkish children's speech errors in consonants as a function of manner of articulation (Year 1)

showed the highest percentage of error among sound classes, and across children. The result with the flap (and to some degree with the lateral approximant) would be expected developmentally. The approximant [ɫ] presented difficulty only for Child D, but inconsistently (Figure 8.5).

Figure 8.6 summarizes the results of the Articulation Test as a function of manner of articulation for the second year of data collection. Child A

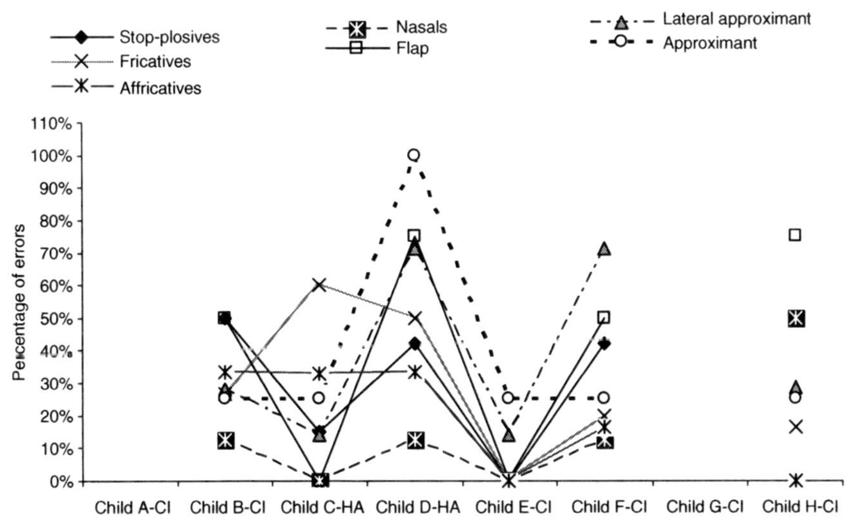

Figure 8.6 Hearing impaired Turkish children's speech errors in consonants as a function of manner of articulation (Year 2)

and Child G moved away and were not available for testing. In comparison to the previous year, a general improvement is evidenced across all the children, with the notable exception of the approximant for Child D. In general, steady increases in performance and decreases in errors over time were evident. The greatest percent change was observed for the lateral approximant and the flap, and for fricatives in implant users. Errors with fricatives seem to have resisted any change within the HA group, as earlier research consistently reports. But some improvement is shown by implant users.

Children's errors as a function of visibility

When analyzed by place of articulation, the data show that in the sound classes of stop-plosives and fricatives, the most visible of each set, that is, [p, b] and [f, v], respectively, were produced with very *minimal errors* for the stop-plosives, and with almost no error for the fricatives by all the children (except Child B) in Year 1 of data collection (see Figures 8.7a and 8.7b).

The *majority of errors* were found with the remaining sounds in each sound class. This finding is consistent with previous reports of better production of bilabial and visible sounds than of other consonants (Gold, 1980; Markides, 1983; Oller *et al.*, 1978). Previous studies regarding the place of articulation used by profoundly hearing impaired children report more accurate production for the visible consonants than for the consonants appearing in the mid or posterior regions of the oral cavity (Geers & Tobey, 1992).

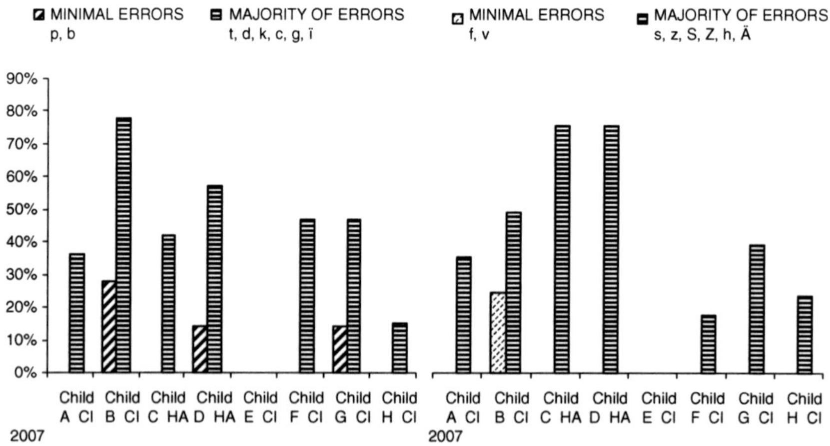

Figure 8.7 (a) Hearing impaired Turkish children's errors in stop-plosives as a function of visibility (Year 1). (b) Hearing impaired Turkish children's errors in fricatives as a function of visibility (Year 1)

Contrasting errors in stop-plosives versus errors in fricatives

When the percentage scores of errors for stop-plosives and those for the fricatives are compared, it is evident that CI users exhibit relatively more errors in the sound class of stop-plosives when compared to the sound class of fricatives, with the exception of Child A who had implant experience for only 10 months and Child H who had implantation at a relatively older age. Figures 8.8a and 8.8b display this finding clearly. Child H had her implant at the age of 6;6 – a relatively late age of implantation among this group. This child's error profile more closely resembles that of the HA users than the younger CI users. These data may be significant in showing the negative effects of later implantation, which usually suggests a later-than-usual adaptation period for learning new auditory stimuli. The reader will remember that her PCC score was 80%, while one child implanted at age 2;6 received 95% on the same test.

Whereas sensorineural hearing impairment particularly reduces acoustical information at higher frequencies, implants are known to provide high-frequency information, enhancing higher frequencies (F2) more than lower ones. The CI users are responding to these stimuli and are exhibiting relatively faster progress with fricatives situated at these frequencies. Although the articulation of these sounds demands more precise movement with the blade of the tongue, the children in this study being older in age have reversed the traditional pattern of acquisition evidenced in HA users and in younger, normally hearing children. They also seem to

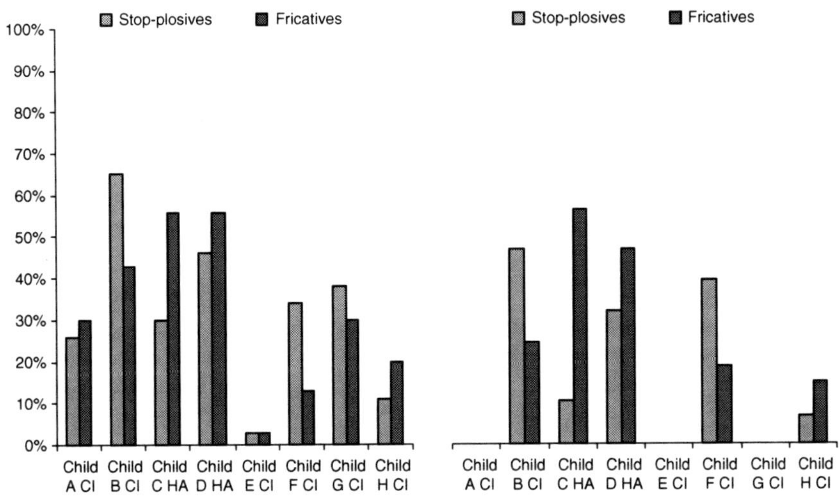

Figures 8.8 (a, b) Contrasting errors in stop-plosives versus errors in fricatives produced by hearing impaired children

proceed with the development of fricatives faster than the stop-plosives, responding to enhanced stimuli.

Conclusion

This study examined the influence of receiving a CI and of using binaural HAs with the combination of auditory–oral training on the speech production achievement levels of children who had auditory stimulation before they were 1;10 years old, on average. Speech production achievement was assessed in spontaneous language samples for consonant inventories. Speech performance on the Articulation Test was analyzed for speech errors. The consonants missing in the inventories of hearing impaired children followed a similar order to the late acquisition pattern outlined by normally hearing Turkish children, with the exception of the consonants [g] and [ɟ], for which the explanations were provided. It seems that the children's rate of development is slower for those consonants which have the lowest frequency of occurrence.

Both CI and HA users showed functionally demonstrable growth in their consonant inventories and considerable decreases in their overall speech errors over a one-year period. The children made errors of substitution considerably more often than errors of omission. A comparison in error patterns was made between the two groups of children. One comparison group consisted of HA users who made the majority of errors in the fricative class, which was consistent with the literature describing the speech characteristics of hearing impaired children. The other comparison group comprised children using CIs who were similar with respect to preimplant hearing status and educational background, and who had CI experience between 10 months and 6 years of age. One striking feature of the data in this study pertains to the relationship between errors in stop-plosives and errors in fricatives produced by CI users. In this study, it was found that those children who had more than two years of CI experience exhibited a higher percentage of errors in stop-plosives compared with errors in fricatives. This finding may imply that their rate of progress in the acquisition of fricatives may have surpassed their rate of progress in the acquisition of stop-plosives, in contrast to the traditional descriptions of hearing impaired children's speech characteristics. If this finding is corroborated by future studies with a greater number of children who have used CIs for more than two years, the descriptions for speech characteristics of hearing impaired children will need to be revised according to the outcomes of this new technology.

Acknowledgments

I gratefully acknowledge Deniz Kazanoğlu for her assistance in data collection with the Articulation Test, Yasemin Yolal and Gökçen Abalı for their assistance in data tabulation at various phases and Gökçen Abalı for her assistance in the graphics work. I would also like to thank my colleague Associate Professor Ümit Girgin for her outstanding work at İÇEM as the principal of the school and the staff and students at İÇEM who participated in the study.

Notes

1. This survey was not repeated in the following years.
2. The numbers are for the year 2008–2009.

Chapter 9

Language Characteristics of Hearing Impaired Turkish Children

UMRAN TÜFEKÇİOĞLU

Introduction

Most children with severe or profound hearing impairment evidence significant delays in the various facets of language comprehension and production (Seyfried-Culbertson & Kricos, 2002). Some common language characteristics of children who are hearing impaired have been described in detail by several researchers (Bamford & Mentz, 1979; Bamford & Saunders, 1991; Blamey, 2003; Blamey *et al.*, 2006; Geers, 2006; Kretschmer & Kretschmer, 1978; Laughton & Hasenstab, 2000; Marschark & Spencer, 2005; Quigley *et al.*, 1974a, 1974b, 1976a, 1976b, 1976c, 1977, 1978; Spencer & Marschark, 2003; Yoshinaga-Itano, 2000). An examination of the literature on the language of hearing impaired children will not only reveal the language characteristics of these children, but also, such descriptions will provide an opportunity to evaluate the linguistic end products of both 'educational and natural influences' and will assist professionals in making evidence-based intervention decisions (Kretschmer & Kretschmer, 1978: 106). In this chapter, for the sake of brevity, only a general discussion on the characteristics of the language structure of hearing impaired children will be given.

Language Characteristics of Hearing Impaired Children

Quigley and his colleagues, in a series of articles between 1974 and 1977, reported their research findings on the development of Standard English syntax in the language of deaf children and adolescents in the United States (Quigley & King, 1980). Linguistic analysis of samples of written language and responses to test items (Quigley *et al.*, 1978) from several hundred deaf students (aged 10–18 years) provided data for identification of common and recurring patterns of distinctive syntactic constructions. The results showed differences from normal standard usage and were initially described as 'deviant' from the accepted norm.

The findings showed gross retardation but a similar, although not identical, order of difficulty of the various syntactic structures for deaf and hearing children. The least difficult structures were negation, conjunction and, to some extent, question formation for both deaf and hearing subjects (Quigley *et al.*, 1977), although Quigley *et al.*, 1974b: 712) reported that in relation to question forms, 'deviant and standard rules coexist, as well as slower rate of development'. The more difficult structures were found to be the verb system, pronominalization, complementation, relativization and passivization. This was true for both groups, although the order was slightly different. The difficulties with the recursive processes of relativization, complementation and passivization were again predictable partly because of the departure from the subject–verb–object (SVO) surface order that deaf students tended to impose on sentences.

In the Quigley *et al.* (1974a) study, deaf students had the most difficulty in understanding medially embedded relative clauses, because they tended to join the noun phrase (NP) of the relative clause with the verb phrase (VP) of the main sentence, thus misconstruing the sentence. Deaf students' responses for this type of relative clauses were 73% incorrect at 11 years of age, and at 18 years, it was still 73%, indicating no improvement over a period of seven years. Problems of this type remained persistent throughout the age range tested. In summary, the 18-year-old deaf subjects performed at significantly lower levels than the 8-year-old hearing subjects on all structures.

Bamford and Mentz (1979) had similar findings with 263 hearing impaired children in the United Kingdom, whose samples of spoken language were analyzed with the LARSP profile (Crystal, 1989). The analysis of the hearing impaired profile showed a marked lack of entries at the word and phrase level, with an even greater delay in the more advanced structures and advanced clause-level entries.

On the basis of the data from Quigley *et al.* (1974a, 1974b, 1976a, 1976b) and Wilbur *et al.* (1975), Quigley and King (1980) assumed that developmental stages in the acquisition of particular syntactic structures were similar for deaf and hearing children, but that the rate of development was greatly delayed in the case of deaf children. An important exception to this was the presence of *certain distinctive syntactic structures* that rarely or never appeared in the language of the hearing subjects but that frequently occurred in the written language of deaf students.

These distinctive structures will be summarized in a list in the following paragraph together with the findings of other researchers. In the summary given below, all the descriptions marked with an asterisk were provided by Quigley and King as reported by other researchers to be found in populations consisting of *normally hearing* people learning English as a second language, but among them there were also some first language learners and language delayed individuals. In conclusion, Quigley and King (1980: 339) stated that these types of distinctive structures do not seem to characterize deaf individuals specifically, but these individuals '... seem to differ from other populations that have difficulties with standard English syntax not in type of difficulty, but in degree. The deaf subjects had all of the distinctive structures shown, had them in profusion, and persisted in their use despite many years of schooling'.

Summary of distinctive structures in the language of deaf students[1]

Language output: Depressed language output, reduced tokens and types of words (Brannon, 1968) reduced the number of sentences and length of sentences (Bamford & Saunders, 1991); lowered output in different words and mean length of utterance (MLU) (Nicholas, 2000).

Sentence construction: Syntactically less complex compositions, single proposition sentences rather than complementation or nominalization, phrase structure difficulties (Kretschmer & Kretschmer, 1978); language delayed and somewhat different in syntactic constructions with respect to the normal-hearing child (Geers & Moog, 1978); virtual absence of conjunctions, fewer connecting devices, a general tendency to use no more than one clause per sentence, also deficits at the phrase level (Bamford & Mentz, 1979); language not acquired at a rate comparable to normally hearing peers, ideas expressed in a telegraphic manner (Geers *et al.*, 1984); delayed syntactic forms (Schirmer, 1985); generally much simpler sentences, complex sentences involving, for example, subordination are rare (Bamford & Saunders, 1991); lower average percentile scores (15%) on the production of complex sentences (Tomblin *et al.*, 2000ci[2]).

Sentence type: Mostly the simple active declarative type in the form of SVO (Brannon & Murry, 1966; Kretschmer & Kretschmer, 1978).

Style of language: Overuse of nouns, and less use of abstract words (Brannon, 1968); generally inflexible and stereotyped (Bamford & Saunders, 1991).

Major sentence constituents: Subject omission or main verb omission (Tur-Kaspa & Dromi, 1998); use of a verb in a noun node (Kretschmer & Kretschmer, 1978).

Word order: Frequent word-order errors (Bamford & Saunders, 1991); a fixed SVO construction (Tur-Kaspa & Dromi, 1998); agrammatical sequential word orders (Sarachan-Deily, 1982); SVO-type word order being superimposed on others that are not SVO, copying, adjective following noun*, negation outside the sentence*.

Content words: Overuse of content words, particularly nouns and verbs; underuse of function words, particularly auxiliaries, conjunctions and prepositions (Bamford & Saunders, 1991).

Morphological rule knowledge: Markedly worse performance in the use of derivational suffixes and inflectional suffixes (Cooper, 1967); problems with verb morphology (Quigley *et al.*, 1976b); incorrect usage of morpho-syntactic markers (Tur-Kaspa & Dromi, 1998); morphological entries only half of those of the control group (Bamford & Mentz, 1979; Nicholas, 2000); morphological development weak compared to semantic knowledge (Young & Killen, 2002ci); deletion of obligatory word forms (Spencer *et al.*, 2003ci).

In the verb system: Verb deletion*, omission of *be* or *have**, confusion of tense markers*; unmarked verb as in *–ing* and *–ed* constructions*, unmarked verb in sequence*, auxiliary deletion such as *be* or *have*, confusion of *be* and *have** (Quigley *et al.*, 1976a); verb constructions deviating from the normal order of acquisition and usage (Pressnell, 1973); time coded through use of adverbs rather than tense (Ivimey, 1976); incorrect verb forms (Kretschmer & Kretschmer, 1978; Spencer *et al.*, 2003ci).

In negation: Difficulty in producing the negative (Boothe *et al.*, 1981); negation outside the sentence*, negative not correctly marked*, nonrecognition of negative marker.

In determiners: Omission of determiners*, confusion of determiners* (Wilbur, 1977); difficulty with use of articles (Kretschmer & Kretschmer, 1978); profusion of determiners.

Prepositions: Prepositions often used incorrectly or omitted (Markides, 1970); not functionally available to the child (Ivimey, 1976); difficulty with use of prepositions (Kretschmer & Kretschmer, 1978).

Plurality and possession: When applying transformations, violation of restrictions such as those related to plurality and possession (Kretschmer & Kretschmer, 1978).

In pronominalizations: Deficient use of pronouns (Brannon, 1968); confusion of case pronouns*, wrong gender* (Quigley & King, 1980; Kretschmer & Kretschmer, 1978).

In conjunction: Marking only the first verb, conjunction deletion*, unusual omissions occurring when test sentences share subject or object (object–object deletion*, object–subject deletion) (Wilbur, 1977; Wilbur *et al.*, 1975).

In complementation: Use of *for* in addition to the infinitive, use of *for* in addition to the gerund*, use of *to* in addition to the gerund, omission of *to* in the infinitive*, infinitive in place of gerund*, incorrectly inflected infinitive*, unmarked infinitive (without *to*) (Quigley *et al.*, 1976b); use of infinitives instead of participle forms (Kretschmer & Kretschmer, 1978).

In relativization: Relative pronoun deletion*, confusion of relative pronoun*, NPs where *whose* is required, object–object deletion, object–subject deletion*, copying of referent unnecessarily, surface reading (Quigley *et al.*, 1974a); extreme difficulty in understanding or producing relative clauses and significant differences in the use of embedded clauses

(Tur-Kaspa & Dromi, 1998); severe difficulty in the comprehension of object relatives, avoiding production of sentences with syntactic movement or producing ungrammatical sentences (Friedmann & Szterman, 2005).

In question formation: Copying the word order of the statement (which is also a word-order violation), failure to apply S-AUX inversion*, overgeneralization of contraction rule with negation and *will**, noun copying, pronoun copying (Quigley *et al.*, 1974b); confusion between *who* and *what*, errors with *where* and *when* (Boothe *et al.*, 1981).

In passive voice: Deletion of *by**, surface reading, greatly depressed scores in tests (Power & Quigley, 1973); no production of passive constructions in 8–11-year-old subjects, adult subjects producing sentences in passive voice with 20% accuracy (Boothe *et al.*, 1981).

In subject–verb agreement: Agreement errors involving subject–verb agreement (Spencer *et al.*, 2003ci), third person marker missing*.

In all types of sentences: Forced SVO pattern in verb processes*, and in relativization*, complementation and nominalization (Quigley & King, 1980); frequent errors of omission, substitution and addition (Bamford & Saunders, 1991); in prelingual deaf children significant delay in grammar before cochlear implantation, and considerable delay following implantation, with distinctive trend toward development (Nikolopoulos *et al.*, 2004ci; Svirsky *et al.*, 2000ci).

The errors reported by Quigley *et al.* were found across ages and across schools that used manual communication and those that did not. The students tested in the Quigley *et al.* studies were tested on the performance scales of the Wechsler intelligence scale for children (WISC), Wechsler adult intelligence scale (WAIS) or other comparable tests of intelligence and all were within the normal range (Wilbur, 1977). Other researchers also reported similar controlled performance. Wilbur also pointed out that Furth's (1966) study of deaf students '... leaves little doubt that their cognitive development is sufficiently normal' (1977: 90) and stated that, since the problem is not cognitive, it is linguistic.

Pressnell (1973) suggested that classroom instruction techniques might underlie some of the differences she found in the syntax of hearing impaired children. Bamford and Mentz (1979) suggested that the special difficulties associated with hearing short-duration morphological structures accounted for the depressed morphological entries. Wilbur, too, reasoned on why deaf students consistently and persistently had these problems with language structure: 'The problem with these structures results from a lack of understanding of *when* and *how* to use them,' which 'most likely arises from the heavy emphasis that is placed on the proper structure of the single sentence in language training programs for the deaf.' ... 'The focus is on the structure of the single sentence, and not on the sentence's use within its larger environment. As long as the modifications in syntax that arise from pragmatic context are ignored in language programs, deaf students' facility with English will continue to be stilted and stereotyped' (1977: 87–91).

More recent research on the language abilities of hearing impaired children took a different turn; research efforts focused on how well children improved with the latest technology, even if the rate was still comparatively slow. Students attending certain programs that utilized a strong Auditory–Oral Approach or an Auditory–Verbal Approach with an effective auditory management program were found to exhibit spoken language performances distinctly better than other 'oral' programs. Pragmatic context was definitely a characteristic of these programs with interaction provided by skillful adults who supplied meaningful language input in rich language experiences (Clark, 1989, 2007). The outcomes were presented as case studies in a series of teaching packs (Clark, 1985, 1986a, 1986b; Estabrooks, 1992, 1994, 2000, 2004, 2006b) rather than research results or descriptive studies because the primary concern of the authors here was to guide professionals, teachers and parents to help the children to learn through the interactional auditory approach.

Apart from these communicative approaches, which have certainly made a difference in the educational methods and techniques for working with children and parents, cochlear implants have become available as a true innovation in audiological intervention and brought further change. Yoshinaga-Itano (2005) summarized the difference between hearing aids and cochlear implants: 'Early-identified profound hearing loss with early cochlear implantation and a high-quality auditory stimulation program results in expectations that are similar to those for early-identified mild-to-severe hearing loss and the use of conventional amplification.' This is mainly because cochlear implants have provided deaf children with access to auditory information that is essential for language development. 'Specifically, a cochlear implant provides high-frequency and temporal information that is not available from a conventional hearing aid' (Bollard *et al.*, 1999: 119).

Because of this access to auditory information, children are expected to benefit from cochlear implants in the acquisition of spoken language. Boothroyd *et al.* (1991: 81) asked whether the expected spoken language benefits are realized for children who do gain access to spectral information via the implant. They report on research conducted by Boothroyd *et al.*, which followed three groups of children in a comparative study, examining whether tactile aids, acoustic hearing aids or cochlear implants provided the greatest benefit for developing spoken language. After the first year of study, the implant users progressed at a greater rate in acquiring auditory speech perception skills. However, in spite of the rapid acquisition of auditory skills, the implantees did not demonstrate an advantage over the other groups in speech production or spoken language. Nevertheless, after 18 months, better progress was observed in speech perception and production for the implantees over the matched groups, although this was not evident in measures of language development. Boothroyd *et al.* (1991: 87) said they had already anticipated that 'as many as 3 years may be necessary to demonstrate the full linguistic consequences of improved auditory capacity'. They concluded that possible effects will only be fully realized when the child is provided with 'spoken language training of the intensity and focus typically (but not exclusively) found in oral programs of education'. Geers (2006: 264) added one comment that is most relevant to what should follow after implantation: 'Research should document when special education is needed, when the child can be most successful in the mainstream, and what support services will allow for maximum academic progress. The importance of early auditory stimulation for spoken language acquisition after cochlear implantation has been documented. Clinical research should examine methods to help parents (and teachers) provide this for their children'.

Research should also examine the topic of wide inter-subject variability in the outcomes of these children, which is a consistent theme in successful outcome reports (Geers, 2004; Miyamoto *et al.*, 1997; Richter *et al.*, 2002; Spencer *et al.*, 2003). As Boothroyd and Boothroyd-Turner (2002) have made perfectly clear, there is no doubt about the immense improvements cochlear implants have brought to the speech and language development of hearing impaired children. Cochlear implants are the most extraordinary recent innovation to positively affect the language learning and quality of life of hearing impaired individuals (Boothroyd & Boothroyd-Turner, 2002; Geers, 2004; Geers *et al.*, 2003; Miyamoto *et al.*, 1997; Nicholas & Geers, 2006; Nikolopoulos *et al.*, 2004; Svirsky *et al.*, 2000; Tomblin *et al.*, 1999). What has to be emphasized is the need for the majority of severely and profoundly hearing impaired children with hearing aids or cochlear implants to receive careful intervention to keep developing speech and language skills at the pace of hearing age peers throughout their school years, especially if the educational settings are not ideal.

Language Characteristics of Hearing Impaired Turkish Children

Research papers investigating language characteristics of hearing impaired Turkish children are few in number for reasons explained in the previous chapter, and therefore the literature review presented here will cover a limited number of studies. Research papers dealing with instruction methods in relation to teaching reading and writing skills, mathematics and science, parent guidance and parent–child interaction studies involving hearing impaired children in this country have been omitted in this section for reasons of brevity. This section will focus on research work that involves studies of morphology and syntax acquisition in hearing impaired Turkish children in order to provide some information on the language characteristics of this population.

One of the earliest studies in this respect is a comparative study of the spoken language performances of students from two distinctively different educational environments (Tüfekçioğlu, 1989). Tüfekçioğlu employed Brown's (1973) MLU measure and Tough's (1981) communicative functions classification system in a comparison of the spoken language of hearing impaired children enrolled in a state residential school for the deaf, and of those in an auditory–oral program. While the auditory–oral program provided earlier diagnosis and intervention including parent guidance, these provisions were, and still are, not available in state schools for the deaf (Tüfekçioğlu, 1992, 1996, 1998). The Auditory–Oral Approach was not known in Turkey then and there was some suspicion of the benefits of a 'Natural Interactionist Approach', which was perceived as not effective for not offering a structure in the form of a recipe to work from. There were disputes among educators as to whether the approach would work better than the structured 'oral method' claimed to be used in the schools for the deaf in the country, where manual communication usually predominated in every setting except the classroom, and perhaps in the classroom as well. The purpose of the study was to determine whether hearing impaired students of an auditory–oral program derived greater benefit in developing spoken language than hearing impaired students of a residential school for the deaf.

The study undertaken was not aimed specifically at a comparison of the two methodologies, auditory–oral versus total communication (TC), mainly because of the many confounding factors existing in the intervention history of the sample of students, but rather dealt with the spoken language outcomes of the two educational settings as their approaches to the management of hearing impaired children were quite different in all aspects. This was particularly important since the latter one was the prevailing methodology and type of provision at the time of the study.

The subjects of the study were 40 students from the auditory–oral program (İÇEM) and 40 students from the school for the deaf, ages 6;5–12;10 years. The subject selection criteria for all students were prelingual, bilaterally profound hearing loss of 90 dB HL or greater, intelligence quotient (IQ) of 81 or higher, no additional handicaps, and no transferral students. Subjects were matched into four groups in terms of age, unaided residual hearing, IQ and socioeconomic groups. Unintelligible utterances, repetitions and imitations were not coded. Only the spontaneous utterances were used for analysis. Spontaneous spoken language samples of 50–100 utterances for each child were analyzed according to three aspects: intelligibility, MLU and the longest three MLUs, based on Brown (1973), and functional use based on Tough (1981). A child's use of language for a variety of purposes or communicative functions is a reflection of normal communicative language development and is a valuable measure from a sociolinguistic point of view. Based on Halliday's (1981) theories, Tough described seven purposes for which a child uses language: self-maintaining, directing, reporting, reasoning, predicting, projecting and imagining. Utterances were coded according to the seven categories listed and reported under the heading of 'The Seven Functions'.

The comparative study found that the language performance of hearing impaired students of the auditory–oral program was statistically significantly more advanced on all three sets of measurements (intelligibility, MLU and communicative functions) obtained on all of the four age groups of children described (either $p < 0.0005$ or $p < 0.005$ for all measures). Figure 9.1 shows the MLU results for the 80 hearing impaired students, 40 from the auditory–oral program and 40 from the school for the deaf. The mean MLU for the oldest group from the school for the deaf was 1.23 morphemes, while the mean for İÇEM was 4.04 morphemes.

The spoken productions of the students from the school for the deaf consisted mostly of single words such as '*adam*' (man), '*araba*' (car), '*çocuk*' (child), '*elma*' (apple) and '*anne*' (mother), the simplest form of vocabulary with almost no morphological suffixes. The longest utterance length was 2.33 for students of the school for the deaf and 9.67 morphemes for students of the auditory–oral program. Apparently, the former group of students had acquired neither the morphological nor the syntactic rules of spoken Turkish and only a very limited vocabulary, consisting of nouns only. Because the language produced was extremely limited, confined to noun use with no morphology (MLU of 1.23 morphemes), syntactic

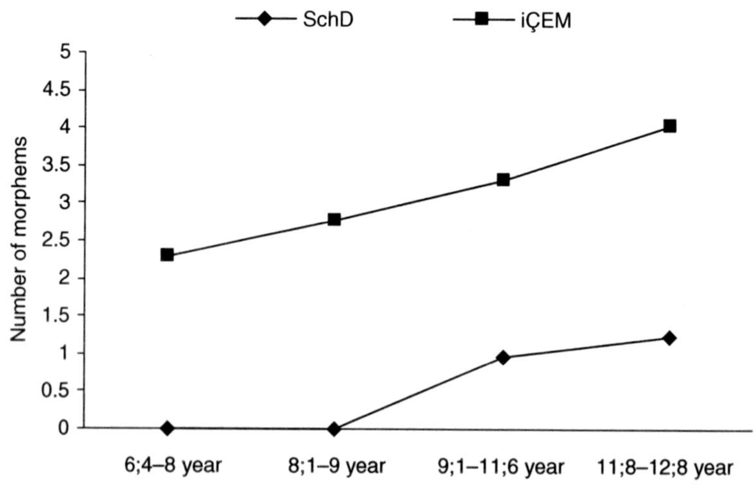

Figure 9.1 MLU of hearing impaired children as a function of educational environment ($N = 80$)

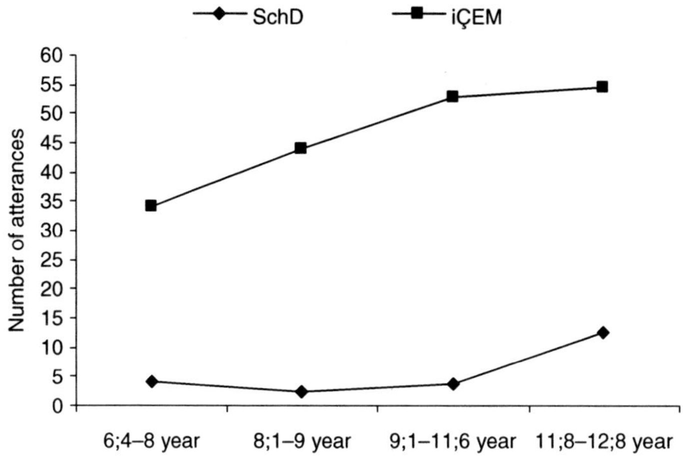

Figure 9.2 The seven communicative functions used by hearing impaired children as a function of educational environment ($N = 80$)

analysis was not carried out. It was not possible to update this study because further permission was not granted to the researchers.

Figure 9.2 shows the number of utterances containing the seven communicative functions – self-maintaining, directing, reporting, reasoning, predicting, projecting and imagining described by Tough (1981) and Figure 9.3 shows the more abstract communicative functions of the seven categories – reasoning, predicting, projecting and imagining for 80 children in the study.

The analysis of the samples showed that, including the more abstract categories of reasoning, predicting, projecting and imagining, the students

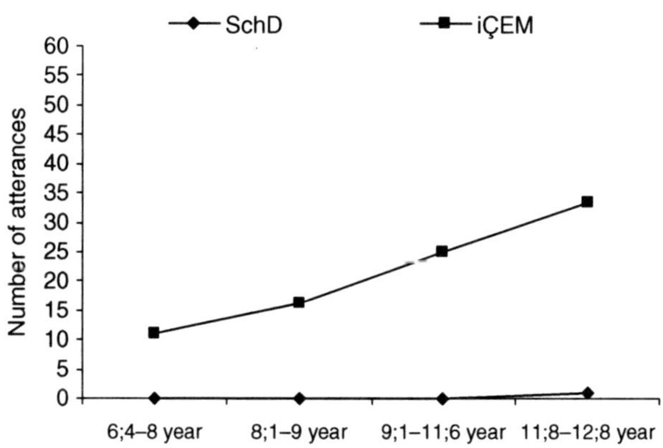

Figure 9.3 The more abstract communicative functions used by hearing impaired children as a function of educational environment ($N = 80$)

of the auditory–oral program evidenced use of these functions in their spontaneous conversations (Tüfekçioğlu, 1989, 1996). The importance of these functions is described by Halliday (1981), Tough (1981) and Tüfekçioğlu (1989, 1998) and the early emerging group of functions by Nicholas (2000). These findings refute the previous findings reported in early studies that deaf children had 'concrete' language and did not exhibit the more abstract forms. As described by Nicholas, the children in the auditory group were 'expanding their communicative function repertoire along with expanding their language skills in other areas' (Nicholas, 2000: 391) as the MLU figures show.

A unique characteristic of the program was its implementation of a progressive curriculum and progressive teaching techniques. Other factors associated with this auditory–oral sample, such as early and consistent amplification, effective management of hearing aids, early education and parental involvement through consistent parent guidance, were also significantly better employed. These findings are consistent with the findings of Geers and Moog's (1992) study on the auditory and speech skills of 227 students who had been educated in oral and TC environments.

In daily interactions with experienced adults throughout the day, each day is 'a way of living' (Clark, 1989). Children with profound hearing impairment showed that they do acquire the necessary vocabulary and grammar but most importantly learn *how*, *when* and *where* to use it for purposes meaningful to them (Tüfekçioğlu, 1989, 1998).

Although there was a marked difference between the comparison groups in favor of children in the Turkish auditory–oral program, examination of the real performance scores reveals that MLU performances of all the subjects were still below those of normally hearing children of the same chronological ages, when compared against the data and prediction lines provided by Ege *et al.* (1998) for Turkish-speaking hearing children. This finding is in parallel with the findings of Geers and Moog (1978), Kretschmer and Kretschmer (1978), Bamford and Mentz (1979) and Geers *et al.* (1984), whose data clearly indicated that 'profoundly deaf children do not acquire language at a rate comparable to their normally hearing peers. This is true for those educated in oral/aural programs as well as for those in total communication programs' (1984: 387). The children in the Geers *et al.* study, ranging in age from 5 to 9 years, did not reach the level of normally hearing 4-year-old children. This delayed development phenomenon proved to be true until the most recent advances in technology were developed, in the form of identification in infancy and cochlear implantation.

The relatively late age of diagnosis and amplification that was prevailing at the time of the study (the mean age for amplification and onset of intervention was three years for the auditory–oral group) could be suggested as one significant factor that led to this delay in MLUs, compared to normally hearing age peers. The evidence for the significance of this factor came from Yoshinaga-Itano *et al.*'s (1998: 1161) study, which found that those children whose hearing losses were '... identified by 6 months of age demonstrated significantly better language scores than children identified after 6 months of age'. It was shown that early identification in the first few months of life followed by early intervention services helped children with even severe hearing loss to exhibit auditory behaviors and speech skills at much earlier age levels (Yoshinaga-Itano, 2001).

The significance of these findings are still relevant today because even now the same approach to the management of hearing impaired children prevails in the many state residential schools in Turkey. Fortunately, not all children are placed in those schools; some are placed in mainstream schools instead. It is the hypothesis of this author that if the research were to be duplicated as of today, the results would not be much different, mainly because the high statistical significance in the study indicated that if the same conditions persisted the same results would be found. A nationwide hearing screening program and a comprehensive early intervention program are not available yet. However, pilot studies for a neonatal hearing screening program have recently started in several hospitals in Turkey.

Because a number of hearing impaired children moved into the mainstream during the following years, another study investigated the spoken language performance, reading comprehension and general academic performance of those students who were placed in their local schools for integration purposes (Tüfekçioğlu, 1992). It is extremely important for professionals to gain an understanding of the situations in educational settings, as these are critical for appropriate placement decisions. The characteristics of the environments into which hearing impaired children are placed can either impose limitations on or enable the development of language. Realistically identifying the problems in a situation is also needed to take the necessary steps toward improvement. The objective of this study was to gather data on language, literacy and academic success of hearing impaired students as outcome measures for successful integration. The sample consisted of all of the 40 hearing impaired students who were in mainstream primary and secondary schools in Eskişehir in 1992. None reported here had any attachments with İÇEM (the auditory–oral program).

Data were collected through the use of interviews with each teacher who taught a hearing impaired child in the mainstream and through dialogues and reading comprehension work with each child. The high-ranking correlation coefficients obtained among the above measures demonstrated the validity of these measures that were derived from three different sources: teacher report, teacher rating and direct observation of the child. The findings showed that as a measure of comprehension of spoken language, the ratings given by the teachers for each hearing impaired child in their class were as follows (in mean percentages): 5% of the children had near-normal comprehension of spoken language; 5% had fairly satisfactory understanding; 17.5% had some understanding; 52.5% had limited understanding; and 20% did not understand spoken language at all, indicating that 72% of the children had limited or no understanding of the language spoken in the class they were placed in. One way to assess language is to group or list children's utterances as single-word utterances, two-word utterances or three-word utterances (Bloom & Lahey, 1978), at least for very young children or for children who have not progressed to a higher stage. A five-point scale was used for teachers to give ratings on the students' level of spoken language ability. The results showed that 32.5% of the students were rated as using simple sentences, 20% using three or more words, 5% using two words, 20% using single words and 22.5% using only vocalizations, indicating that half of them had severely delayed language. This level of language did not evidence any use of morphological and syntactic rules for the group.

Reading performances were assessed individually by using a set of simple comprehension questions. With the child's teacher present and providing a reading text that she had used with the child previously, each child was asked individually to read the text and answer some comprehension questions about it. The results showed that 0% could discuss the main idea, 0% could give satisfactory short answers, 7% could give short answers, 52% could only do decoding but no comprehension and 41% could neither decode nor read or answer (Tüfekçioğlu, 1992). In short, the great majority of the students were not equipped with language to be able to read and understand a simple text. These results were not surprising given the background information for the students in this study. Most of the subjects were enrolled directly into mainstream classes without prior intervention of any type, most of the hearing aids were in bad working condition and no support services were provided. These are not conditions conducive to learning and developing language in the mainstream for hearing impaired children.

As Geers (1990) pointed out, laws in some countries require that handicapped children receive education in 'the least restrictive environment', which is often interpreted to mean mainstreaming as quickly as possible. However, there are prerequisites to successful integration of children with hearing impairments, such as being at a language level that enables the child to at least follow the classroom teaching, as well as displaying some intelligibility in order to be understood for social interaction. Learning through direct experience and with scaffolding adults is another enabling method, in contrast to direct instruction that occurs in environments where the language and previous experiences of the child are limited. These children need good audiological management and communication-enabling environments that should address language development (Tüfekçioğlu, 2000). The results of a further study conducted by Girgin (1997, 2000), using a different and more detailed technique for reading assessment, were consistent with the above results and showed very low levels of reading comprehension, due to minimal intervention.

On the request of the State Planning Office, a large-scale investigation of the situation of deaf education in Turkey was conducted by Tüfekçioğlu *et al.* (1992), who examined the technology, methods and facilities provided at the time. The findings pointed to late diagnosis, late onset of intervention and education for hearing impaired children starting in general at age 5 or 6, the age of starting school. Early intervention, parent guidance and preschool education were not among the services provided. The prerequisites for successful integration into regular classrooms, such as well-developed language and reading skills (Geers, 1990), were not satisfied. The state of spoken and written language, reading comprehension and academic performance was poor, as reported by Tüfekçioğlu (1992, 2000). This should not be surprising considering the predictive factors for successful outcomes in the education of severely or profoundly deaf children, such as early identification and amplification, early and consistent intervention, parental guidance, use of the latest technology for improving the signal-to-noise ratio, an interactionist Auditory–Oral Approach (Clark, 1989, 2007), an aggressive audiological management and emphasis on the development of audition (Estabrooks, 2006a). The findings and suggestions were reported for the information of the State Planning Office in a comprehensive report.

The following years saw research aimed at analyzing communicative acts and/or communicative intents employed by young hearing impaired Turkish children in interactions with their hearing mothers. Researchers were also interested in the strategies used by normal hearing mothers during group play (Uzuner, 1997) and repair strategies used by mothers (Uzuner, 1999).

Only a few studies have focused on the language characteristics of hearing impaired Turkish children, and most of these studies have been conducted in recent years. One such study is by Ekinci (2007), who investigated the production of case suffixes in this population. The study was conducted with 42 hearing impaired students attending schools for the deaf, and 42 normally hearing children, all of whom were either third-, fourth- or fifth-grade students. The results showed that hearing impaired students' use of nominal suffixes was significantly lower than the control group. In fact, the most frequently produced case by the hearing impaired group was the nominative, which takes no suffixes. There was no difference between spoken and written language performances. A study by Topbaş *et al.* (1997) showed that very young Turkish children are sensitive to marking cases appropriately. Based on this study, one can say with confidence that normally hearing young Turkish children have no difficulty in acquiring case suffixation and that this group of hearing impaired children had difficulties that were similar to those reported in earlier studies in the United States and the United Kingdom. It needs to be pointed out that, most likely, the late onset of intervention and ineffective practices in the management and education of these children contributed to the reported results.

Recently, a number of other studies have also focused on the spoken language performance and acquisition of certain structures by hearing impaired Turkish children. A series of studies examining the acquisition of certain morphological and syntactic structures in hearing impaired Turkish children was recently conducted by Tüfekçioğlu (2008b–2009c), and preliminary findings will be discussed here in an effort to portray the language characteristics of some hearing impaired Turkish children who have been attending an auditory–oral program at İÇEM. Language measures of interest were mean syntactic length (MSL), verb inflections, coordinating and subordinating conjunctions, complementation, relativization and passivization.

Language measures of interest were derived from spoken language samples collected at one-year intervals as part of an ongoing study, and from a syntax test devised by the researcher herself. For eliciting spoken language, children's teachers used two sets of sequenced picture cards that depicted two stories, a picture about a family picnic or playhouse toys in order to motivate children to produce spontaneous spoken language and engage them in conversation. Continuous spoken language during the conversations was videotaped and transcribed following procedures explained by Brown (1973). Criteria for including the utterances for analysis followed the procedures outlined for such analysis. All imitations and repetitions of the teacher's utterances or the child's own utterances were excluded from the analysis to ensure spontaneity of language. As can be seen from the speech measures given in the previous chapter (Chapter 8, this volume), most of the utterances of the younger children and all of the utterances of the older children were intelligible enough for analysis. The rules that were used for separating utterances in the conversation samples were in agreement with Blamey *et al.* (2006: 95). A total of 100 spontaneous utterances were used as samples for the analysis of MSL, tense and aspect inflections in verbs, coordinating and subordinating conjunctions, and the use of complex syntactic structures, and for identifying errors for grammatical correctness.

MSL in the spontaneous utterances of hearing impaired children

One widely used index of children's early grammatical development is MLU (Brown, 1973; de Villiers & de Villiers, 1973). Although there are debates on how to measure the construct of linguistic complexity, it is widely accepted that children's spoken utterances become longer and more highly subordinated with age. Scott and Stokes (1995: 310) report that sentence length measures are thought to be useful indicators of syntactic growth only in young preschool children, 'but research documents a slow, steady increase in the average length of spoken and written sentences throughout the elementary and secondary school years'. Aksu-Koç and Slobin (1985), Özcan (1996) and Ekmekçi (1982, 1979) have shown that normally hearing young Turkish children do use suffixation in their spoken language even when their utterances are short in length. Therefore, a study of sentence length in morphemes seems justified for a morphologically more complex language such as Turkish.

Although MLU seems to be a very useful index for the Turkish language and has already been used with hearing impaired children in an earlier study (Tüfekçioğlu, 1989), in this study, the researcher preferred to use the index of MSL 'to eliminate a possible pragmatic influence upon mean utterance length imposed by single-morpheme responses (e.g. *yes, no, cat, there*)' (Klee & Fitzgerald, 1985: 255). This influence was observed to be present especially in the older children's samples in the form of elliptical responses or on account of teenage moodiness. In examining the language samples of the children, it was observed that single-morpheme utterances of this type occurred more frequently in older children's replies to questions. Because these children were beyond the stage of single-morpheme utterances, as Klee and Fitzgerald suggested, such a procedure was adopted to control a pragmatic variable that distorted the value of MLU (Tüfekçioğlu, 2009b). Single-morpheme responses, only elicited because of teacher questions demanding single-morpheme pragmatically correct answers, were not included in the calculations. Those single-morpheme answers that could have instead been supplied with more than one morpheme were included in the calculations. The results are shown in Figure 9.4 as the MSL for eight hearing impaired children under study for the years 2007 and 2008.

Figure 9.4 illustrates an accelerating growth in syntactic sentence length when the data are plotted over the one year of data collection. Note that the younger children tend to have lower MSL than older ones. The imaginary line of rate of growth shows quite a steep line of growth, indicating that all children are developing at a good rate, without a plateau effect as was reported in earlier studies with deaf children, and this promises further growth. Profoundly deaf children, who were orally trained but not given cochlear implants at an early age, continued to demonstrate a much lower level of lexical and syntactic skills even in the most recent studies (Nicholas, 2000). Child C, who is a hearing aid user, demonstrates delayed MSL compared to the two younger children with cochlear implants. One other possible explanation could be her late start into the auditory–oral program. The hearing aid users also evidence fast

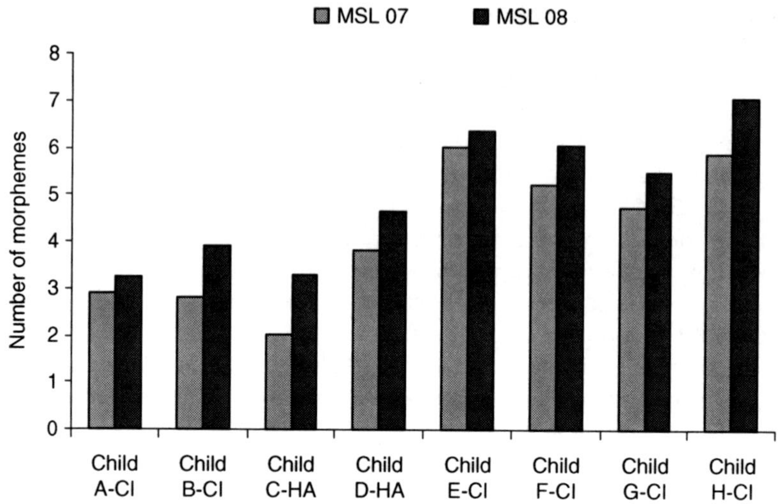

Figure 9.4 MSL for hearing impaired children over one year

rates of growth and are quite comparable to the cochlear implant users, possibly because they are making good use of the auditory–oral training they are consistently receiving, coupled with effective hearing aid management and attention to signal-to-noise ratios in the educational setting. Another explanation would be that the cochlear implant users started life and the program with more profound hearing losses, as can be seen in Table 8.1, and need more time with implant use to show its effectiveness over hearing aids. One explanation for Child E exceeding the MSL of the next two older children, F and G, might very well be the age of implantation: 2;9, 3;10 and 4;8, respectively. Child E is the youngest to have had an implant of all the children, a finding in agreement with researchers Nicholas and Geers (2007) and Connor *et al.* (2006) who, among others, have identified age of implantation as the most significant factor for positive outcomes.

Tense, aspect and modality in spoken language productions of hearing impaired Turkish children

Earlier studies with English-speaking children in the United States and the United Kingdom consistently reported that deaf students had considerable difficulty with the verb system of English, and this difficulty was mostly found in the formation of tense and voice, but also in tense and number agreement (Quigley *et al.*, 1976a; Quigley & King, 1980).

The verb system of Turkish is more complex than the English verb system. Turkish children have to master how to mark verbs for aspect as well as tense and modality, among other functions. Several researchers have described the complexity of the Turkish verb system (Aksu-Koç, 1988a, 1988b, 1986; Gencan, 2007; Underhill, 1986). Aksu-Koç (1986: 249) describes Turkish as an 'agglutinating language where the invariant verb stem is followed by a string of affixed particles agreeing with the stem in vowel harmony and marking the following functions: voice, modality, negation, aspect, tense, mood, person, and number'.

Figure 9.5 summarizes data on the production of verb inflections by the children under study (Tüfekçioğlu, 2008b). Without exception, all of the children used the present progressive [*-Iyor*] most frequently in their spoken language in the context described. The second most frequently used tense varies with each individual child, but tends toward the simple past/past of direct experience [*-DI*] and narrative past [*-mIş*]. This finding for the first three is consistent with Aksu-Koç (1988a, 1988b) who reported on young normally hearing Turkish children's acquisition of verb inflections.

Although the study is neither longitudinal nor cross-sectional over a large sample size, the number of utterances for spontaneous spoken productions and the number of inflections used were large enough to make inferences for a tentative/possible order of acquisition for the most frequently used inflections realized by the children in the study. The three most frequently used are the present progressive, then the definite past and the narrative past and, finally, the future, abilitative and the aorist. The imperative, the narrative progressive, the past progressive, passive voice, the past perfect, the necessitative and the narrative future are used much less frequently, and because they were used less frequently within the context described earlier, an order of acquisition should not be inferred for these from these data. However, it would be safe to infer that, with the exception of the imperative, they are likely the later acquired ones. The

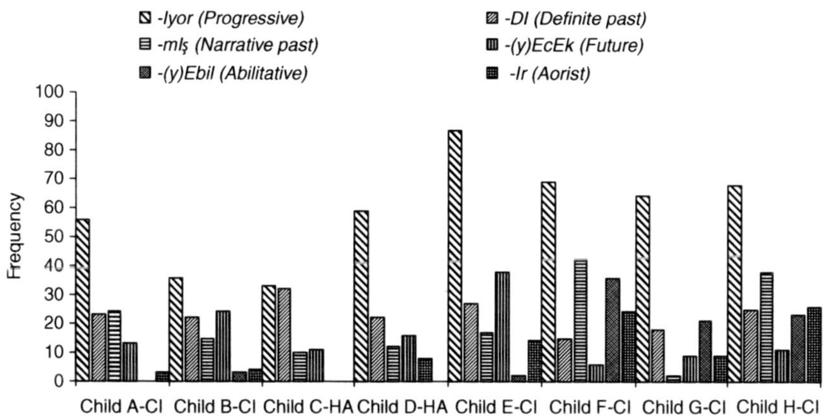

Figure 9.5 The distributional use of tense–aspect–modality inflections in the spoken language productions of hearing impaired Turkish children

imperative may belong to the first group but it is possible that the pragmatic context of the conversation did not allow opportunities for its use. Interestingly, the first two tenses are also consistent with Brown (1973) and de Villiers and de Villiers (1973), who have reported only on the first two tenses for English-speaking normally hearing children.

Coordinating conjunctions used by eight hearing impaired Turkish children

As children mature, so does their language, and as a result they comprehend and produce increasingly complex language. Coordination, complementation and subordination are devices for increasing the complexity of language, allowing for the production of an infinite number of different sentences. Figure 9.6 displays the most frequently used connectives as coordinating conjunctions by eight hearing impaired Turkish children under study (Tüfekçioğlu, 2008c). The conjunction used most is the *DA* clitic *-dE* (and, too), followed by *sonra* (then). Other frequently used ones are *ama* (but), *çünkü* (because) and *ve* (and). The use of these five conjunctions is seen much less frequently in the younger group and more frequently in the older group. The less frequently used ones, which are observed in children's samples starting from Child D on are as follows: *onun için* (because of), *yani* (I mean), *veya* (or), *hem ... de* (that too), *ki* (so), *demek ki* (in other words), *ondan* (that's why) and *mesela* (for example).

In the study by Özcan and Topbaş (1996), *sonra* (then) was also among the most frequently used conjunctions in the spontaneous speech of young Turkish children. This, as well as *çünkü* (because) and *ama* (but), was also among other more frequently used conjunctions, all three having parallels

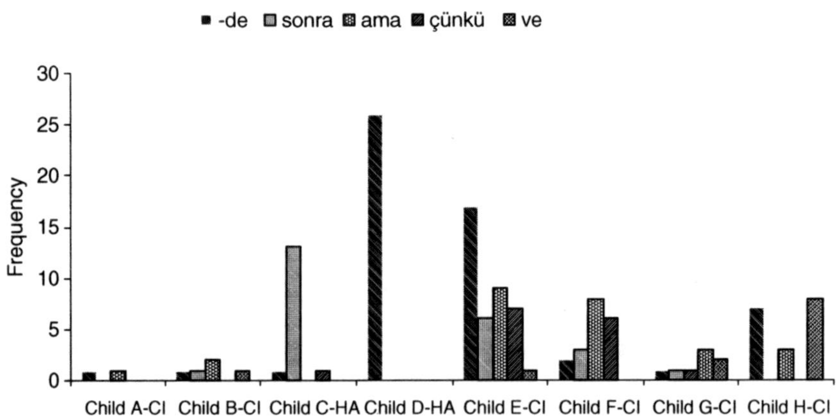

Figure 9.6 Types of connectives used as coordinating conjunctions by hearing impaired Turkish children

with normal hearing data. Among the less frequently used ones, *veya* (but) and *demek ki* (in other words) came up in both studies.

Verbals used for complementation or as subordinating conjunctions by eight hearing impaired Turkish children

The previous study on verb inflections showed that the children acquired a variety of tense–aspect inflections of Turkish and were using them in their spontaneous productions. The acquisition of verbals that are used for complementation or as subordinating conjunctions would developmentally follow the acquisition of verb inflections in Turkish. As Aksu-Koç (1986: 252) stated for the order of acquisition of adverbs, 'It is clear that the acquisition of adverbs and adverbials for temporal reference follows the acquisition of verb inflections in Turkish'. In this case, the question to be answered was whether the children were acquiring any verbals, and if so, which ones (Tüfekçioğlu, 2008d). As S+odowicz (2007: 127–128) pointed out, Turkish makes intensive use of nominalizations in subordination, and suffixes 'form verbal nouns which function as predicates in complement clauses', also allowing for 'modification by means of adverbials of manner', forming adverbial clauses, or by suffixation forming relative clauses. Verbals also '... must be marked for possessor agreement and case, as the example in (7) demonstrates' (S+odowicz, 2007: 129).

'Nurhan Sevgi'ye [para al – acağ – ın – ı] bil – dir – di.
N. S. – DAT money get – GER-3SG.P-ACC know-CAUS-PST.3SG
"Nurhan informed Sevgi that s/he would get the money."'

Figure 9.7 displays the types and frequencies of verbals as a function of individual children. In total, 11 different types of verbals were found in the samples.

The actual number of verbals used is inconsistent from one year to the next across all children. Therefore the numbers for the two years have been collapsed into one sum for each verbal seen in Figure 9.7. It seems that the use of verbals is highly context- and interlocutor-dependent and pragmatically variable. Therefore, statistical analysis might be more reliable for 200 or more utterances and over several recordings. However, the data here show a considerable and a consistent increase in the number of verbals used, starting with Child E and increasing with the older children. As can be seen from Figure 9.7, there is a significant difference between the first four children and the rest, the cut-off point being Child E with the earliest implant, earliest amplification and better MSL compared to those similar in age. The oldest child, Child H, uses all of the verbals quite frequently in her sentences, consistent with her MSL finding as well as the scores on the Test of Syntactic Structures for Turkish (TSST).

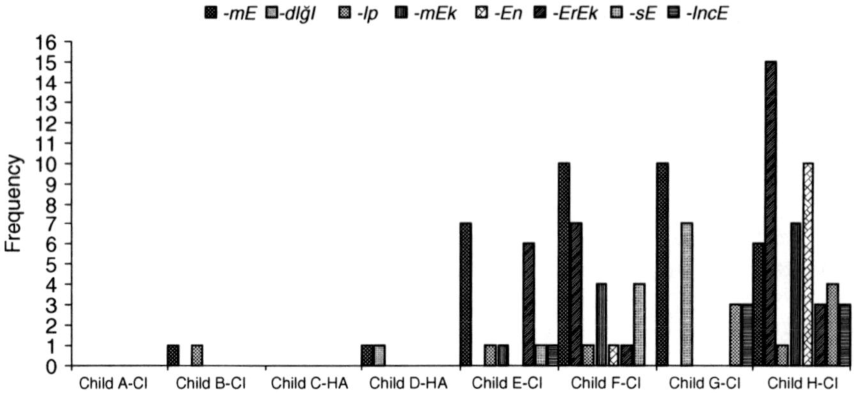

Figure 9.7 Types of verbals used for complementation or as subordinating conjunctions by eight hearing impaired Turkish children

The most frequently used three verbals were '*-mE* and *-dIk, -diye* and *-sın diye*' and the rest of the verbals '*-mEk, -Ip, -sE, -An, -ErEk* and *-IncE*' were used in varying degrees and comparatively less frequently by the older children. The verbals *-mEdEn, -mEk için* and the connective device for a pseudo-clause '*hani … ya*' were too few in number, used only by the oldest three and were not included in Figure 9.7 for the sake of clarity. The verbals '*-dIk, -mEk* and *-sın diye*' are also among the most frequently used connectives on the list of Özcan and Topbaş (1996).

As can be seen in Figure 9.7, the most frequently used verbal functions is complementation, which is to be expected given a language universal principle that the syntactic–semantic function and difficulty of the structure rules the order of acquisition, namely that the less difficult and semantically more accessible structure precedes the more difficult one. This finding is consistent with S+odowicz's (2007: 127) remark that complementation is used very often in Turkish. It is also consistent with the results of the TSST, as will be seen in Figure 9.8, that the highest scores were obtained for complementation, the results of which will be discussed in the following section.

Comprehension of complex structures by hearing impaired Turkish children

The suffixation requirements on verbals that act as verbs of subordinate clauses as well as connecting devices for the subordinate clause to the main clause must place high demands on children. Data on acquisition of Turkish show that '… the means for expressing case relations are acquired rapidly and without error by Turkish children. Before the age of 2, the entire system of agglutinative morphology on nominals has been mastered. On the other hand, the means for subordination and complementation are not easily acquired at all, and 5-year-olds are still sorting out the various participial and nominalized forms for clause and sentence embedding' (Slobin, 1986: 273–274). This is quite challenging for Turkish children as Slobin observed, yet even more so for those with hearing impairment, who have to deal with the short auditory duration of particles in the form of suffixes. Word order is also more complicated in subordination, yet the hearing impaired children under study were using these structures in their spoken language. Whether they were up to the challenge of a test for comprehension of sentences containing complementation, subordination and passivization was the purpose of the next investigation.

Earlier studies indicated that deaf children's productions and grammaticality judgments of sentences containing complex structures such as complementation, relative clauses or passive voice were significantly poorer than those of hearing children of even younger ages (Bamford & Mentz, 1979; Boothe *et al.*, 1981; Brannon & Murry, 1966; Kretschmer & Kretschmer, 1978; Power & Quigley, 1973; Quigley *et al.*, 1974a, 1976b; Tur-Kaspa & Dromi, 1998). A study by Tüfekçioğlu (2009a, in progress) examined hearing impaired Turkish students' comprehension of sentences that each contained complex structures of complementation, relativization or passivization.

The three subtests of the *TSST* (Tüfekçioğlu, 2009a, in progress) were administered to the children under study. The test was also administered to a control group of hearing children, aged between 7;7 and 10;8 years. Since work on the test is still in progress, only the results for normally hearing children up to the age of 10;8 are available at the time of writing this chapter. All were students at a public primary or secondary school in the neighborhood.

Figures 9.8 and 9.9 display the results of the complementation, relativization and passivization subtests, each one being part of a receptive language measure employing sentences of a moderate degree of complexity. The subtests required the comprehension of a test sentence with the target structure, and four multiple-choice short sentences of which three distractor sentences are designed to be perceived as correct if a 'surface order reading' strategy or a 'connecting the nearest NP with the VP' strategy is used as reported in earlier studies or if the test sentence's morphology for complementation and subordination is not understood by the child. The test was challenging for these children as well as for their normally hearing counterparts, as the scores show. The test was also administered to 12 college-level students to check the key and level of the test. The average scores of college-level students for the subtest for complements was 97%, ranging between 94% and 100%; for relative clauses 92.6%, ranging between 92% and 94%; and for sentences in the passive voice 95.6%,

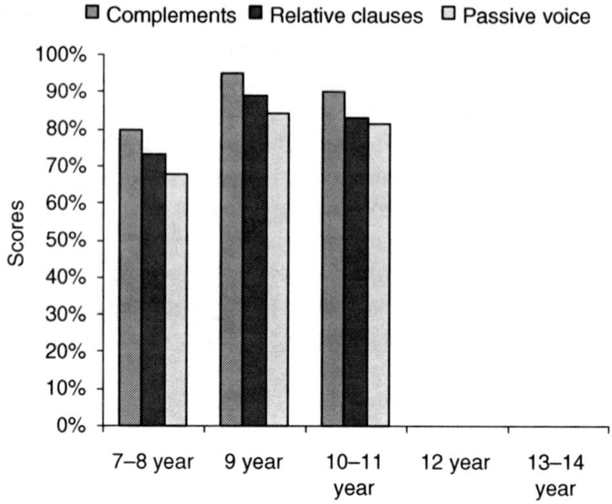

Figure 9.8 Performance scores of hearing children on the TSST ($N = 74$)

ranging between 94% and 97%. For this test group, the highest scores were obtained for complements, followed by relative clauses and then the passive voice.

Figure 9.8 shows the average percentile scores for hearing students for each subtest as a function of their chronological age. Figure 9.9 shows individual scores for six of the eight hearing impaired children under

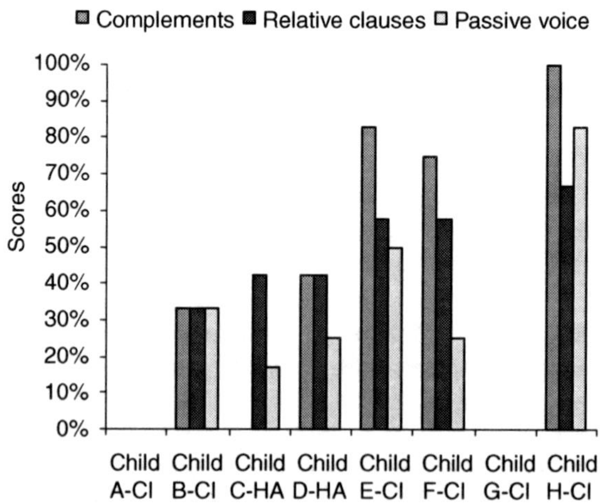

Figure 9.9 Individual performance scores for profoundly hearing impaired children on the TSST ($N = 6$)

study. Two of them, Child A and Child G, moved elsewhere at the time of testing and therefore did not participate in this study. All the participants in the control group scored above chance on all sentence types. Lower average scores were found on the relativization and passivization tests. This analysis shows that on each test, the percentile scores for the normal hearing children are systematically higher for the older children than for the younger children; the normally hearing children scored lower than the college-level students, as expected, since they are younger.

The low scores of the hearing impaired children B, C and D are consistent with their performance on the verbals, that is, minimal usage. The scores of the older children E, F and H, who use cochlear implants and who have been in the educational program for a longer period of time, are relatively higher than those of the younger hearing impaired children. It should be noted that the oldest child had maximum scores on complementation, which is higher than some of the hearing children. As seen in Figures 9.8 and 9.9, although the average scores for the normally hearing children are higher than that for the hearing impaired children of the study, the older hearing impaired children are within the same range for complementation. The oldest child's score for the complementation subtest was at ceiling level, showing a performance equal to or better than the normally hearing group of age 10;8 years, and this was true for the passive voice as well. On relativization, the oldest child was similar to 7–8-year-old normally hearing children.

This study presents several interesting findings. Higher scores found for complementation are consistent with the natural language used by adults and the fact that complementation is used often in Turkish (Rodowicz, 2007). Slobin's finding that Turkish children develop relative clauses later (Slobin, 1986) is also consistent with the performance of the control groups of (1) normally hearing children and (2) normally hearing young adults. The relative level of performance of the hearing impaired group compared against the normally hearing children shows a much better performance than what Quigley and his colleagues have reported in earlier studies. Although the tests were not the same in kind, still they should be regarded as measuring the same construct. Considering the performances of the normally hearing children as well as the college-level students, the task was somewhat difficult, even for the normally hearing ones, as only a few displayed ceiling-level scores.

Hearing impaired Turkish children's comprehension of relative clauses as tested with the subtest of the TSST shows lower scores compared to the complementation subtest. In his cross-linguistic studies with Turkish children, Slobin (1986) found much less use of relative clauses in young Turkish children's speech samples compared with American children's speech samples recorded in similar settings. He also collected samples of conversations between Turkish adults and found 118 relative clause in

English and 49 in Turkish. In both age groups, English speakers used relative clauses more than twice as much as Turkish speakers. Slobin's data showed that Turkish children learned to use relative clauses considerably later than their English-speaking age peers. This relatively late acquisition is consistent with the infrequent use of relative clauses by Turkish adults when speaking among themselves but also when conversing with children.

The scores were lowest for passive voice constructions. These findings have parallels with the Power and Quigley (1973) study, which also reported lower scores for deaf students in the comprehension of passive sentences. Apparently, hearing impaired children have difficulty recognizing the marker for the passive in the Turkish language, namely *–Il*, as in *yapıldı* (do PASS+past3rdper). Another difficulty must be the reversal of the canonical SOV order of Turkish into OSV order as in the following sentences: *Adam kadını kovaladı (SOV) (The man chased the woman)* >>> *Kadın adam tarafından kovalandı (OSV) (The woman was chased by the man) or Kadın kovalandı (The woman was chased).* Power and Quigley (1973: 8) supplied information on hearing children, based on data from research with normally hearing English-speaking children that the passive voice is a relatively difficult structure for young children to learn and its comprehension and production may not be fully mastered until the age of eight or nine years.

These data demonstrate that the utilization of a strong auditory–oral educational program together with effective use of amplification at an early age, and specifically the use of cochlear implants, enable children with profound hearing loss to obtain comprehension and production skills for complex structures that exceed the levels reported by previous research with English-speaking (Power & Quigley, 1973; Quigley & King, 1980) or Hebrew-speaking hearing impaired children (Friedmann & Szterman, 2005; Tur-Kaspa & Dromi, 1998).

Morphosyntactic errors of eight hearing impaired Turkish children

The investigation of hearing impaired children's comprehension of syntactic structures considered only complementation, relativization and passivization, rather than an analysis of errors (Tüfekçioğlu, 2009a, in progress). Another study conducted at the same time focused on morphosyntactic errors from the perspective of correct grammatical usage (Tüfekçioğlu, 2009c). Analysis for grammatical correctness involved identifying errors in the spoken language productions of the eight hearing impaired children under study. An *error unit* was defined after Hughes *et al.* (1997: 253) as 'the omission, inappropriate use, or overuse of a language variable'. The grammatical correctness of word order, of the ordering of a number of suffixes and appropriate use of all markings in these language samples are judged against adult language. Error units were coded as shown and Table 9.1 summarizes data on grammatical errors of the eight children under study.

The errors are shown as the percentage of errors of the total morpheme count for each individual child. Since Turkish is a morphologically complex language with case suffixation, as well as affixed particles marking the functions of voice, modality, negation, aspect, tense, mood, person and number (Aksu-Koç, 1986; Underhill, 1986), the ratio of errors to the total output of morphemes was considered to be a more valid calculation when comparing one child with another who had a different amount of output.

The results of the analysis showed that the children were using the suffixes and inflections as the grammar of Turkish dictates, with minimal errors, the highest being 4.7% of that child's total morpheme count. The most frequent error type occurring *across* children, in order from the most frequent to the least (the highest percentage of error for an individual for each type is given in brackets) was: omission of inflections (3.5%), tied with fragmented (unfinished) sentences (4.3%), verb tense tied with possessive markings (4.7%) and subject–verb agreement in number (2.8%), plural markings (2.6%) tied with redundant inflections (1.2%). Those errors that had a ratio of less than 1% are not included in this listing in the interest of brevity. Table 9.1 and also the above listing show that the percentage of each type of error never exceeds approximately 5%, which should be considered quite low considering the long history of deaf students' errors consistently reported as abundant.

Word order: The language productions observed in the younger hearing impaired children's spoken language samples, specifically children A, B, C and D in the present study, were dominated by SV and SOV simple syntactic constructions in Turkish canonical word order (Tüfekçioğlu, 2009c). The earlier study also evidenced such an order, although MLUs were shorter and constructions simpler (Tüfekçioğlu, 1989). Tur-Kaspa and Dromi (1998) had a similar finding, except that the word order of Hebrew is characterized as SVO and their subjects displayed this order. Word-order violations were rarely observed in the present Turkish samples.

Omission of a central structure: Tur-Kaspa and Dromi (1998) reported the omission of a central node of a sentence such as the subject or the main verb to be a serious syntactic deficiency and that it was the most frequently recorded error in the productions of their Hebrew subjects. Such an omission was not observed in this sample of hearing impaired Turkish children.

Order of inflections: No errors or minimal errors were observed in the categories of order of inflections.

Negation: No errors or minimal errors were observed in the use of negation in simple sentences.

Table 9.1 Morphosyntactic errors of eight hearing impaired Turkish children

	Child A-CI		*Child B-CI*		*Child C-HA*		*Child D-HA*		*Child E-CI*		*Child F-CI*		*Child G-CI*		*Child H-CI*	
	2007	**2008**	**2007**	**2008**	**2007**	**2008**	**2007**	**2008**	**2007**	**2008**	**2007**	**2008**	**2007**	**2008**	**2007**	**2008**
WO	0	0.3	0	0	0	0	0	0	0.8	0	0	0	0.2	0	0	0
IO	0	0	0	0	0	0	0	0	0	0	0	0	0	0	0	0
SV	0	0	1.5	0	2.8	0.7	0.8	0.6	0.1	0	0.3	2.3	0.9	1.8	0	0.1
O-W	1.1	0	1.9	0	0.5	0.3	0.2	0.2	0	0	0	0.1	0	0.2	0.1	0.1
O-In	2.6	0.3	3.5	0.8	1.6	0.7	1.6	0.4	0.1	0.3	0.3	0.1	1.3	0.6	0.3	0.4
RI	0.3	0.3	0	0.2	0	0.7	0.8	0	0.8	0.3	1.1	0	0.2	0.6	0.6	0.7
VT	1.5	0.9	1.1	0	1.6	2.6	1.3	0.4	0	0	0	0	0.2	0.2	0	0.2
PL	2.6	0	0	0	2.2	0	0	0.2	0	0	0.1	0.3	0.9	0.2	0.1	0
PS	1.5	0.9	4.6	0	0	0	1.1	1.3	0	0.3	0.5	0.3	1.1	1.1	0	0.1
Neg	0	0	0	0	0	0	0	0	0.1	0	0	0	0	0	0	0
FRAG	0.7	0.9	4.2	0.2	3.9	2.6	1.1	0.6	0.1	0	0.1	0.5	2	0.9	0.8	0
SE	0	0	0	0	0	0	0.2	0.4	0.5	0.1	0.9	0	0.2	0	0.1	0.1

WO: word-order error; IO: inflectional-order error; SV: subject–verb agreement error; O-W: omission of key word error; O-In: omission of obligatory inflection error; RI: redundant inflection error; VT: verb tense error; Pl: plural error; Ps: possessive error; Neg: negation; Frag: fragment error; SE: series error-connective overused.

Fragmented sentences: Some fragmented sentences were seen in older children when producing complementized or relativized clauses. It seemed that once the clause was produced, the child came to a stop, possibly to collect his or her thoughts for the connecting clause, but at that point the teacher would offer a comment or a 'Hımm' sound to motivate the child to go on. Because the criteria for transcription of utterances ruled 'a stop of two seconds' or 'a turn to the other speaker' as utterance boundaries, these types of utterances were coded as fragments. In a real-life situation when conversing with the same child, one does not take so much notice of these rules of boundaries and the dialogue seems more fluent.

Tense and aspect in verbs: Apart from verbal tense and aspect acquisition being a learning process, one other explanation for the relatively higher number of errors in this category may be that the adult and the child were taking different perspectives in interpreting a scene of events. The situation from the adult point of view might not be a shared situation from the child's perspective or vice versa. 'That is, situation types are associated with different aspectual forms and meanings in different languages. Speakers of a given language relate an actual situation to an idealized situation type by using the linguistic forms, or, aspect markers associated with that situation-type in their language, and thereby present it as a particular instance of it' (Aksu-Koç, 1988a, 1988b: 180). Aksu-Koç (1988a, 1988b: 178) in that respect describes the three early acquired inflections and, in the language of the children under study, the most frequently used inflections as follows: '*-DI* with change of state verbs in contexts where an action or event reaches completion', which in this study is identified as simple past/past of direct experience, '*-Iyor* with activity verbs in reference to ongoing processes in time, and *-mIş* with stative verbs in reference to existing states or in narrative frames'. Most of the errors coded under 'verb tenses' were the result of disagreement on the inflections used in the teacher's question or comment and the child's reply to it. The coding for errors followed a very stringent criterion and searched for agreement, taking the teacher's corrections as a clue as well. It might be possible that, at least in some of the dialogues, the teacher may not have taken into consideration that the child could have had a different viewpoint as to the state of the event as an ongoing process or an event that reached completion from the child's perspective, or in the case of *-mIş* inflection used in reference to existing states as described by Aksu-Koç. We would know this only if the analysis had been carried out at the time of the dialogue. The coding system marked it as an error each time an inconsistency occurred. After the conversation came to an end, there was no possibility of checking it through probing questions to determine whether the child was taking a different viewpoint or if it was indeed an erroneous inflection. One point that has implications for educators/therapists is that when working or conversing with a child, extra care ought to be taken to be sensitive and check which viewpoint the child has taken as he/she tells his/her story of the scene, and then proceed with corrections.

Subject–verb agreement: A possible explanation as to why children and, sometimes even adults, use subject–verb agreement in number inconsistently is the many – more than 20 – rules (Gencan, 2007: 126–132) that govern the proper use of number in subject–verb agreement in Turkish. Perhaps the child needs more time to construct his/her knowledge in relation to this rather perplexing grammar rule of Turkish.

Possessive markings and plural markings: The errors in marking possessive and plural signify a stage that represents a significant developmental phenomenon, because, as Cazden (1968: 436) pointed out, 'systematic errors and overgeneralizations provide convincing evidence that the child has a productive rule'. The same viewpoint is in fact also true with omission of inflections and redundant inflections.

Omission of inflections and redundant inflections: Omission of inflections was mostly observed in younger children, which would be expected developmentally. A quantitative examination of morphosyntactic errors in the structure of the language system of older children showed that there was an increase in the number of redundant inflections where a decrease would be expected as children had more time in education and with device use. A qualitative examination of errors of older children revealed that the structure of their language system was more complex than the structures used by younger children, which was consistent with the results of the MSL measure and the syntax test. It appears from these data that, as the child's MSL grows as it did in this study, the diversity of syntactic constructions in spontaneous language also grows. For example, in Turkish, verbal nouns that function as predicates in complement clauses 'retain the ability to express negation' (S+odowicz, 2007: 128). Across eight children, a qualitative analysis showed that there was only one error in negation in simple sentence constructions for both years. This showed that the children had mastered negation. However, errors of negation were present in complex syntactic constructions. This could have been described statistically, but erroneously, in the formulation of: 'as age increases, errors of negation (and others) increase'. Similar types of errors occurred in the marking of verbals for possessor agreement and case. The errors were made in the strings that constituted subordination and embeddedness in the sentences produced. In fact, the older children were initiating advances in semantic–morphosyntactic communication complexity. This pattern of development recalls Piaget's cognitive theory and explanation of 'accommodation' and 'assimilation'. It was as if the children, during their efforts to establish the new structure, went through a phase of restructuring, which defaulted the system for the time being – hence the increase in number of errors while during this phase lasted. Once a structure was established, as seen in the simple sentences in which almost no grammatical errors occurred any longer, assimilation had taken place in the linguistic database. It is the hypothesis of this author that the same kind of incorporation process is expected to happen at an upper level now with these markings, resulting in fewer and fewer errors, given time but most importantly opportunities for meaningful interactive communication that stimulates the reception and use of these constructions at a semantic–syntactic level that the child is ready to receive and accommodate.

Conclusion

It is well documented that most hearing impaired children have errors of omission, substitution and redundancies in their spoken and/or written language. This research work documents that education in a progressive auditory–oral program enables hearing impaired Turkish children to develop a spoken language system that also contains the more complex structures such as complementation and subordination with complementized and/or relativized subordinate clauses. The morphosyntactic errors present in these constructions can in no way be described as bizarre, aberrant or deviant. In fact, the children display very few errors relative to their output, and the errors that do exist represent attempts at more complex structures. The children's comprehension scores are consistent with this finding, in that the older children's scores are identical or similar to the scores of children who are three years younger. This also indicates normal language development in the sense that children are developing comprehension abilities of these complex structures in a similar order to hearing children, as well as developing production abilities.

There is, however, another picture to be portrayed, since there are other hearing impaired children in the country, who are receiving different types of intervention or who are unfortunately not receiving any intervention at all. The case of one child in his late teens will help to illustrate this. This case is described here as an example representing a large number of hearing impaired children educated, as he was, in schools for the deaf and thereafter in vocational schools for the deaf until the age of 18 (Tüfekçioğlu, 2009a, in progress). This case will be coded here as Child M, who is a prelingual, possibly congenitally hearing impaired youth with bilateral profound hearing loss. Child M's father requested an evaluation of his child and a second opinion for considering cochlear implantation. Child M started wearing hearing aids only at age 16. Upon evaluation, he exhibited no perception of speech, a very limited spoken and written language consisting only of single words of a limited vocabulary, no use of syntax or morphology and no evidence of comprehension of reading even at the primary level. He communicated with his friends with signs and with his parents and others by writing in single words. Otherwise, he was intelligent and well behaved, and his father announced proudly that he was one of the best students at the school. This was possibly because Child M had excellent memory and could copy writing without comprehension. It was not possible to get a spontaneous spoken language sample based on conversation; therefore no further analysis was carried out. He was tested for comprehension of syntactic structures with the TSST and scored below chance level. He was not granted candidacy for implantation on grounds of minimal language and no experience of auditory stimulation.

The purpose of including him in this summary of recent research on the language characteristics of hearing impaired Turkish children is to portray the other end of the continuum. İÇEM, the auditory–oral program, is recognized in Turkey for providing the best practices for these children and their parents. There may be isolated cases of other excellent practices as well. However, this researcher had no access to them and therefore İÇEM students' language was described in these pages as to what might be possible for Turkish children at present with similar histories. This may constitute one end of the continuum of possibilities. Child M's condition signifies the other end of the continuum, and one can expect to find many variations in between, perhaps most of them displaying the language characteristics described in the earlier section; those that were observed in earlier studies of deaf children in the United States and United Kingdom, and possibly in other countries as well. The majority of hearing impaired Turkish children fall somewhere in the lower-mid section of this continuum.

The research work in relation to the auditory–oral sample summarized in this section did not provide a detailed and sophisticated statistical analysis that would give grounds for more definite conclusions, but rather data that point to some specific issues in relation to the type of intervention for possible positive outcomes, that positive outcomes are possible, and also possible errors in the process of acquisition. It is the hope of this author to have shown what are or might prove to be problems when dealing with the language development of children with hearing impairments acquiring morphologically complex languages, but most importantly, that even the profoundly hearing impaired children can and do develop language at a level of complexity that was never before possible.

Because the sample of children in this study was limited to those in a strong auditory–oral educational setting that utilizes progressive teaching methods, it is unknown whether or not these results would generalize to children who are in settings that utilize other language-teaching methods, such as TC or bilingual or structured oral, or to children with or without cochlear implants who are in mainstream settings that utilize more traditional teaching methods.

More than ever, professionals in this field are in a position to welcome the days to come, because research indicates what type of intervention works for better outcomes, and technological advances such as neonatal hearing screening, modern hearing aids and cochlear implants make these improvements possible. All that is needed is the implementation of these practices at the earliest possible age for all hearing impaired children.

Acknowledgments

The author gratefully acknowledges Yasemin Yolal, Ayşecan Tüfekçioğlu and Gökçen Abalı for their assistance in data tabulation at various phases and Gökçen Abalı for her assistance in the graphics work. She would also like to thank her colleague Associate Professor Ümit Girgin for her outstanding work at İÇEM as the principal of the school and the staff and students at İÇEM who participated in the study.

Notes

1. Parts of the list were adapted from Quigley and King (1980: 340–343).
2. Findings relating to children with cochlear implants are marked with 'ci' abbreviation.

Chapter 10

Characteristics of Aphasia in Turkish

İLKNUR MAVİŞ

Introduction

Most researchers in the field accept the premise that the patterns of language breakdown in brain-damaged patients reflect some degeneration of a universal language processing system. On the other hand, the 'same' aphasic syndromes look very different from one language to another, which makes some scientists attempt to distinguish between the universal symptoms of the disorder and those that are language specific. Those who focus on cross-linguistic research on aphasia, while searching for language specificity, base their studies either on *Syndrome-dominant models* (e.g. The Closed-class Theory of Agrammatism) or on *Language-dominant models* (e.g. The Competition Model). Syndrome-dominant models predict differences between patient groups, whereas language-dominant models predict differentiation as a function of language type (Bates & Wulfeck, 1989).

It is only very recently that researchers and clinicians have documented the language specificity of aphasia symptoms. The characteristic manifestations of aphasia symptoms in 14 languages (African American English, Afrikaans, Basque, Catalan, Czech, Farsi, Finnish, Friulian, Greek, Hebrew, Hungarian, Polish, Spanish and Swedish) have illustrated how the symptoms are interpreted in terms of specific traits linked to the language spoken by the person with aphasia (Paradis, 2001).

This cross-linguistic evidence has shown that the relationship between symptoms and mechanisms is much less direct than that which one might infer from the literature on aphasic speakers of English. The Competition Model, for example, accounts for findings across an array of different languages that vary widely in the nature and richness of their morphological systems (Bates & MacWhinney, 1987).

Agglutinative languages (e.g. Hungarian, Basque, etc.) are said to be an excellent testing ground for research in some of the key issues in lexical and/or morphological access. Turkish, being rich in morphology, is another agglutinative language and much research has been undertaken on Turkish stems of two major categories: nouns and verbs. To each of these categories, there belong distinct inflectional paradigms and sets of derivational suffixes, all of which are strictly specified for affixation to their own particular category (Haig, 2003).

There has been a debate on the underlying disorder of agrammatic production in which explanations with respect to a syntactic/morphological deficit or a limitation in processing capacity have been proposed. Under either type, a deficit may lead to the reception or production of incomplete (or ungrammatical) sentences and agrammatic performance, mainly restricted to concrete nouns with high frequency. Several studies have reported that Broca's aphasics display specific deficits in the production of main verbs, when compared to their production of object names. These patients often omit verbs in their spontaneous speech. A complementary profile has also been reported for fluent patients, including Wernicke's aphasics and some anomic patients. These patients display fewer problems with verbs and more severe problems in the production of names for common objects in their spontaneous speech, resulting in an overuse of pronominal forms and circumlocutionary frames (Chen & Bates, 1998). However, the distributed lexical access in patients with aphasia is often not so clear cut as is proposed in the literature since studies in Turkish aphasia present varying results for noun and verb dissociations.

Agrammatism in Turkish

The studies we mention in this chapter have focused on the characteristics of Turkish agrammatism and paragrammatism as compared to the prototypical Broca's or Wernicke's aphasia in other languages (especially in English). The pioneering work on aphasia in Turkish was done by Slobin (1991) who studied 7 Broca's and 10 Wernicke's aphasics. Patients were assessed by a battery of measures, which included a naming test, a lexical comprehension test, a sentence comprehension test and spontaneous speech elicited through the use of a 'cookie theft' picture from Boston Diagnostic Aphasia Examination (BDAE) (Goodglass & Kaplan, 1983). The battery of measures also included the given/new task presenting nine series of three pictures each. The task included the assessment of two subject-verb (SV) (a bunny is crying/a boy is crying), three subject-verb-object (SVO) (a monkey is eating a banana/a boy is kicking a dog/a girl is eating an apple), two subject-verb-locative (SVL) (a dog is in a car/a cat is on a chair) and two subject-verb-object-dative (SVOD) structures (a lady is giving a present to a girl/a cat is giving a flower to a boy). The data showed the appropriate use of nominal morphology for both groups. Although produced in a limited set of verb forms, Broca's patients' verb suffixes were contextually appropriate. Wernicke's patients used a wide range of verb forms, all morphosyntactically correct. The basic subject-object-verb

(SOV) word order of Turkish was observed to be preserved in fluent and non-fluent aphasics and indeed may have been overused by aphasic patients (especially Broca's), when these data are compared with the word order variations produced by the control group. In Slobin's article, it was reported that both study groups were quite similar with regard to subject omission and locative omission, both of which are grammatical and pragmatically normal in Turkish. Nouns were correctly marked with suffixes in Turkish where a case marked form was required. What is of interest among the results was that Broca's aphasics omitted verbs more frequently than Wernicke's aphasics and normal individuals; second, Wernicke's aphasics omitted both direct and indirect objects more frequently than the control group. Slobin (1991: 151–155) concluded that 'the grammatical features of aphasic speech in Turkish do not conform well to the standard textbook descriptions of these two patient groups' and he added that 'if agrammatism is defined as the absence of closed class elements, it is clear that Turkish patients of aphasia cannot be classified as agrammatic'. Studies on other inflectional languages (such as Finnish, Polish, Serbo-Croat and Icelandic) also confirmed the preservation of case marking, as was mentioned in Menn and Obler (1990: 1370). There, Menn and Obler (1990: 1370) claimed that 'the features of agrammatism, especially the omission of bound grammatical morphemes and the use of infinitive verb form, appear to vary in accord with differences in the grammars of different languages'.

Subsequent studies on aphasia have extended the investigation of agrammatism to 'closed class elements' and 'noun–verb' production in Turkish (Maviş, 2000/2004). The case study was designed to observe the expressive language of two patients with aphasia in 15–20-min intervals of free conversation. The subjects of this study, a 70 year-old male (MA) and a 55 year-old female (KK), were selected from among the inpatients at the Neurology service of the University Hospital. They were diagnosed as mild to moderate Broca's aphasics, whose sub-cortical regions may possibly not have been affected. The patients were observed for five months from the onset, during which time they met with a speech and language pathologist (SLP) once a month. The patients did not wish to attend therapy sessions for various reasons, but were scheduled to meet the SLP each month who was to follow them during the spontaneous recovery period. At the end of the fifth month, it was observed that at each of the five data points, KK and MA produced more verbs than nouns, but in varying proportions (Table 10.1).

The table shows that both KK and MA produce more verbs than nouns in their spontaneous speech, but there is not a large difference in the proportions of verbs and nouns.

The second task in the same study was designed to require simple SV utterances to be produced, including a noun that bears an appropriate case marking in relation to 20 pictured semantic relations. The two patients were tested each month. Below is the speech sample between the patient

Table 10.1 The distribution of noun and verb productions of the patients over five months

	First month (March)	*Second month*	*Third month*	*Fourth month*	*Fifth month (July)*
CASE-1 (KK)	%	%	%	%	%
Noun	7.06	2.51	5.65	8.08	5.49
Verb	14.3	6.91	9.8	13.5	8.4
CASE-2 (MA)					
Noun	1.61	4.3	8.3	7.5	7.1
Verb	2.9	6.1	12.2	13.3	9.9

and the therapist during the second month of elicitation. The expected sentence was 'adam araba-*y-ı* itiyor' ('the man pushes *the car*', with the required accusative case marker).

P: araba
P: car (nominative use).
T: evet..araba..adam böyle yapıyor (arabayı itme hareketini yapar)
T: yes..car..the man is doing like that (animates the action)
P: evet, biliyorum..arkadan..adam..itiyor
P: yes, I know..at back.. man…pushing
T: evet..neyi?
T: good ..what?
P: arabayı
P: the car (accusative use in Turkish)

The number of correct responses for the expected cases produced out of the 20 trials in the five-month period did not exceed 25%. However low this amount was, it was concluded that KK correctly produced the accusative, locative and ablative cases more often than the other two cases.

The performance differences between the patients might be due to factors related to their individual characteristics: age, perhaps gender and/or lesion localizations. Willmes and Poeck (1993) claim that possible agrammatic symptoms become apparent in the majority of patients during the chronic rather than the acute phase of recovery, that is, not earlier than six months post-onset (Springer *et al.*, 2000); consequently, the data collected from the task was limited to the early onset period during the acute phase of recovery.

Another study done by Maviş and Tunçer (2007) presented data in favor of noun retention, and therefore, did not support the previous

Table 10.2 The frequency of nouns, verbs and suffixes for the study groups

Groups	*Total word*	*Total noun*	*Total verb*	*Related noun*	*Related verb*	*Nominal suffix*	*Verb suffix*	*Total suffix*
Control ($n = 21$)	1334	321	229	258	152	231	168	399
Non-fluent ($n = 12$)	126	53	21	39	14	14	36	50
Fluent ($n = 11$)	497	69	75	40	37	27	24	51

Type token ratio of the nouns: number of related nouns divided by the total number of nouns.
Type token ratio of the verbs: number of related verbs divided by the total number of verbs.

results. The study was undertaken with a larger number of patients with aphasia. The subjects of the study consisted of 23 aphasic adults (11 fluent and 12 non-fluent) and 21 non-aphasic adults. The purpose of the study was to find out the differences between aphasic or non-aphasic adults in terms of content units and grammatical morpheme production through an 'accident' theme picture description task (Topbaş, 2004/5: Item 6). Also, the frequency of picture relevant nouns and verbs was compared to the total word production (Table 10.2).

A significant difference was found between aphasic and non-aphasic adults; that is, the frequency of nouns, verbs and inflections produced by the non-aphasic adults was, as hypothesized, greater than those of adults with aphasia. Contrary to the findings of the earlier study, the type token ratio of the picture-related nouns for non-fluent aphasic adults was 31% (it was 11% for verbs). The type token ratio of the picture-related nouns for fluent adults with aphasia, on the other hand, was 8% for nouns and 7.4% for verbs. The type token ratio of the verbs for the control group was 11.3% (almost the same as the non-fluent group) and 19.3% for the nouns. The non-parametric Kruskal–Wallis analysis found significance between the groups for all the variables in the study. The fluent and non-fluent groups with aphasia also differed from each other, especially in total word ($U = 17.5$; $z = -2.992$; $p < 0.01$) and total verb productions ($U = 18, 50$; $z = -2.953$; $p < 0.01$), as calculated by a Mann–Whitney U test.

The dominant verb forms in the picture elicitation procedure for Broca's aphasic patients in the study were 'present progressive (-yor) and non-witnessed past (-mış)', which were the same for the Wernicke's patients. Regardless of the type of aphasia, the patients favored genitive/possessive and plural endings more often, whereas they rarely used ablative forms. LaPointe (1985) reported on the production of verb forms in an agrammatic output, both in spontaneous speech and in sentence construction task. His conclusion was that agrammatics show a strong tendency to use less marked verb forms, that is, infinitive (V), V + *s*, V + *ing* and *be* V + *ing* (for English). Saffran *et al.* (1989) found more or less the same phenomena as did LaPointe; however, Bastiaanse *et al.* (1995) showed that these results might be task dependent.

What we deduced from the last two studies was that the patients did not demonstrate omissions of nominal or verbal cases as long as they retrieved the required nouns or verbs; therefore, they cannot be called agrammatics in this sense. Second, the patients used more verbs than nouns in spontaneous speech but more nouns than verbs in the picture tasks. Bastiaanse *et al.* (1995) found that the verbs belonging to the pictures are more problematic in action naming tasks. Task-dependent results were also reported by Hillis and Caramazza (1994) on the performance of a neurologically impaired patient who made far more errors on nouns than on verbs in spoken output tasks, but made far more errors on verbs than on nouns in written input tasks.

Originally, it was believed that verb retrieval was impaired in agrammatic patients (Bates *et al.*, 2001); however, in recent years, researchers have preferred to be cautious in their opinions due to the findings of subsequent studies. The presumed distortion concerning the highly preserved verbs in the aforementioned Turkish aphasic patients might be due to an inappropriate instrument of assessment or the misdiagnosis of patients. Yet when considering Turkish with its specific typology, one can predict why verbs and nouns are somehow preserved in an aphasic language. This prediction gets its support from child acquisition in Turkish.

In verbs, there are more inflectional categories than in nouns in Turkish. Despite this, children acquiring Turkish develop verb forms quickly (Aksu-Koç *et al.*, 2007). For example, the mini paradigm criterion for verbs and their inflections has been observed to be acquired for Turkish between age is 1;7 and 2;4, with the first verb oppositions at 1;5, whereas for English these do not occur until after 2;5. Further, in Turkish, nouns and verbs constitute the largest categories in parental language input. Analyses conducted on the speech directed at four Turkish children between ages is 1;1 and 2;0 (including 15,000 utterances produced by parents and other adults) showed that the distribution of verbs is regular and better than chance according to the immediate contexts. In noun distribution, however, there is no significant regularity in any context (Aksu-Koç & Ketrez, 2003b). The developmental curve for the mean size of the paradigm for verbs is far steeper for Turkish (showing faster development). This is mostly related to language-specific properties, such as the transparency of inflections and the salience of nouns and verbs in Turkish sentences. For example, verbs appear particularly in the highly salient sentence final position in the SOV word order in Turkish (Kauschke *et al.*, 2007). Kauschke *et al.* (2007: 1047) added that regular and transparent verb morphology increases the accessibility of verbs, as does a pragmatic focus on actions in spontaneous speech. Consequently, in Turkish, there is less of a difference in the abilities of children to produce and perceive verbs than in other languages (Broschart, 1991).

The results of the data with Turkish patients indicate the retention of nominal and verbal case markings whenever they are able to retrieve the lexical item; that is, the majority of verbs and nouns produced by Turkish patients were affixed even though retrieval was low. Word form frequency is likely to influence the production of verb and noun inflections in agrammatic aphasia (Druks & Carroll, 2005). Based on the results of their study, Miceli *et al.* (1984) state that the agrammatics' difficulties with verbs occur due to problems in retrieving the correct lexical form of the verb from the lexicon.

Additional speculative considerations about noun and verb production were suggested for agrammatics in the literature. Although studies on the production of verbs in aphasia are relatively rare, some researchers claimed that verbs taking *more* arguments (such as unaccusative) are *more difficult* for agrammatic patients to produce (Luzzatti & Chierchia, 2002). Some have found that Broca's aphasic patients could name transitive verbs better than intransitive verbs (Davidoff & Masterson, 1996; Jonkers & Bastiaanse, 1998; Jonkers, 2000), whereas some proposed just the opposite difference both in Broca's patients and in language acquisition (De Bleser & Kauschke, 2003). In Maviş and Tunçer's study, verbs were not considered in terms of their frequency, neither were the types of verbs considered.

So far, it seems that having more aphasic participants in research made the results more consistent with data from other languages; that is, nonfluent patients seemed to preserve nouns more than verbs. It is not evident yet whether task demands might have made this difference. We should consider further if the data elicited through spontaneous conversation or more structured picture tasks influenced the difference in noun and verb productions. It is expected that patients should feel freer to talk on given topics that are familiar to them or of daily interest to them in spontaneous speech samples, whereas they would be more limited by the required vocabulary in picture elicitations. In fact, the selected picture themes could be another factor that might have affected their productions.

Considering that patients demonstrated a favorable tendency toward noun-listing for the 'accident' picture theme, another theme (hospital) was added in the following study. A group of children was also included in order to revisit the regression hypothesis (Maviş, 2008). This hypothesis is another issue which is currently being readdressed in the literature. Jakobson (1971) stated that aphasic regression has proved to be a mirror of the child's acquisition of speech sounds and exemplifies the child's linguistic development in reverse. Furthermore, instead of being solely confined to phonemic patterns, he proposed to extend the search for the order of acquisitions and losses to the grammatical system. The hypothesis claims that certain vocabulary items learned at the final stages of the learning process tend to be forgotten first. De Bot and Weltens (1995) underlined that this vocabulary is supposed to be lost fairly easily, as are syntactic aspects of a language that have been acquired late in the process. While Caramazza (1994) assumes that there is a noun bias in language acquisition (De Bleser & Kauschke, 2003), Cohen (1989) detected evidence for loss in the productive lexicon, especially for nouns. It was mentioned previously that early vocabularies of Turkish children are balanced between nouns and verbs (Aksu-Koç, this volume: Chapter 4). Regarding the production tendency, Küntay and Slobin (2001) reported that there is a noun bias in terms of variety, but a verb bias in terms of frequency in Turkish children.

Accordingly, the study investigated a possible correspondence between the acquisition and breakdown of the ability to name nouns, verbs and their sub-categories. In view of these considerations, children at different ages of acquisition were referred to in the study in comparison to aphasic patients in regression. The groups established for the present study were comprised of a control group of neurologically intact adults ($n = 21$), a group of typically developing children still acquiring language ($n = 15$), and a group of adults with mild to moderate aphasia ($n = 26$). The neurologically intact adults and the patients with aphasia were almost the same mean age (58;1 and 58;9, respectively), and the children ranged from 24 to 40 months old. The data, elicited through two pictures (designed with accident and hospital themes), were classified in order to measure the subjects' tendency to name picture elements. Enumerative words (EWs) consisted of the nouns and verbs produced by the participants, and content words (CWs) were the words that were relevant to the picture. The language data were compared on the basis of the amount of information conveyed in CWs (Nicholas & Brookshire, 1993).

For each speech sample, the number of words and the number of correct information units were calculated (Table 10.3).

Table 10.3 Frequency of the production of CWs and their inflections

Accident + Hospital	*CWs*				*Inflections*			
	Noun	%	*Verb*	%	*Noun*	%	*Verb*	%
Adults	77	60	52	40	544	59	371	41
Aphasics	57	65	31	35	195	49	202	51
Children	41	60	27	40	214	34	417	66

CWs are the picture-related nouns and verbs.

A one-way analysis of variance (ANOVA) analysis revealed a significant difference between the groups in terms of total CWs ($F = 29.2$ (2), $p < 0.001$). The significance was looked at for three groups: between the neurologically intact adults and the children, between neurologically intact adults and adults with aphasia, and between the adults with aphasia and the children. Accordingly, the variations were high enough to reach significant differences for noun production between the groups of participants. Similarly, the Kruskal–Wallis one-way ANOVA on ranks revealed that there was a significant difference in the total number of verbs produced by the groups ($H = 30.2$ (2), $p < 0.001$). Save for the non-significance between 'neurologically intact adults and the children' ($p > 0.05$), the differences were large enough to reach significance for the other two. Total nominal inflections appeared to be significant in the analysis ($H = 26.8$ (2), $p < 0.001$), except for the non-significant difference between the aphasics and the children in the *post hoc* test ($p > 0.05$). Total verbal inflections were significant ($H = 29.1$ (2), $p < 0.001$) as well between the aforementioned groupings.

It is obvious that the children in the study (between 24 and 40 months) were the ones who produced fewer nouns and verbs in frequency when compared to the adults and aphasics, yet children produced more noun inflections than aphasics and more verb inflections than the adults and aphasics. The data imply that verb morphology develops far faster than noun morphology in Turkish. In accordance with this claim, nouns may have a priority in lexical development, but verbs follow in development a relatively short time after. These findings seem to be parallel to the results given by Slobin and Bever (1982) on the acquisition of cases by Turkish children. Unlike children acquiring case in Indo-European languages, Turkish children already have most of the adult case system under control in both comprehension and production by 2–2;5 years of age. Slobin and Bever attribute this early mastery of case to two factors: (1) Turkish case suffixes are extremely regular and semantically transparent (e.g. there are no arbitrary distinctions based on gender and/or morphophonological class); (2) the inflections carry stress and are therefore quite easy for children to perceive. The same semantic and phonological factors may serve to 'protect' case inflections (even though fewer case endings occur in the language of brain-damaged adults, owing to a general shortage of nouns and verbs). Processing factors seem to play a major role in determining degrees of sparing and loss within the grammar. Accordingly, the findings presented so far appear to be quite as expected.

In sum, the productions of aphasic patients regarding nominal inflections did not reach significance as compared to the children. However, aphasic individuals produced much fewer inflections than did the children. What attracts attention as a result of the study was that aphasic patients produced more nouns with fewer inflections but fewer verbs with more inflections. The patients tended to list the objects or produce nominative nouns for what they saw in the pictures; yet they could not produce verbs without tense and subject inflections. As seen in the following sample, referents are not clear and a subject can be omitted, which is semantically normal; yet they do not use verbs in their infinitive forms.

Some of the aphasic speech samples elicited through picture narration are as follows:

Accident	TR	doktor, ambulans, trafik feneri, bunlar lastik, ev, adam, adam..adam..adam gidiyo, çocuklar, anne
	ENG	doctor, ambulance, traffic torch (light), these are tires, house, man....man...man is going, children, mother
Hospital	TR	Bu iğne yapıyor..bu da ikisi konuşuyo..çocuk yatakta..ayağı sarılı..dişçi
	ENG	this...injecting, this is ..both are talking, doctor.. child.. in bed..his leg bandaged...dentist
Hospital	TR	Çiçek görüyom, şırınga görüyom..boğazına bakıyo.. kırık..masa var..masada şişe var..kaşık var
	ENG	I see flower..ı see injection..looking his throat... broken (pointing to leg)..there is table..bottle on the table..there is spoon...

The most frequent nouns and verbs were very similar among the three groups. For example, in the elicitations of the picture 'accident', the adult control group and the aphasic group produced 'car, accident, police, ambulance and traffic' as the most frequent nouns. The children shared most of the words (such as car, police, ambulance and accident) with the previously mentioned groups. In the elicitations from the picture 'hospital', all three groups of participants produced 'patient, doctor, injection and flower' in common. It also was noted that the verbs highest in frequency were about the same for the adult control group and the aphasics; however, the children differed from the other groups in this respect. The children employed the verbs 'to die', 'to be broken' and 'to stop' for the accident picture and repeated some synonymous verbs for the hospital picture. In Kauschke *et al.*'s study (2007), it is obvious as well that Turkish children produced general all-purpose verbs such as 'have', 'make' or 'be' to a lesser extent rather than more specific verbs as mentioned in Maviş' study. On the other hand, studies investigating verb types claim that light verbs (by definition, specified by fewer semantic features than heavy verbs) are more difficult for agrammatics to retrieve (Gordon & Dell, 2003); however, in this study, aphasic patients produced light verbs such as var/exist, olmak/be, demek/say and the like frequently.

When the amount of nominal and verbal inflections produced was considered, the results between the groups seemed to support the regression hypothesis, most notably at the inflectional level. The average difference between the typical and atypical adults was 27% CIUs (content information units), while the average variation between the children and the aphasic group was 12% CIUs. The data verified that aphasics produced far fewer CIUs than the children; however, in the production of nominal inflections, the differences were not large enough to produce statistically meaningful significance between aphasics and developing children. On the other hand, the difference was highly significant between groups in the production of verbal inflections.

Researchers have also found that non-fluent individuals tend to have more agreement errors than omission errors in highly inflected languages (Bates, 1995). Word order and verb inflection have been investigated in several recent studies on Turkish agrammatic aphasia. In sentences with a derived word order (sentences that deviate from SOV order), patients produce both word order and morphological errors (see Yarbay-Duman *et al.*, 2007 for object scrambling (OSV); Yarbay-Duman *et al.*, 2008 for relative clauses). The data of Yarbay-Duman *et al.* (2008) on the production of relative clauses show that when Turkish agrammatic speakers fail to produce the right order, they accommodate case to the different order they produce. For example, in object relative clauses (adamın diktiği ceket/the jacket that the man has sewn), when the object moves to a post-verbal position within the noun phrase, the constituent order changes as does the case of the subject: it changes from nominative to genitive (ceketi diken adam/the man who has sewn the jacket). Apparently, there is an interaction between word order and case that Turkish agrammatic speakers are aware of when producing sentences. However, the authors suggest that the difficulties with sentence production are not restricted to problems with derived word orders (hırsızları polis vuruyor/the thieves, the policeman shoots). For example, in another study, Yarbay-Duman and Bastiaanse (2009) also show that the patients have problems with time reference, which is also reflected in participles. Not only is time reference in general difficult, but reference to *remote* structures that express the past is even more problematic for them. The authors argue that the deficit relates to an integration problem: integrating morphological (verb inflection) and semantic information is difficult for the patients.

It has long been noted that agrammatic aphasia is not a deficit which only affects the production of language but also affects its comprehension. If the grammatical symptoms of Broca's aphasia were restricted entirely to expressive language, one might accept the classic argument that 'telegraphic speech' reflects an effort to economize language (primarily because of motor problems in speech production). However, there is now a large number of studies showing that Broca's aphasics also have difficulty in a variety of receptive language tasks (if those tasks require them to rely primarily on grammatical morphemes and on various syntactic structures).

Yolcu-Kamali (2004) investigated the comprehension of several different types of sentences by Broca's aphasics using a picture-matching task. 54 sentences were used in her experiment, in which she selected types of truncated passive (adam öpülüyor>The man is being kissed), the object relative clause (Burada bir kadının öptüğü bir adam var>here, there is a man whom a woman is kissing), the subject relative clause (Burada bir adamı öpen bir kadın var>here, there is a woman who is kissing a man) and the object fronted sentence (OSV: Adamı kadın öpüyor>The woman is kissing the man) alongside the canonical active SOV sentence types (Kadın adamı öpüyor>The woman is kissing the man). The subjects of the study were six men and a woman (with 2.5 year post-onset) between the ages of 49 and 68 and a matched number of control subjects.

The findings indicate that for all participants, the most difficulty occurs with the OSV sentence type. The comprehension of the second most problematic type, the passive, varied among subjects considerably. All the other sentence types were comprehended above 'the chance level', but again with individual variation.

The finding that relative clause comprehension is relatively spared in Turkish aphasic patients is an interesting one. Kükürt-Özge (2004), using a slightly larger number of participants and tokens, confirmed this finding with subject relative clauses. These clauses are comprehended as well as simple canonical active sentences, even though they have the non-canonical linear word order 'OVS (Kadını öptü adam)'.

Combining the data from both studies, Kamali *et al.* (2006) argued that the impairment in the OSV sentence type – compared to the reliably above-chance performance of the OVS subject relative clause – must be due not only to syntactic movement, but also to the morphemes themselves, which can contribute to comprehension. In the problematic OSV sentence, the only cue for correct comprehension was the accusative marker -(y)I on the object. On the other hand, in the OVS relative clause, there was one additional aid to comprehension: the relative clause marker -(y)An. Kamali *et al.* hypothesized that the uninterpretable nature of the structural case (e.g. accusative) makes the case marker more vulnerable to impairment than the fully specified relative clause marker.

To be clearer, we should mention Kükürt-Özge (2004), who tested two hypotheses in her thesis: the first concerned the nature of deficit and comprehension strategies employed in Broca's aphasia (namely the Trace Deletion Hypothesis, or TDH), and the second, Regression Hypothesis concerned the similarity between child and aphasic language. A psycholinguistic test was designed in which the comprehension of Turkish relative clauses (RC's) was tested via a sentence-picture matching tasks. The same test was applied to 17 children ranged from 41–52 months, 15 neurologically intact control participants and 11 Broca's patients. The test consisted of 30 sentences, 10 for each set (i.e. subject RC's, object RC's and simple SOA sentences). There were three pictures for each sentence, and each picture described an event in which both NPs could act as a performer of the action or a recipient of it. Only one picture, among the three, represented the correct thematic roles. There was another picture showing the reversed thematic roles, and the last one represented a totally irrelevant activity (in order to test the comprehension of the basic words and actions in the sentences). The participants were asked to indicate the picture appropriate to the one the experimenter described.

The TDH mainly suggested that the cause of the difficulty was the deletion of traces and the default strategy was to assign the agent role to the first NP without a theta-role. In English TDH would expect above chance performance in subject RCs and chance performance in object RCs. Kükürt-Özge (2004) argued that Turkish, being a head-final language, should yield the opposite pattern if the first NP is selected as an agent. As in the first NP in an object RC is marked in the genitive case and it is already in the subject role [adamın öldürdüğü kadın/the woman whom the man killed] whereas the first NP in a subject RC is marked in the accusative case and is in the object role as in [adamı öldüren kadın/the woman who killed the man]. As for the Regression Hypothesis, one would expect a similar performance from children and adults with Broca's aphasia.

The results were not compatible with the TDH hypothesis; that is, the patients did not show any comprehension deficit in subject relatives, but they did have problems with object relative clauses, which led to the conclusion that TDH was not offering a cross-linguistic suggestion for the compensatory strategy in the comprehension of relative clauses. Kükürt-Özge proposed that Turkish patients might be committing to two possible strategies namely the pre-verbal strategy, which selects the NP that is in the pre-verbal position as the patient and the *accusative-object strategy*, which assigns the patient role to the NP with the accusative case (see also Özge, 2007; Özge *et al.*, in press).

Besides, the researcher believed that the complexity in object RCs in Turkish was due to the morpho-syntactic complexity, namely the genitive-possessive agreement morphology, in those structures rather than due to the deletion of traces. This study is compatible with the Regression Hypothesis since both the patients and children exhibited similar patterns in the comprehension of object RCs.

Despite the fact that their overall comprehension appears to be normal, Broca's aphasics perform well below age-matched non-aphasic adults on tasks like these. Since such findings parallel the telegraphic nature of speech output in the same patients, they support a definition of agrammatism as a central processing deficit (Caramazza & Berndt, 1978, 1985;

Zurif & Caramazza, 1976). From this point of view, Wernicke's aphasia could also be reinterpreted as a mirror image syndrome: difficulty with both the comprehension and the production of CWs, suggesting that there is a selective impairment of semantics along with a selective sparing of grammatical structure. Fluent types of aphasia are generally associated with comprehension-deficit varieties, fluent speech with grammatically tangled sentences, and impaired repetition and naming abilities.

The other cited hallmark is the paragrammatic aspect of patients' speech, characterized by the substitution of grammatical morphemes. Maviş (2005) aimed to describe the language characteristics of Turkish fluent aphasic patients and their performance in the aforementioned skills. The results related to paraphasic characteristics of Turkish fluent aphasics also demonstrated some morphophonological characteristics. In that study, Turkish fluent aphasic patients were given task sets in auditory comprehension, verbal fluency, repetition and naming (since these are suggested to be the main areas of language functioning). The researcher aimed, in general, to describe fluent-type language impairments in terms of the correlational relationship within task sets. Participants in this study were eight fluent aphasics (three women and five men ranging in age from 33 to 84 years: the mean age being 57.5 + 17.69). They were clinically defined as exhibiting 'sensory aphasia' in the university hospitals both in Istanbul and in Eskişehir. All patients were evaluated during the first year of their infarcts (mean months post-onset 4.8 + 2.59 months), within a range of 3–10 months. The education levels of the patients ranged from 5 to 8 years, which was sufficient for them to be literate.

In the assessment, every correct response from each 10-item task was allotted one point for a maximum possible of 10 points (over 100 in total). Results showed that the means for the measures of repetition ($\bar{X}$ = 26.2 ± 30.6) and confrontational naming ($\bar{X}$ = 23.7 ± 34.6) were seriously lower than was mentioned in the literature, whereas measures for category comprehension were the highest ($\bar{X}$ = 75 ± 28.2). The age of the patients and the time post-onset were added as variables to describe the existing situation more clearly. It was clear that the time post-onset was positively correlated with the recovery of language ability; however, a negative correlation was observed between age and time post-onset (although, this was not very large). The negative correlation between age and time post-onset might be a product of the sample's wide range of demographical characteristics.

The Turkish fluent aphasics in this study were rated as severe in repetition (7%) and low to moderate at auditory comprehension (45.2%). Their verbal fluency (17.6%) did not reach the expected high rates mentioned in the literature. They were observed to be poor in verbal fluency, probably due to their severe word-finding deficiencies (19.9%). As observed from their performance profiles, most of the Turkish fluent patients failed, especially at repetition (7%) and confrontational naming (6.3%) when immediate

Table 10.4 Classification of paraphasia types

Lexical level	*Sub-lexical level*
Semantic paraphasia: may relate to the target in meaning (semantic error; e.g. van/bus)	Phonemic paraphasia: when the relation to a target is obvious (ghost: /goθ/)
Formal paraphasia: may relate to the target in sound (formal error; e.g. train/tree)	Neologistic paraphasia: neologisms when the relation is more remote (cane: [tʌ])
Mixed paraphasia: may relate to the target in both meaning and sound (mixed error; snail/snake)	
Unrelated paraphasia: they may bear no relation to the target (unrelated error; e.g. banana/drum)	

responses were taken into consideration. They were a little more successful at responsive naming (13.6%).

Çıtav (2004) assessed the verbal performance of the aforementioned fluent aphasic patients. It was obvious that language deviations dominated their speech. The number of paraphasic errors produced, especially in repetition and naming trials, was taken into consideration as proposed by Davis (2000). The type of the errors and where they occurred in a word was determined. Accordingly, paraphasia samples were transcribed phonetically and grouped into formal verbal/phonemic (e.g. pear/dare), semantic verbal, neologistic or off-target utterances. Following the classification of Dell *et al.* (1999), the data were studied in two broad categories as shown in Table 10.4: (1) lexical errors (verbal paraphasias), in which one word is substituted for another, and (2) sub-lexical errors (e.g. phonemic paraphasias, neologisms), in which the phonological structure of a recognizable word is deformed by substitution, addition, deletion or transposition of segments or syllables, the distribution of which is shown in Figure 10.1 for the fluent type of Turkish patients with aphasia.

In naming tasks, paraphasic errors were mainly neologistic, whereas in repetition they were phonemic, both of which belong to the sub-lexical error type (Figure 10.2).

The error types are closely associated to Wernicke's and the conduction aphasic individuals, as noted in the literature.

The mixed type of paraphasia has been the least-observed error type. Errors in Turkish paraphasias occurring toward the end of words was another finding of the study; that is, these errors involved a phonological change to the root, with only a phoneme substitution/addition and/or omission, such as *çatal* (fork) to *çatır* (a cracking noise), *sar* (bind) to *say* (to count), *sar* (bind) to *sarı* (yellow), *köpük* (foam) to *köpek* (dog), *göz* (eye) to

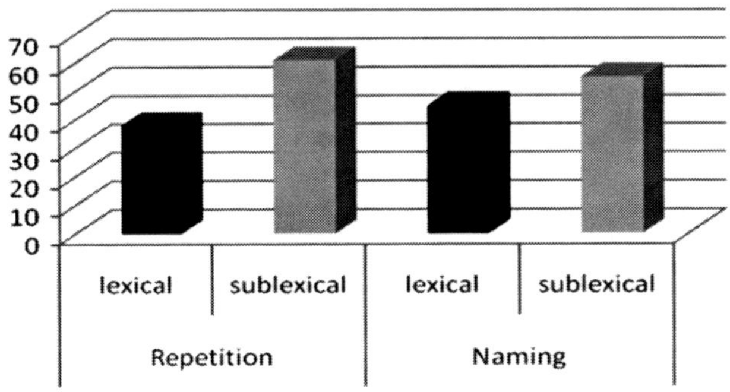

Figure 10.1 Levels of paraphasia in Turkish fluent aphasia

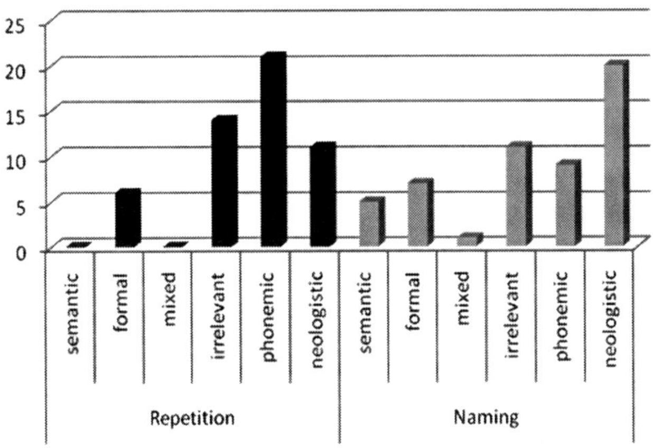

Figure 10.2 Types of paraphasias in Turkish fluent aphasia

göl (lake), etc., which resulted with form-related real words, as suggested in the literature (Dell *et al.*, 1999).

Standard Measures of Aphasia in Turkish

Aphasia assessment is the first step toward a well-founded language therapy. Language tests need to consider in detail the cultural as well as the typological linguistic aspects of a given language.

The Gülhane Aphasia Test (GAT) (Tanrıdağ, 1993) was a version of the BDAE (Goodglass & Kaplan, 1972) adapted for the Turkish population, with the aim of detecting aphasia in general, but not to classify aphasics typologically, for which a fully comprehensive test was required. GAT, validated by a narrow sampling, has been widely used in Turkey as a clinical assessment of language and cognitive deficits in hospitals or medical centers by neurologists since the 1980s. The original GAT included sub-tests of auditory comprehension, written sentence comprehension, paragraph comprehension, fluency of speech, yes–no questions and complex questions, reading and writing, repetition, numerical skills and shape copying.

Nonetheless, a simple direct translation from the original into the target language (Turkish being very different typologically from English) was reported as not being suitable since it was not evaluated for equivalence. Consequently, Tanrıdağ declared his wish for the test to be modified and redesigned according to the changing situations in aphasia assessment and therapy (personal communication) and therefore to be revised on the basis of normative data from a large number of healthy individuals. Consequently, the Gülhane Aphasia Test-2 (GAT-2) has been developed and includes means to assess speech disorders accompanying aphasia, such as apraxia and dysarthria, and to supply more reliable data about aphasic patients (Maviş *et al*., 2006).

The GAT-2 includes seven sub-tests consisting of six language areas, such as spontaneous speech, auditory comprehension, reading comprehension, automatic speech, repetition and naming (which determine the *language score*), and another area of oral-motor assessment (which determines the *motor score*). All other sub-tests in the original GAT (namely complex questions, color naming, writing, numerical skills and copying) were removed. This extensive shortening was made feasible by the high degree of redundancy in the original version. Test and sub-test items were all replaced by items with more relevant content (which were also considered to be more culturally appropriate).

GAT-2 was standardized on 134 non-aphasic individuals. Further, 30 individuals with aphasia and 11 individuals with right brain injury were included in the validation study. The mean years of education for healthy individuals was 8.2 (SD = 3.9), for patients with aphasia it was 7.2 (SD = 3.2) and for patients with right brain injury it was 9.1 (SD = 4.8). '7–9' years of education corresponds to the junior high/middle school in Turkey. The mean year of age among the healthy individuals was 49.6 (SD = 12.8), for patients with aphasia it was 63.2 (SD = 11.4) and for patients with right brain injury it was 64.9 (SD = 10.5). Each participant from the non-aphasic adults group was screened for any neurological dysfunctions at the University hospital and was administered a mini mental test to exclude any possible cognitive deficit.

The inter-group GAT-2 score differentiations and the effects of age, years of education and sex difference were all observed. GAT-2 cutoff scores were calculated by tabulating the scores from the non-aphasics group. Test–retest reliability (with 32 individuals) and inter-observer reliability for GAT-2 were calculated. The GAT-2 scores for healthy individuals significantly differed from the scores of aphasic patients, especially in reading comprehension and naming (but not from the scores of the right brain injured patients). Furthermore, ANOVA statistics reported a significant difference between healthy individuals and patients with aphasia in each of the two sub-tests for total language and motor scores ($p < 0.001$). Healthy individuals' GAT-2 scores were not affected by sex and age differences, but they were affected by the number of years of education; hence, the cutoff scores were determined on this difference alone. The cutoff scores for 1–8 years (low education) was determined as 65 and for above nine years (higher education) it was 68. GAT-2 scores of aphasic patients were not affected by age, sex and years of education. Test–retest ($r = 0.85, p < 0.001$), inter-observer reliability ($r = 0.88, p < 0.001$) and internal consistency ($\alpha = 0.91$) analysis showed that GAT-2 is a highly reliable aphasia screening test for Turkish stroke patients.

Another test adopted for aphasia in Turkish is the Ege Aphasia Test (EAT) (Atamaz *et al.*, 2007), which consisted of nine sub-tests, including spontaneous speech, praxis, auditory comprehension, visual comprehension, production of language, repetition, naming, reading and writing, picture tasks and calculations.

The EAT was administered to 133 volunteers, between the ages of 20 and 80 years. All the subjects were native Turkish speakers living in the Aegean region. The respondents were divided into four groups according to their educational level: illiterate (no schooling, no reading or writing skills or non-completion of elementary school), low (completion of elementary school: 5–8 years of schooling), mid (completion of high school: at least 11 years of schooling) and high: university degree (at least 15 years of schooling). Three age groups were formed: young (between 20 and 39 years), middle-aged (between 40 and 59 years) and old (between 60 and 80 years). Twenty-five subjects were tested twice to collect test–retest reliability data. Educational level was the demographic variable that most influenced the performance on the test. The EAT showed a significant test–retest reliability for the overall score (ICC = 0.99). Test–retest correlation coefficient ranged from 0.84 for praxis to 0.99 for naming, reading and understanding what is seen (visual comprehension), and writing and picture tasks. As a result, normative data demonstrated that the EAT is influenced by demographic variables, particularly education; thus, adjustments in the test scores based on a particular patient's characteristics should be made, and precise indicators of the sociocultural reality of the country should be considered in the test design. Atamaz *et al.* (2007) mentioned that the requirement of diagnostic validity and acceptability for the test would be determined in further studies on aphasic patients.

Although bedside examination usually reveals the type of aphasia a patient may have, formal language evaluation by an SLP is important to determine fine levels of dysfunction, to plan therapy and to assess the patient's potential for recovery. This assessment must be broad enough to detect subtle language disorders in patients in whom aphasia is suspected. Each component of language should be tested individually and thoroughly

(Yavuzer, 2001). For this reason, many tests were developed and standardized for each 'cluster' area for languages in other countries. These tests are required for an SLP in meeting documentation requirements for reimbursement, and compare the performance of the individual being tested according to select populations. No adapted or translated tests from another language can achieve these goals in Turkish, because of language and cultural differences.

Consequently, a study was designed to determine the standardization, validity and reliability of a unique 'Afazide Dil Değerlendirme Testi (ADD)' (Language Assessment Test for Aphasia in Turkish) (Maviş & Toğram, 2009; Toğram, 2008), which consists of eight sub-tests including spontaneous speech and language, auditory and visual comprehension, repetition, naming, reading, grammar, pragmatics (use of speech acts) and writing.

A sample of 282 healthy participants (145 women and 137 men) and 92 persons with aphasia (38 women and 54 men) matched by age, education and gender groups was examined with the ADD. The ADD was administered to healthy adults in four age groups (23–44, 45–59, 60–74 and 75+), and in five educational levels (0, 1–5, 1–8, 1–11 and 12 years or more). The distribution of gender was balanced between the aphasic and the healthy adult groups. The mean age was 51.9 ± 13.7, and the mean education level was 7.9 ± 4.1 years for the healthy individuals. The mean age was 57.3 ± 14.1 years and the mean education level was 7.2 ± 4.6 years for the patients with aphasia. The patients were tested on the ADD (Maviş & Toğram, 2009) in order to discriminate among the aphasic types. The results showed that the number of patients with fluent aphasia was 26, the number of patients with non-fluent aphasia was 46 and that with global aphasia was 20. The mean post-onset for the patients was 29.2 ± 50.1 weeks (almost seven months). Any individual with a history of psychiatric or neurological diseases (or with reported head trauma, abuse and/or other illnesses that were assumed to have an influence on performance) was excluded.

Language quotient was calculated by the sum of spontaneous speech, auditory comprehension, repetition and naming sub-tests. The language quotient calculated for the aphasic patients was expected to be lower than the language quotient of the normal group (to distinguish aphasia from normal language). As expected, a significant difference was found between the two groups' general test scores [$t(372) = 31.7$, $p < 0.0001$] and the language quotient scores [$t(372) = 31.3$, $p < 0.0001$].

It is evident that the Pearson coefficient shows a positive high correlation between the test scores and the sub-test scores [spontaneous speech and language ($r = 0.76, p < 0.01$), auditory comprehension ($r = 0.77, p < 0.01$), repetition ($r = 0.50$, $p < 0.01$), naming ($r = 0.31$, $p < 0.01$), reading ($r = 0.99$, $p < 0.01$), grammar ($r = 0.56$, $p < 0.01$), speech acts ($r = 0.28$, $p < 0.01$) and writing ($r = 0.97, p < 0.01$)], which is a good indicator of construct validity.

There is no significant high correlation between the normal control group and the patient group in terms of test scores and sub-test scores

(–0.05 and 0.22). A low correlation between test scores and sub-test scores demonstrates a high criterion-related validity of the ADD.

The internal consistency of the ADD is significantly high since the means of correlation coefficient is above 0.30 (varying from 0.36 to 0.96 for the ADD in general, and from 0.51 to 0.86 in all sub-tests). There is a significant internal consistency in the ADD as shown by the fact that Cronbach's α coefficients are above 0.90 for the normal control group. The split-half reliability coefficient of ADD was calculated as 0.87, which implies the internal reliability of the ADD is significantly high. Test–retest reliability was assessed via the ADD on 30 normal controls and seven aphasic individuals. The test–retest reliability coefficient of the ADD is significant ($r = 0.88$, $p < 0.001$). Inter-rater reliability coefficient of the ADD is also significant ($r = 0.97$, $p < 0.001$). In short, the ADD was found to be a highly reliable and valid aphasia test for Turkish-speaking aphasics either in Turkey or in other Turkish-speaking communities around the world.

The mean test score for healthy participants was 280.8, and for the aphasics it was 111.3. The mean language score was 158.6 for healthy participants, whereas for the aphasics it was 76.1. The ADD test scores and the language scores of the healthy group were significantly correlated by age ($r = -0.49, p < 0.01$ and $r = -0.59, p < 0.01$, respectively) and educational level ($r = -0.51, p < 0.01$ and $r = -0.55, p < 0.01$, respectively), but not correlated by gender. This means that the general test, sub-test and language scores of healthy participants increase with higher education and younger age levels. Considering education levels, the reference values for the cutoff scores were presented. Accordingly, the cutoff score for the participants between the 23 and 59 years age levels, having a 1–8 year education, is 277; for the ones having 9+ years of education it is 272. The cutoff score for the participants over 60 years old and for the participants who are illiterate is 161; for the ones having a 1–8 year education it is 229, and for the ones having 9+ years of education it is 239. Therefore, only patients who have had a stroke will be diagnosed as aphasic within the aforementioned cutoff values.

Considering age levels, the reference values for the cutoff scores were presented. Accordingly, the cutoff score for the participants between the 23 and 59 years age levels, having 1–5 years of education, is 152; for the ones having six years of education and more it is 155. The cutoff score for the participants over 60–74 years of age and for those who are illiterate is 127; for the ones having 1–5 year education it is 145 and for the ones having more than six years of education it is 152. The cutoff score for the participants over 75 years old and for those who are illiterate is 63; for the ones having 1–5 years of education it is 118. In short, only patients who have had a stroke will be diagnosed as aphasic within these cutoff values.

The purpose of this study was to contribute to the generation of a unitary clinical diagnostic instrument for the assessment of aphasic language impairment in Turkey. It aimed at gathering a reliable classification of the aphasic symptoms of Turkish bilingual aphasics living in Europe or other countries while adding specific data to the cross-linguistic data corpus.

Therapy Considerations

Occurring in 175 of every 100,000 people in Turkey, stroke is the third leading cause of death, after heart attack and cancer, and is the leading cause of physical disability among people in Turkey, which is consistent with the statistics of other countries in the world (Göksan, 2005). Following Germany (127,000 people with strokes each year), Turkey appears as the second country in Europe in terms of frequency of strokes (Özdemir, 2000). Sixty to sixty-five percent of stroke survivors were diagnosed as having a permanent physical disability.

Relevant literature advocates that defining aphasia only in terms of neurology should not necessarily mean that we should ignore the social and personal aspects of the patient (Parr *et al.*, 1997). Since it is a communicative obstacle, aphasia not only prevents the development of the individual's personality and community life but also impedes his/her relation with his/her family and others, which in turn, threatens the quality of the individual's life. The community is thought to have a joint responsibility for detailed environmental arrangements, in which caregivers – as part of the individual's environment – are perceived as either 'facilitators' or 'blockers' of communicative success.

Rehabilitation is not confined only to language functions; instead, it also includes other goals such as developing acceptance and emotional stability, and raising positive attitudes toward the problem in both the aphasic patient and others in his/her environment. If the members of the family take part in this process, it may accelerate rehabilitation. Four diagnostic categories (namely biographic, medical, language and personal/social variables) determine how much of an appropriate candidate the patient is for rehabilitation and what the possible future results might be (Tompkins *et al.*, 1990). Forming the personal and social variables in this group, the attitudes of the individual with aphasia and those of his/her family members are especially valuable in terms of prospective outcomes in rehabilitation (Chapey, 1994). Personal and social problems cover a series of reactions from sudden and major changes brought about by the stroke, including feeling incompetent in adapting to and coping with social problems, a decrease in self-confidence, and/or potential depression. Interviews held with aphasic patients and with their caregivers reveal that the social outcome of aphasia is what most concerns primary caregivers (Van den Heuvel *et al.*, 2002). The first decision taken by family members in order to adapt to the patient and to the new situation is to undertake the role of the caregiver. This role assigns the daily responsibilities of the patient and some other serious duties to the caregiver. Accordingly, an investigation was conducted to describe the role of caregivers with an aphasic family member, the obstacles that have changed their lives and the variables that affect their opinions (Maviş *et al.*, 2005).

Forty primary caregivers, sons, daughters, and sons- and daughters-in-law (22 females and 18 males) participated in the study. The mean age of the primary caregivers was 38 (with a range between 20 and 63 years). Most of the caregivers were graduates of either primary school or high school. The patients with aphasia included 19 women and 21 men with a mean age of 71. Seven of the female patients were married and the rest of the patients were widows or widowers.

The 'Pre-interview Form for an Analysis of the Nonlinguistic Behaviors of an Adult Aphasic Patient from His Child's Perspective' (Chapey, 1986) was administered as the data collection instrument for this study. The 'non-linguistic behaviors' refer to topics such as 'role shift, uneasiness, feelings of guilt, economic status, denial and acceptance, ignoring school/work, changes in social life and health'. The tool also contains three other sequential items that ask caregivers to prioritize their problems concerning 'uneasiness, feelings of guilt and changes in social life'. The reliability studies of the 39-item scale showed that the Cronbach α value of the scale was 0.80.

The subsequent analyses showed that primary caregivers scored between 75 and 166 in the scale. It is possible to say that primary caregivers generally have negative feelings and opinions about the situation the aphasic patient is in ($X = 115.12 <$ total mean score $= 117.00$).

The caregivers were observed to have many negative feelings about the items under the topics of 'role shift/responsibility, change in social life, health and denial and acceptance'. For instance, the participants stated that their social lives changed after the stroke, and that the care of their parents took up most of their time; that their parents desired to be with them for a longer period of time than ever before. Yet they also expressed that they never thought about getting professional help to cope with the stress on account of their parents' situation, but rather preferred sharing and discussing the problems within the family.

A one-way ANOVA showed that the caregivers with a graduate or post-graduate degree were more positive about the situation of having an aphasic parent with paralysis [$F(2, 34) = 6.97, p < 0.05$]. *T*-test results indicated that the views of caregivers significantly differed in terms of the gender [$t(38) = 3.69, p < 0.05$] and the marital status [$t(38) = 2.41, p < 0.05$] of the patient. The results demonstrated that female caregivers hold a more negative perspective regarding the personal care of a female aphasic patient. The most frustrating factors about dealing with an aphasic patient appeared to be 'being responsible for the personal care of their parents', 'making decisions about the health of their parents' and 'making monetary decisions for their parents'. In short, primary caregivers expressed that they could not spare any time for their own personal lives, and that their participation in outside activities and the number of their friends was decreasing, because their roles in the family had changed. They often feel lonely since their social activities and personal time have been affected negatively, while their responsibilities have increased. Many of the results obtained from the study were confirmed by studies in related literature (Le Dorze & Brassard, 1999; Zemva, 1999).

This study provided indications as to why caregivers are so reluctant to take on this additional role after the event of a stroke. It is very obvious that taking their aphasic family members to a center for therapy is yet another burden on the caregivers' part, especially if they are working full time and have a hard time getting permission for time off from work. Therapy fee is another problem for the caregivers since the patients are not supported by the government. Therefore, time or money limitations prevent caregivers from taking their parents to therapy sessions. In fact, another study (Maviş, 2007) explains a more important problem regarding the issue, that is, that neither caregivers nor patients are aware of the consequences of stroke and aphasia.

Of the estimated strokes that occur each year, 75–85% of the cases are ischemic infarcts and 25% of them are hemorrhagic. How many of these strokes resulted in aphasia is not yet known; however, the expected incidence is high. Cerebrovascular accident potentially causes physical, visual, sensory and perceptive impairments, as well as aphasia. Stroke-related aphasia is more common than that caused by Parkinson's disease, cerebral palsy or muscular dystrophy. But many people have not even heard of it.

Recent studies on awareness have drawn attention to the fact that aphasia is a relatively unknown disorder to the public, in spite of all the publicity about this frequently occurring neurogenic language disorder (Elman *et al.*, 2000; Simmons Mackie *et al.*, 2002). Being a very new concept, studies on awareness are rare in Turkey. Awareness research in the literature has raised interest among researchers in Turkey about the current situation in the country. The study by Maviş (2007) assessed the extent of public awareness of neurological disorders (including stroke and aphasia) and of information sources that could be consulted about such disorders. A survey questionnaire was designed with 22 brief questions, 14 of which were divided into three sections on awareness: awareness of neurological disorders, awareness of aphasia and awareness of information sources. The survey was administered to a convenient sample of 196 adults at a university hospital in 2004 in Eskişehir, a city in the central region of Turkey.

The results indicated that *epilepsy and dementia* are 'the most well-known' and *Multiple Sclerosis* (MS) is 'the least well-known' among the surveyed diseases or disorders. Aphasia awareness was also low. It was declared by 65.8% of the respondents that they had never heard of aphasia by name (mean = 51.65, SD = 5.47). Statistical tests were carried out to demonstrate if the sex, age or education of the respondents affected their awareness of aphasia. Chi-square analysis indicated that sex and education, but not age, were significant factors in familiarity of the term 'aphasia'. Further, females were more likely to have heard of aphasia than males (41 females compared with 26 males). There was a greater tendency for educated people (15+ years) to have heard of aphasia. Participants did not have much of an opinion about the causes, the most affected age groups, or its related characteristics. Sixty percent of the sample reported that they had no knowledge about the causes of aphasia. Almost half of the respondents thought that they would need neurologists or doctors initially. Respondents were most likely to cite doctors as a source for general health information as well. SLPs and psychologists (PSY) were determined to be the subsequent referral sources during the recovery and rehabilitation processes. The other choices reflected that respondents considered radio, television and newspapers as the secondary and tertiary sources of information. This widespread lack of knowledge about the needs of individuals with communication impairments makes life even more difficult for them, restricting their ability to regain control of their affairs in many areas of everyday life. Likewise, it is unfortunate that many people with aphasia are unaware that this disorder has a name or that treatment for the disorder exists.

Organized stroke unit care has recently been provided in hospitals by nurses, doctors and allied health professionals (namely occupational, physical and speech therapists) in a high-functioning team to encourage positive stroke outcomes in Turkey. These professionals work to deliver high quality patient care services, especially for the identification, prevention and treatment of diseases, disabilities and disorders. It is a well-known fact that allied health professionals working in a coordinated team achieve a greater recovery rate among stroke patients with or without aphasia (Berry *et al.*, 1996; Indredavik *et al.*, 1991, 1999; Langhorne *et al.*, 1993). The advantages of working as a team can be better realized when team members have some knowledge of each member's professional role. A pilot study was conducted to determine the perceptions and knowledge about allied health professionals in the existing teams who were working together and their wishes concerning any other disciplinary team (Tuncer & Maviş, 2008). A total of 54 allied health personnel, including 18 PSY, 18 physical therapists (PTs) and 18 SLP who work in Eskişehir, İstanbul, Bursa, Ankara and İzmir, were administered the survey.

A survey developed by Felsher and Ross (1994) and adopted and used by Insalaco *et al.* (2007) was translated and adapted into Turkish. The questionnaire includes three sections. The first section asks for biographical information. The second section elicits information on the participants' knowledge of rehabilitation and their perceptions about teamwork. The third section specifically asks about the role of SLPs in treating a series of impairments in terms of appropriateness. Some minimal changes were made to the original Felsher and Ross (1994) and Insalaco *et al.'s* (2007) versions. Descriptive percentages were measured by the non-parametric chi-square test. For the current study, significant differences were not taken into consideration.

Eighty percent of all the participants of the study had worked with stroke patients before. Almost all SLPs and all PTs have stroke rehabilitation experience. The PSY have the least experience (44%) with stroke patients. SLPs, PTs and PSYs all agreed that the currently existing teamwork approach is interdisciplinary (45%), but they said that there was a tendency for transdisciplinary teamwork (22%). SLPs' preferred teamwork approach was constant; they would rather work in a transdisciplinary team (together with doctors and other health personnel during assessment and maybe even during treatment too) for diagnosis, treatment, communication management, family training, research and speech and language therapy. However, PTs preferred the transdisciplinary team (28%) for diagnosis, and speech and language therapy, but the interdisciplinary teamwork for communication management and family training, and the multidisciplinary team for research. PSY preferred transdisciplinary teamwork (23%) for every intervention except for research. In general, participants preferred shared leadership.

In general, participants believed that teamwork is beneficial and that they generally are aware of the primary areas of responsibility for SLPs. SLPs expect to be a part of a transdisciplinary team in which they can share leadership.

The results reflected not the current situation, but the desired situation in Turkey. Allied health personnel seem to work in collaboration within a stroke unit in order to take care of patients; however, very few therapists are able to work in hospitals now. The hospital management discharges stroke patients as soon as they recover neurologically (so, there is not enough time for sufficient speech and language therapy). Besides, the health system does not cover SLP therapy for stroke patients in either hospitals or private clinics. Considering that aphasia therapy takes a long time, the families of stroke patients cannot afford either physical or language therapies. As we have deduced from the previous study, caregivers give their priority to the physical therapy, since they have a difficult time dealing with a paralyzed patient at home. They want their family members to be able to be mobile and take care of themselves without the help of others. They ignore other therapies and may leave their afflicted family members speechless most of the time. Consequently, the number of referrals for language therapy sessions is often insufficient for the clinicians.

In this chapter, we have reviewed the past and the present situation of aphasia in Turkish studies. Speech–language pathology is an emergent field of research and clinical practice in Turkey. Increasingly, dedicated researchers and therapists are making important contributions to the quality of life of persons with aphasia and their families.

Acknowledgments

I am grateful to Bülent Toğram (PhD), A. Müge Tunçer and Özlem Doğramacı-Diken, who are SLPs working as research assistants at the Center for Speech and Language (DİLKOM) at Anadolu University. They, as coauthors of some articles, contributed a great deal during the data collection and data coding process of the studies. Many thanks to Kemal Colay, a graduate SLP, trained at DİLKOM.

Chapter 11

Semantic Relatedness Judgments in Normal Turkish-English Adult Bilinguals

İLKNUR MAVİŞ and SWATHI KIRAN

Introduction

One of the main questions in bilingualism research concerns the representation of words in the two languages of the bilingual individual. Several recent models of bilingual memory generally agree that bilingual individuals have a shared semantic/conceptual system and that there are separate lexical representations of the two languages. However, the models differ on how the lexicons interact with the conceptual system and the influence of language proficiency on the varying strengths between the two lexicons. For instance, the word association model, first described by Potter *et al.* (1984), assumes that second language (L2) words gain access to concepts only through first language (L1) mediation. The L1, on the other hand, has direct connections to the conceptual system. In contrast, the concept mediation model also proposed by Potter *et al.* proposes that the second language lexicon directly accesses concepts. Kroll and Curley (1988) examined the premise of these two models using translation and picture naming tasks and found evidence for the word association model in low proficiency bilinguals and evidence for the concept mediation model in high proficiency bilinguals.

Another model proposed by De Groot (1992), the 'mixed model', suggests that the lexicons of a bilingual are directly connected to each other through a bidirectional connection as well as indirectly connected by way of a shared semantic representation. Finally, Kroll and Stewart (1994) proposed the revised hierarchical model, which accounts for differences in language proficiency to be reflected in differential strengths between L1, L2 and the central concept. In bilingual individuals with a dominant language, the lexicon of the L1 is generally assumed to be larger than that of the L2 since more words are known in the dominant language. Lexical associations from L2 to L1 are assumed to be stronger than those from L1 to L2. Conversely, the links between the conceptual system and L1 are assumed to be stronger than those from the conceptual system to L2.

The models of bilingual language generally explain the interaction between the two lexicons. They, however, are not directly developed to explain the process of lexical access in each of the two lexicons. Further, the relative language proficiency also influences the extent of lexical access in each of the two languages. The issue of lexical access has been examined using the *Boston Naming Test* (BNT), a confrontation picture naming task (Goodglass *et al.*, 1983). For example, Kohnert *et al.* (1998) tested 100 young, educated Mexican-American Spanish/English bilingual adults, who learned both languages before age 8. They found that 75% of their participants named poorer in Spanish than in English, and the progression of difficultly on the BNT normally seen in English monolinguals was not evident in Spanish. The authors argue that age of acquisition of the languages learned by bilinguals may have less to do with language proficiency later in life than language use. In a related study, Roberts *et al.* (2002) tested English monolingual, Spanish/English bilingual and French/ English bilingual groups on the BNT. Roberts *et al.* found that the bilingual groups scored significantly lower than the monolingual group in English.

Another approach to examine lexical access has been the use of category generation. Several studies reveal that bilinguals generate fewer words than monolinguals for given semantic categories (Hernandez & Kohnert, 1999; Rosselli *et al.*, 2000). For instance, Roberts *et al.* (1997) examined category generation for two categories, animals and foods, in 40 French-English participants. Results revealed that there was no language effect on the number of correct responses across languages. However, for *animals*, French-English bilinguals recalled more subcategories (*birds, insects, etc.*) in French than in English. The authors suggested that some semantic fields may have similar types of semantic organization across languages, whereas others may differ among languages even in balanced bilinguals. Rosselli *et al.* (2000) examined 82 healthy older participants who were English monolinguals, Spanish monolinguals or Spanish-English bilingual speakers. Participants were asked to provide a verbal description of a picture and generate words for given phonemic letters and semantic categories. Results revealed that bilingual speakers were similar to monolingual participants on picture description and on phonemic letter generation. However, bilingual speakers produced significantly fewer items than monolingual speakers on the category generation tasks. In a follow-up study, Rosselli *et al.* (2002) compared the performance of Spanish-English bilinguals with monolinguals on phonemic or semantic category generation. Again, bilingual participants produced a significantly smaller number of items on the semantic category (animal) task but performed similar to monolingual participants on the phoneme category generation tasks.

Gollan *et al.* (2002) investigated 30 Spanish/English bilinguals and 30 English-speaking monolinguals in a category generation task comprising 12 semantic categories, 10 letters and two proper name fluency categories. They found that bilinguals produced significantly fewer responses in all tasks, and the difference was larger for semantic categories than it was for the letter and proper name fluency categories. Finally, Bethlehem *et al.* (2003) examined category generation of animal names in 35 Zulu-English speakers. Results revealed no significant differences between performance in English, in Zulu and in the bilingual mode. Participants who learned English later than Zulu still performed better in English than in Zulu.

In general, studies have suggested that bilinguals produce fewer items than monolinguals because of cross-language interference between the two languages. On the other hand, studies that have compared the language output in the two languages of the bilingual have found no differences between the two languages. Further, Roselli *et al.* (2000) suggested that semantic categories are more vulnerable to the effects of cross-language interference because concrete items are produced more often in semantic categories and concrete translation equivalents share more overlapping features relative to abstract words in semantic memory. Although these studies suggest that performance during category generation in the two languages is influenced by semantic factors, it is not clear whether differences between the two languages in category generation are consequent language differences or are due to differences in semantic processing. One way to address this issue is to examine if lexical–semantic processing in the two languages is similar across a range of tasks such as picture naming, category generation and semantic judgment. Such an approach will permit differentiating between language-specific differences in semantic processing and participant-specific abilities related to their relative proficiency in the two languages.

In a recent study, Edmonds and Kiran (2004) examined the relationship between naming and semantic relatedness in 23 Spanish-English bilinguals. Participants were involved in a confrontational naming task and were asked to complete a semantic relatedness questionnaire in Spanish and in English. Participants were divided into three groups (*balanced, English dominant* and *Spanish dominant*) depending upon their naming performance in the two languages. Participants were more accurate in English than they were in Spanish. On the semantic relatedness task, no significant difference was observed between the ratings of word pairs in each language across participants or items in any group.

The Present Study

The proposed project extended the methodology employed by Edmonds and Kiran (2004) to include category generation and further examine the nature of semantic processing and lexical retrieval in Turkish-English bilinguals. Specifically, the present study investigated the relationship between confrontational naming, category generation and semantic representation (as measured by a semantic relatedness judgment task) in Turkish-English bilingual adults. The overall goal of this study was to obtain comparable data across language combinations.

Learning L2 in Turkey: English

The unusual link between English and Turkish, due to syntactic and morphological differences makes learning English exceptionally difficult for native speakers of Turkish. In addition, a highly centralized education system also likely influences the relatively lower proficiency in English. Before 1997, Anatolian high schools offered strong education in English with a prep class in which students had the opportunity of taking 24 hours of English language courses per week for a whole year. After 1997, Anatolian high schools and other schools decreased the amount of course time dedicated to foreign language learning. Therefore, unless individuals are born in a bilingual family or situation, they start learning a second language (i.e. English, German or French) in secondary schools when they become 13 years old. The age or the amount of time that is invested in young peoples' learning of English are both considered to be factors for insufficient levels of English in Turkey.

Aim

In the present study, we examined three tasks, each designed to investigate one aspect of lexical analysis. First, we administered a confrontation picture naming task to examine the nature of lexical access between the two languages when semantic information in the form of a picture was provided to participants. Second, we examined category generation across nine semantic categories. A category generation task was chosen due to its relative simplicity in terms of administration and analysis as well as the easy comparison to extant category generation studies in other language combinations. Lastly, in order to understand the conceptual system in both languages, a semantic relatedness judgment task was chosen. The purpose of this task was to investigate whether participants rated word pairs differently across the two languages.

Method

Participants

Twenty-two Turkish-English bilingual individuals participated in this study. Participants' ages ranged from 25 to 57 years, with a mean age of 43 years (STD: 9.03). All the participants were recruited from the Anadolu

University staff in Eskişehir. Most of the participants had at least a PhD degree; seven of them were faculty members from the English teaching program in the Education Department. All were of Turkish origin and were born in Turkey; however, some had traveled overseas for varying times for educational purposes. Participants had normal vision and no known reading or learning disorders. None of the participants had a history of neurological problems. Handedness was not controlled in these individuals. See Table 11.1 for further description of the participants.

Language profiles of the participants

In the first session, questions were asked about participants' usage and self-evaluation of language skills. Their current language abilities were rated by a language use questionnaire that is currently under development (Kiran *et al.*, under development). The participants were asked to write down the languages they used at home, in social situations, and at work and in what modalities. All responses were provided in Turkish. All participants were born in a Turkish-speaking city in Turkey; therefore, they acquired their native language at the expected age. On the other hand, they learned English as a second language only when they started secondary school at either 11 or 13 years of age. Thus, all were late learners of English, having acquired English at an average age of 12.5 years (STD: 3.97). All the participants rated their speaking and comprehension in English as almost bilingual. All the participants are academic members of the university and all but three had earned their doctorate in various fields. Eighteen of them had earned their degrees in the USA where they spent 4–7 years during their education. Three of them lived in the USA for more than 10 years while they were taking their PhD courses. Two of them had not gone abroad for their education; however, they had been to the USA or various European countries several times. They identify their English level as proficient in all aspects of language in their CVs as well.

Stimuli

Stimuli to be used for oral confrontation naming, semantic relatedness judgment and category generation tasks were developed for this experiment.

In total, 152 items were selected for the oral confrontation naming task based on the following criteria. Cognates (e.g. *balloon, potatoes*) were eliminated in order to avoid facilitation of naming across languages. Some pictures such as *'trunk, cane* and *cod'* were extracted from the original corpus since the first two have too many meanings with different names in Turkish and the third is an unusual fish type not available in Turkey. The pictures for the words were selected from search-motor visuals and had a clear white background. The pictures were presented in a random order to prevent participants from using a self-cuing strategy.

Table 11.1 Demographical characteristics of the participants

Participants	*Sex*	*Age*	*Eng. learning age*	*Staying abroad (year)*	*TR speaking*	*TR comprehension*	*Eng. speaking*	*Eng. comprehension*
1	F	59	11	12	5	5	5	5
2	F	54	11	–	5	5	4	5
3	F	48	11	5.3	5	5	5	5
4	F	48	11	5	5	5	5	5
5	F	43	11	4	5	5	5	5
6	F	46	13	15	5	5	5	5
7	M	32	14	–	5	5	5	5
8	F	45	11	4	5	5	4	4
9	M	35	23	5	5	5	5	5
10	M	33	21	7	5	5	4	4
11	F	51	7	1.5	5	5	5	5

(Continued)

Table 11.1 *Continued*

Participants	*Sex*	*Age*	*Eng. learning age*	*Staying abroad (year)*	*TR speaking*	*TR comprehension*	*Eng. speaking*	*Eng. comprehension*
12	F	56	11	14	5	5	4	5
13	F	51	11	2	5	5	4	4
14	F	39	13	4.2	5	5	5	4
15	F	43	10	7	5	5	5	5
16	M	40	11	2	5	5	4	4
17	F	49	11	–	5	5	5	5
18	M	28	13	1	5	5	4	4
19	F	40	5	1.6	5	5	5	5
20	F	26	14	6	5	5	5	5
21	F	38	11	–	5	5	4	4
22	M	28	9	6	3	5	4	4
	$\overline{X}$	41.5	12.35	4.9	4.9	5	4.57	4.62
	SD	8.82	3.69		0.44	0	0.51	0.49

For the category generation task, three broad categories were employed (*food, animals and clothing*). In addition, these categories were further examined for taxonomic or thematic information. For instance, for the category *'food'*, participants were asked to list food items for lunch and food items at a birthday party. This resulted in a total of nine semantic categories that were tested and analyzed.

A total of 117 word pairs (e.g. purse–wallet, house–barn, etc.) across various semantic categories were selected from an original amount of 150 words for the semantic relatedness judgment task developed by Edmonds and Kiran (2004). The Turkish version was presented as the rote translation of word pairs. None of the word pairs were excluded from the original corpus.

Procedures

Each task was conducted across two sessions that were at least two days apart with the order of language and tasks counterbalanced. Therefore, in each session, each task was only administered once in each language. First, the naming task was conducted. Participants were required to sit in front of a computer screen on which pre-selected pictures were shown one by one. After naming the pictures, in separate L1 and L2 sessions, participants were asked to generate names for nine categories, namely *food for lunch, clothing when it is warm, animals, clothing when it is cold, meals at a birthday celebration, animals in a zoo, food, clothing* and *animals on a farm*. Participants were not limited in time while generating names.

Lastly, participants were given a semantic relatedness task. Items for the Turkish version were translated from English into Turkish. English words were matched with the primary translation equivalent in Turkish. A group of native Turkish speakers evaluated the Turkish translations for appropriate translation meaning and correct spelling. Word length was matched as closely as possible in the English word list. The semantic relatedness questionnaires in both languages were mailed to participants who were asked to assess the degree of relatedness of the words on a four-point rating scale. For this task, participants were required to rate how similar they considered the meanings of pairs of words by circling the appropriate number on a scale of 1, indicating 'very similar/related' to 4, indicating 'not similar/related'. Each of these concepts can usually be described by a number of attributes or features. The instructions in the English version were translated and no other instruction was added before the questionnaires were given to participants. The questions related to which attributes of the concepts (physical descriptions like color, shape and composition or function, purpose and role) they were going to consider. The time the participants spent on the task was not controlled.

Scoring

For the oral naming task, the total number of correct responses in each language was calculated. An item was considered incorrect if it did not exist in either English or Turkish. Further, some alternative responses with lexical variations for the same object were credited as they have more than one name (e.g. *salyangoz/sümüklü böcek* for *snail*; *salatalık/hıyar* for *cucumber*, etc.) which may differ from region to region.

For the category generation task, an item was counted as correct as long as it belonged to the category. Since it was difficult to say if some words in Turkish were labeled as a cognate or had cross-language interference, all the listed words were included. The translation words that were produced in both languages were also listed and statistically analyzed. Further, because it was not clear whether certain words were 'borrowed' or were cognates (e.g. *television-televizyon, tactic-taktik*, etc.), these words were labeled in the study as translation equivalents of the target words.

For the semantic relatedness task, scores were assigned to word pairs irrespective of the nature of their polysemy (i.e. how many senses they have) or the particular senses in which they have been used. Subjects were asked to rate the given word pairs on a scale of 1 to 4 as per their relatedness, which ranged from very similar and almost synonymous to unrelated. Each pair was judged by 22 participants (a collection of 2574 relatedness scores for 117 word pairs, which were averaged for each pair to produce a single relatedness score). The analyses were run in SPSS 13 using parametric 3 × 2 analysis of variance (ANOVA) or non-parametric Kruskal–Wallis scalings.

Results

Grouping of participants

Based on their naming performance (Table 11.2), participants were divided into groups. Dominance for each subject was calculated by comparing the difference between their naming performance in both languages against the main difference in naming for all of the participants (mean: 12.2).

Naming accuracy

The goal of the naming task was to examine the nature of lexical access between the two languages when semantic information in the form of a

Table 11.2 Naming accuracy scores for Turkish and English items

Participants (n = 22)	*TR naming (152 items)*	*TR naming (%)*	*Eng. naming (152 items)*	*Eng. naming (%)*	*/TR/–/Eng/*
$\overline{X} \pm$ SD	148 ± 3.7	97.07 ± 2.25	130 ± 13.7	84.8 ± 9.49	12.2 ± 8.06

Table 11.3 Groups of dominance according to naming accuracy

	Turkish		*English*		*/TR/ /Engl/*
	$\overline{X} \pm SD$	%	$\overline{X} \pm SD$	%	%
Balanced (n = 11)	149.5 ± 2	98.3 ± 1.3	140 ± 5.2	92.2 ± 3.4	6.1 ± 2.7
Less-balanced (n = 7)	145.7 ± 4	95.8 ± 2.8	125 ± 7.3	82.2 ± 4.8	13.5 ± 2.3
TR dominant (n = 4)	145.6 ± 2	95.8 ± 1.1	105 ± 3.5	69.2 ± 1.8	26.6 ± 1.5

picture was provided to participants. Table 11.2 shows that Turkish pictures were named with 97% accuracy whereas English pictures were named with 85% accuracy.

In order to assign the subjects to proficiency levels in each language based on their naming accuracy in both languages, dominance for each subject was calculated by comparing the difference between their naming performances. The mean difference in naming for all of the participants was 12.2 ± 8.06. Participants who fell within 1 standard deviation (SD) were deemed as balanced ($n = 11$). Another group called the less-balanced group ($n = 7$) was created, because even though this group also fell within 1 SD (with a mean difference of 13.5), performance in Turkish was notably higher than performance in English. Finally, a third group, labeled TR dominant ($n = 4$) showed a clear advantage for Turkish responses with a mean difference of 26.6. Table 11.3 and Figure 11.1 show the distribution of the participants into groups of dominance according to their naming accuracy.

A 3 × 2 ANOVA on Turkish naming accuracy revealed no significant effect on the three groups, ($F(2) = 4.85$, $p > 0.05$). Differences in English naming accuracy were significant ($F(2) = 58.2$, $p < 0.01$). A Bonferroni *post hoc* analysis across groups revealed a significant difference between the balanced and the less-balanced groups ($p < 0.01$), the balanced and the Turkish-dominant groups ($p < 0.01$), and the Turkish-dominant and

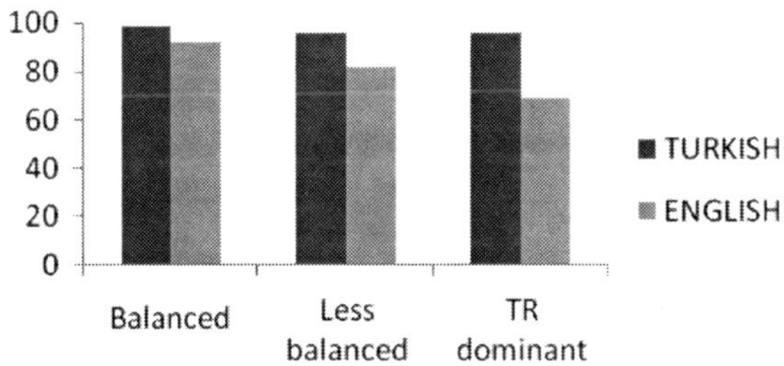

Figure 11.1 Naming accuracy for all groups across participants in percentages

the less-balanced groups ($p < 0.01$) (the mean difference is significant at the 0.05 level).

Semantic relatedness judgments

The aim of the semantic relatedness judgment was to examine conceptual representations of words in both languages using a judgment task. A 3 × 2 ANOVA was conducted with factors 'language' and 'groups' on the semantic-related pair ratings, the means and SDs of which are demonstrated in Table 11.4.

A 3 × 2 ANOVA demonstrated that the effect of neither groups [$F(2) = 0.813$, $p = 0.45 > 0.05$] nor languages [$F(1) = 1.72$, $p = 0.19 > 0.05$] was significant on semantic pair ratings.

One-way ANOVA compared groups for English and Turkish, respectively, to test for significant differences in the mean values among the groups. An ANOVA showed that the effect of English [$F(2) = 1.81$, $p = 0.190 > 0.05$)] or Turkish [$F(2) = 0.087$, $p = 0.917 > 0.05$)] was not significant. The differences between the mean values of the three groups, however, suggested that the TR-dominant group rated words in English as being more related to each other ($x = 2.02 \pm 0.2$) but in Turkish as being less related to each other ($x = 2.82 \pm 0.8$) (Figure 11.2).

Table 11.4 Mean ratings of word pairs between languages and across proficiency groups

Groups		***Eng***	***TR***
	Languages	***X ± std***	***X ± std***
	Balanced	2.69 ± 0.57	2.81 ± 0.50
	Less-balanced	2.52 ± 0.75	2.68 ± 0.82
	TR dominant	2.02 ± 0.28	2.82 ± 0.87

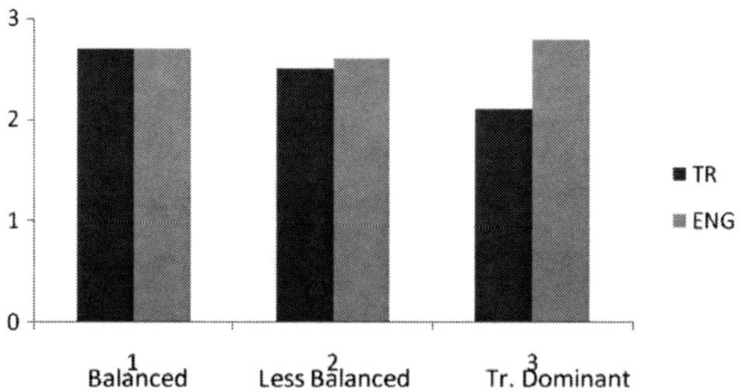

Figure 11.2 Semantic relatedness judgments across items for all groups

Category generation

The aim of the category generation task was to examine similarities and differences across different taxonomic and thematic categories. The frequencies and the average of the items for each category for both languages are presented in Table 11.5.

As evident by the total frequencies presented in Table 11.5, there were more responses for the taxonomic categories than there were for the thematic categories. Specifically, Turkish-English bilinguals generated more for the 'food' category in both languages ($\overline{X}: 18.3 \pm 8$ for TR and $\overline{X}: 14.9 \pm 7.2$ for Eng), followed by the 'animal' and 'clothing' categories, respectively. Participants generated fewer words for 'food at a birthday party' in both languages ($\overline{X}: 5.1 \pm 2.2$ for TR and $\overline{X}: 5.7 \pm 2.3$ for Eng). The dominant groups of participants differed in some categories generated both in English and in Turkish (Table 11.6).

Specifically, the three groups were different on the category of food in Turkish ($F = 3.67$, $p < 0.05$) and the category of clothing in English ($H = 9.7, p < 0.05$). Bonferroni post-hoc analysis revealed that the balanced group produced significantly more items for food ($p = <0.05$) than the less-balanced group in Turkish and the balanced group produced significantly more items than the TR-dominant group for clothing in English ($p < 0.05$).

Translation equivalent items

Translation equivalent items were determined for each participant; that is, the items produced the same in both Turkish and English (e.g. *elma-apple*) were conceptually scored in every category. For instance, if they produced *elma* and *apple* in the same category, they were credited once for getting conceptually matched words. Table 11.7 demonstrates that the translation equivalent words were higher in frequency in the 'animals' category and lower in the category of birthday food.

Table 11.8 shows the distribution of translation equivalent words for each category among dominance groups.

When conceptually matched translation equivalent words were analyzed, it should be noted that overall, the balanced group had a higher number of translation equivalents than the other two groups across the nine categories. On a non-parametric Kruskal–Wallis test, a significant difference appeared for animals ($H = 10.5$, $p < 0.05$), animals on a farm ($H = 14.5$, $p < 0.05$) and clothing categories ($H = 8.8$, $p < 0.05$). A post-hoc analysis (Dunn's test) revealed that the balanced group produced significantly more *translation equivalent items* in the 'animals' category than the less-balanced group. The balanced group produced significantly more *translation equivalent items* in the 'farm animals' category than the TR-dominant group, and the balanced group produced significantly more *translation equivalent items* in the clothing category than the less-balanced group.

Table 11.5 The frequencies and the average of the items for each category for Turkish and English

TR		*Yiyecek*	*Öğle Yemeği*	*Doğum Günü*	*Hayvan*	*Hayv. Bahçesi*	*Çiftlik*	*Giyim*	*Yazlık*	*Kışlık*
	Total	404	206	113	335	292	197	305	145	214
	$\overline{X} \pm SD$	18.3 ± 8	9.3 ± 5.2	5.1 ± 2.2	15.2 ± 7.6	13.2 ± 4.7	8.9 ± 2.7	13.8 ± 3.7	6.5 ± 1.5	9.7 ± 3
Eng		*Food*	*Lunch*	*Birthday*	*Animals*	*Zoo*	*Farm*	*Clothing*	*Warm*	*Cold*
	Total	328	194	127	297	270	150	280	133	173
	$\overline{X} \pm SD$	14.9 ± 7.2	8.8 ± 3.1	5.7 ± 2.3	13.5 ± 4.8	12.2 ± 2.7	6.8 ± 1.9	12.7 ± 2.9	6.0 ± 1.6	7.8 ± 1.8

Table 11.6 Significantly produced categories in Turkish and English

Categories	*Language*	*Balanced*	*Less-balanced*	*Turkish dominant*	*F*	*p*
		$\overline{X} \pm SD$	$\overline{X} \pm SD$	$\overline{X} \pm SD$		
Food	Eng	19 ± 9.3	11.8 ± 6	9 ± 2.82	$F(2) = 3.30$	$p = 0.058$
	TR	23 ± 10.4	12 ± 5.4	21.2 ± 6.8	$F(2) = 3.67$	$p = 0.045 < 0.05$*
Food for lunch	Eng	6	8	10.5	$H(2) = 2.41$	$p = 0.29$
	TR	11 ± 6.08	8.57 ± 4.2	6.5 ± 1.91	$F(2) = 1.41$	$p = 0.26$
Food for birthday	Eng	7	4	4	$H(2) = 5.53$	$p = 0.063$
	TR	6.18 ± 2.5	4.14 ± 2.79	5 ± 2.1	$F(2) = 1.39$	$p = 0.27$
Animals	Eng	13	11	15	$H(2) = 3.55$	$p = 0.169$
	TR	19 ± 11.6	11.1 ± 3.33	15 ± 5.35	$F(2) = 1.88$	$p = 0.17$
Animals at zoo	Eng	12	10	10	$H(2) = 1.84$	$p = 0.39$
	TR	15 ± 8	9.14 ± 2.7	18 ± 5.3	$F(2) = 2.90$	$p = 0.07$
Animals at farm	Eng	8 ± 3.43	5.85 ± 2.26	5.25 ± 1.25	$F(2) = 1.95$	$p = 0.16$
	TR	10	7	8.5	$H(2) = 4.94$	$p = 0.08$
Clothing	Eng	14	11	7.5	$H(2) = 9.77$	$p = 0.008 < 0.05$*
	TR	17	12	12.5	$H(2) = 5.26$	$p = 0.07$
Clothing for warm weather	Eng	6.72 ± 2.14	5.14 ± 1.34	5.75 ± 2.06	$F(2) = 1.52$	$p = 0.24$
	TR	7.27 ± 2.19	6.28 ± 1.11	6 ± 1.63	$F(2) = 1.00$	$p = 0.38$
Clothing for cold weather	Eng	8.72 ± 3.06	7.42 ± 0.97	6.25 ± 2.63	$F(2) = 1.57$	$p = 0.23$
	TR	11.3 ± 3.95	8.71 ± 1.79	8.25 ± 2.36	$F(2) = 2.18$	$p = 0.14$

*$p < 0.05$.

Table 11.7 The frequency and means of translation equivalent words among categories

	Food	*Lunch*	*Birthday food*	*Animal*	*Zoo*	*Farm*	*Clothing*	*Warm*	*Cold*
Total	115	71	54	162	145	101	146	76	87
$\overline{X}$	5.2	3.2	2.4	7.3	6.5	4.5	6.6	3.4	3.9
SD	6.6	4.3	1.9	6.7	6.1	2.6	5.5	1.5	2.6

Table 11.8 The distribution of translation equivalent words for each category among dominance groups

	Food			*Food for lunch*			*Food for birthday*		
	Balanced	***Less-balanced***	***TR dom.***	***Balanced***	***Less-balanced***	***TR dom.***	***Balanced***	***Less-balanced***	***TR dom.***
Tot.	79	23	13	44	19	8	35	10	9
$\overline{X}$	7.1	3.2	3.2	4	2.7	2	3.1	1.4	2.2
SD	9	1.2	2.7	6	1.1	0.8	2.4	0.9	1.5
	Animals			*Animals at a zoo*			*Animals at a farm*		
	Balanced	***Less-balanced***	***TR dom.***	***Balanced***	***Less-balanced***	***TR dom.***	***Balanced***	***Less-balanced***	***TR dom.***
Tot.	111	24	27	95	32	18	66	23	12
$\overline{X}$	10	3.4	6.7	8.6	4.5	4.5	6	3.2	3
SD	8.5	1.5	2.2	8.1	1.5	2.3	3.1	0.4	0.8
	Clothing			*Clothing for warm weather*			*Clothing for cold weather*		
	Balanced	***Less-balanced***	***TR dom.***	***Balanced***	***Less-balanced***	***TR dom.***	***Balanced***	***Less-balanced***	***TR dom.***
Tot.	97	31	18	52	26	12	41	23	9
$\overline{X}$	8.8	4.4	4.5	4.7	3.7	3	3.7	3.2	3
SD	7.1	1.5	1.2	3.3	1.1	1.1	1.8	1.2	10.8

Self-ratings across groups

Finally, the self-rating scores that the participants gave themselves on their formal speaking and comprehension abilities in both languages were also analyzed. The non-parametric Kruskal–Wallis one-way ANOVA test across groups revealed a significant difference in self-ratings for only English comprehension ($H = 6.14$ (2), $p = 0.046 < 0.05$) (Table 11.9).

Discussion and Conclusion

In order to understand how a bilingual speaker uses and comprehends two languages, researchers find it necessary to find out how different types of linguistic knowledge such as lexical-semantic information in both languages are accessed and maintained. Therefore, the current study sets out to examine Turkish-English bilinguals using single word naming, semantic relatedness and category production tasks.

Participants, before being grouped, named 152 items with 97% accuracy in Turkish and 86% accuracy in English. Based on their naming performances, three groups were determined. The balanced group was the most accurate in naming items both in Turkish and English, whereas the Turkish-dominant group was the least accurate in English (69.2%). As expected, the less-balanced group showed an advantage for naming Turkish items (95%); besides, English naming was relatively high (82%) as well. The reduced accuracy on English stimuli in all three groups can be explained by their relative lack of familiarity with the stimuli in English. In fact, Segalowitz and Almeida (2002) state that 'less than native-like fluency in a language usually results from having had less experience and practice with the language'.

In bilingual speakers, it is known that it is very difficult to select the target lexical node in picture naming experiments since many synonymous lexical representations become activated to roughly equal levels (Finkbeiner *et al.*, 2006). This was confirmed in our study as well. More synonyms were uttered in Turkish such as *yatak/şilte* for bed, *zil/çıngırak* for bell, *keçi/oğlak* for goat, *fener/lamba* for lantern, *oturak/tabure* for stool, *çengel/kanca* for hook, *kadeh/kupa* for cup, etc. In English, however, responses were varied in error types. For example, participants named *sink* as *basin*, which is acceptable, but *cleaner, tap, faucet* or *washed up* is not. Also, responses such as *ring* for *bell*, *spade* for *shovel*, *rat* for *mouse*, *capricorn* for *goat*, *spectacle* for *eyeglasses* or *bunny* for *rabbit* were accepted. Finkbeiner *et al.* called those words that share a common semantic representation 'translation equivalent lexical nodes'. Participants also made a few phonological errors such as *chain* for *chin*, indicating some confusion in the activation of the phonological form of the target word.

In the second task, participants rated the degree of semantic relatedness of 117 associative word pairs. Semantic relatedness is based on a

Table 11.9 Self-ratings of the dominant groups for their English and Turkish proficiency

	Balanced	*Less-balanced*	*TR dominant*	*H*	*p*
	$\overline{X}$	$\overline{X}$	$\overline{X}$		
Eng comprehension	5	5	4	6.14(2)	$0.046 < 0.05$*
Eng speaking	5	5	4	3.79(2)	$0.150 > 0.05$
TR comprehension	5	5	5	2.14(2)	$0.343 > 0.05$
TR speaking	5	5	5	2.14(2)	$0.343 > 0.05$

*$p < 0.05$.

semantic system in which similar concepts tend to cluster together by virtue of their shared attribute structure (Kiran, 2007). Conceptually related objects usually share a high number of physical features (Damian, 2000). The more the two words are semantically related, the more common co-occurring words they will have, such as in *doctor–operate* or *doctor–nurse*. However, certain word pairs have a special relation with each other, which cannot be explained by an intuitive competence. Mohammad and Hirst (2005) gave an example of *strawberry and cream* as words which are not similar physically or in properties but still are related semantically. The criteria for a semantic relation between the two might come from their inseparable use in the culture where they are eaten preferably together. However, the relation differs according to the cultures. For example, in Turkey, strawberries are eaten with powdered white sugar. Ontology-based measures will correctly identify the amount of semantic relatedness only if such relations are inherent in the ontology. In the study, regardless of ontology, bilingual participants were expected to interpret the specific wordings in the much larger context of their background knowledge and experience and to determine to what extent the given pairs of concepts are semantically related. In the present study, relatedness judgment showed no major differences between the groups. The only finding of interest was that the Turkish-dominant group had a tendency to rate English pairs as more related (being very similar). It may be possible that the Turkish-dominant group was unable to decide the appropriate relatedness for stimuli in English, reflecting an apparent lack of familiarity with the words in English.

Finally, a category generation task was conducted to examine participants' lexical access across nine categories. One animate (animals) and two broad inanimate categories (food and clothing), as well as two subcategories for each, were used in this study. Participants were asked to provide as many instances of the nine categories as possible. Several findings of interest emerged from this task. First, overall differences in the processing of category production frequencies were observed, in which there were more responses for food than for other categories. This difference reflects an interaction between the nature of the category studied and the influence of culture. Therefore, there are far more instances of food than of animals that can be generated and that span across two cultures (Turkish and Western-English speaking).

Second, when the data were separated and analyzed by participant group, results revealed significant effects for category generation tasks in English. Specifically, the balanced group produced more items than the other two groups for food, food at a birthday party, animals, animals at the zoo and clothing. While it would be expected that the balanced group would produce a greater number of English responses than the other two groups by virtue of the fact that they have greater access to lexical targets in English, it is interesting to note that these participants also produced more items in Turkish across most categories. Therefore, the present results suggest that balanced bilinguals may have greater access to lexical items in both languages than their counterparts who are more proficient in one language. Notably, items generated in Turkish were higher in the balanced group relative to the groups more proficient in Turkish.

Finally, items produced in both languages were marked as translation equivalents (e.g. *elma, apple*) and analyzed. It is clear that the balanced group produced notably higher translation equivalent responses than the less-balanced group and the Turkish-dominant group across all nine categories, although only three categories survived the statistical criteria. Nevertheless, these results provide an interesting window to understanding lexical–semantic abilities in Turkish-English bilinguals who present with varying levels of English proficiency. Based on the theoretical models described in the introduction (de Groot, 1992; Kroll & Stewart, 1994), the results for the balanced group can be accounted for by strong connections between the semantic system and the L1 and L2 lexicons. Consequently, lexical targets active in L1 (Turkish: elma) correspondingly activate targets in L2 (English: apple) due to the higher proficiency in English. In contrast, both the less-balanced and the Turkish-dominant groups have relatively fewer translation equivalents suggesting that access to English targets may be relatively more difficult. Within a theoretical framework, we can posit that connections between the semantic system and the L1 are strong but connections between the semantic system and the L2 are weak (to a relative degree). Taken together, results from translation equivalents in the three subject groups illustrate the influence of relative language proficiency (in L2) on lexical–semantic abilities in the two languages.

Finally, analysis of the participants' self-ratings on the language use questionnaire reflected an apparent disconnect between perceived ratings on proficiency in a given language and actual performance in that language. All participants rated themselves as being rather fluent in their production, save for comprehension of English. In fact, subjects' self-ratings were assumed to reflect their naming abilities in both languages. However, when self-ratings were compared to their naming scores in English, the results implied that not self-ratings but naming tasks may be a good indicator of overall language proficiency. These results are notable, because they underscore the need to obtain objective measures of language use and proficiency such as naming or category generation.

To conclude, results of the present study provide important preliminary information regarding the nature of lexical–semantic processing abilities in Turkish-English bilinguals. First, they highlight the variation of L2 (English) proficiency that exists in the Turkish-English bilingual population. Additionally, when the results of the present study are integrated with theoretical models of lexical–semantic processing, they provide an important insight into probable mechanisms underlying lexical processing in this bilingual population.

Acknowledgments

I am grateful to Nida Şanlı-Colay, a graduate SLP trained at the Department of Speech and Language Pathology (DILKOM) at Anadolu University. She contributed a lot during the data collection and data coding process of the study.

Part 3

Communication Disorders in Multilingual Settings

Chapter 12

Aspects of Acquisition and Disorders in Turkish-Dutch Bilingual Children

KUTLAY YAGMUR and ELMA NAP-KOLHOFF

Introduction

Specific language impairment (SLI) is a highly specialized area for speech therapists and linguists. In general, the diagnosis of SLI includes children with normal intelligence and extremely weak language skills (Verhoeven & van Balkom, 2004). Most Turkish immigrant children start school with very little competence in Dutch. In most cases, the Turkish language proficiency of such children is assumed to be higher than their Dutch skills (Extra & Yagmur, 2004). Given their low proficiency levels in Dutch, most Turkish immigrant children encounter problems at school. In most cases, they cannot understand their teachers' instruction. Because the submersion education model is the dominant approach in schools, there is no specialized assistance to facilitate Dutch acquisition, which leads to further delays in the socio-emotional and cognitive development of the immigrant children. On the basis of small vocabulary and incomplete grammar, such children are mostly identified as linguistically impaired and, even worse, as mentally underdeveloped. Given their very low levels in the mainstream language, such children are slow in language production and in most cases they can express themselves neither in their first language nor in their second language. Instead of questioning the role of subtractive environment and submersion education on children's first language and second language development, policy makers and school practitioners blame children's first language use as an obstacle to second language development. In more serious cases, even though they have normal cognitive skills, some immigrant children with delayed language skills are identified as having language deficits and impairment, as a result of which they are sent to special education schools.

In this chapter, we argue that what is identified as impairment might simply be a deviation from monolingual development. We will also show that using monolingual assessment instruments might be misleading in the case of bilingual children. By using the Turkish Systematic Analysis of Language Transcripts (SALT) (Acarlar & Johnston, 2006), we will document the differences between the results of monolingual and bilingual Turkish children.

Can limited bilingualism be identified as SLI?

Researchers increasingly focus on immigrant minority children's development of second language proficiencies in the European context. Mostly based on single or multiple case studies, researchers and school practitioners claim language deficiency and/or subtractive bilingualism on behalf of immigrant minority children. In most multilingual settings, schools only measure immigrant minority children's mainstream language skills rather than their home language skills. On the basis of proficiency levels in the second language, sizeable numbers of immigrant children are considered to be language-impaired. In order to provide appropriate schooling for such children, bilingual assessment is vital. Mostly on the basis of monolingual assessment instruments, most immigrant children are placed in special classes which are also attended by children with disabilities. Such schools are called *sonderschulen* in Germany and *bijzondere scholen* in the Netherlands. Even though most immigrant children do not have any physical or mental disabilities, they are placed in such special education classes due to their lower mainstream language skills. In most cases, immigrant children are stigmatized as having language impairment simply on the basis of ineffective assessment instruments. By separating and segregating such students, educational policy makers construct social inequality early in the lives of many immigrant children. Bilingual children must be assessed in their respective languages so that accurate assessment of their linguistic competence can be made. If the children are dominant in Turkish, then their Turkish skills need to be assessed before labeling them as having a deficit in language development. In this volume, Jan de Jong *et al.* (Chapter 13) provide a detailed analysis of SLI in the Dutch context. In this study, we will focus on unbalanced bilingual development, which is sometimes mistakenly identified as SLI.

Regarding bilingual competence, one of the most discussed theories related to the cognitive effects of bilingualism is the threshold hypothesis (Cummins, 1979). It is commonly accepted that cognitive development is essential for academic achievement. The relationship between language development and cognitive growth has certain implications for bilingual children's school achievement. Cummins (1977: 10) proposed that 'there may be a threshold level of linguistic competence which a bilingual child must attain both in order to avoid cognitive deficits and allow the potentially beneficial aspects of becoming bilingual to influence his cognitive growth'. A threshold explains the difference between a balanced bilingual and a dominant bilingual. Each threshold is the level of language competence that has consequences for a bilingual child. In order to avoid the negative consequences of bilingualism, the child has to reach the first threshold of his or her respective languages. If the child reaches the second threshold in both languages, he or she will be able to obtain cognitive benefits from bilingualism. Concerning language competence, bilingual speakers might be equally dominant in both languages, or more dominant in one language only and/or insufficiently competent, *limited bilingual*, in either of the languages (Baker, 2006). Discussions seem to concentrate on the language ability of bilingual children; yet, there is a close relationship between the larger linguistic environment and the language competence of immigrant children. It appears that a subtractive bilingual environment adversely affects immigrant children's cognitive and scholastic progress. Cummins (1976) suggested that linguistic minorities undergo native language attrition and that the level of linguistic competence attained by a bilingual child may mediate the effects of his bilingual learning experiences on cognitive growth. Given the submersion model in the Dutch context, native language skills of immigrant children are denied both in schools and in the larger public arena, which has serious implications for the cognitive and social–emotional development of such children. Even though some of Cummins's theories are disputed, the general principle that there exists a relationship of interdependence between the first language and the second language, and knowledge and skills learned through the respective languages, has achieved common consensus among bilingual specialists (Francis, 2000). In the US context, academic instruction in a child's native language has been shown to be associated with outcomes superior to those resulting from English-only instruction (August & Hakuta, 1998). However, due to the prevalent submersion model, immigrant children's home languages are not utilized in Dutch schools.

School success and language competence

People of Turkish descent constitute the largest immigrant group in Western Europe. The majority of them originate from rural areas in Turkey. Most of the parents have very little or sometimes no schooling at all. Even though Turkish families value education, they are unable to provide guidance and support to their children at home. Low skills in Dutch as well as cultural differences between the mainstream school system and the home culture act as barriers to parents' involvement in their children's schooling process. Involvement in children's schooling is mostly connected with the parents' educational level, rather than with their ethnicity. Both in the

German context and in the Dutch context, Turkish immigrant children are shown to lag some years behind native children. For instance, Driessen *et al.* (2002) showed that at the end of primary education, Turkish and Moroccan children are approximately two years behind in their language development compared with children of *highly educated* Dutch parents. This finding is not surprising at all because the majority of Turkish and Moroccan parents in the Netherlands belong to the working class and in most cases they have very little or even no formal schooling. If low Socio Economic Status (SES) Dutch children's examination results were compared to high SES Dutch children, the same differences would have emerged. Instead of pointing out the role of social differences in test results, some researchers prefer pointing out the ethnic differences. Concluding from such results, most policy makers claim that immigrant Turkish and Moroccan children perform worse at schools because 'they speak another language at home'. Nevertheless, there are also studies that approach the matter from a more linguistic perspective; for instance, Klatter-Folmer's (1996) study has shown that Turkish children's Turkish and Dutch language proficiencies are closely related to their educational achievement. She has also shown that the level of proficiency in the first language goes hand in hand with the level of proficiency in the second language. Those students who perform the best at school had high proficiency levels both in Turkish and in Dutch.

Driessen *et al.* (2002) provided some evidence to the discussion of home language proficiency versus second language proficiency. They conducted a large-scale longitudinal study into the development of language proficiency of Dutch primary school pupils aged 7–10. On the basis of their findings they show that Turkish pupils, whose parents speak Turkish at home, perform significantly lower than the children of Dutch-speaking parents. Driessen *et al.*, however, do not report any findings or differences between the language proficiency of Dutch-speaking Turkish parents and Turkish-speaking Turkish parents. Availability of such findings might provide more conclusive evidence on the matter. Nevertheless, Driessen *et al.* (2002) contribute further evidence to the discussion. Concerning Dutch language proficiency differences, they show that dialect speakers perform even better than the native Dutch speakers. They conclude that children in dialect-speaking families find themselves in a diglossic situation in which they have mastered both languages (e.g. Dutch and Limburgish dialects are not always mutually intelligible) but use them in different domains. Immigrant parents do not show this type of bilingualism or at least not to a similar degree. These findings point to the fact that due to insufficient command in the first language, there is no positive transfer possible to the second language. Driessen *et al.* (2002: 191) conclude that 'Our analyses also show that the children's use of a language other than Dutch does not need to have any negative consequences for language proficiency. Limburgish-speaking children use Dutch the least, but they have the highest language proficiency score; whereas Turkish and Moroccan-speaking (i.e. *Arabic*) children speak Dutch more often, yet they have a much lower language proficiency score'. (*Italics* authors' note.)

As opposed to public discourse, Driessen *et al.* (2002) with their findings, show that home language use does not have any negative effects on the dialect-speaking children's Dutch language skills. Preparing language minority children for more successful school careers ideally requires a balanced bilingual approach in which children's greater proficiency in the home language is utilized to promote general cognitive development and acquisition of the school language (Leseman & van Tuijl, 2001: 309). However, given the widespread use of the submersion model in most European schools, immigrant children's first language skills cannot be further developed.

The submersion model is the most common bilingual approach in the Dutch school system. Bilingual education as a form of coordinated language teaching and learning has seldom been regarded as necessary. Even though there is a general reluctance to refer to migrant students as bilinguals and to develop bilingual programs for them, there is widespread support for native Dutch students in various bilingual programs. Bilingual programs in high-status languages such as English and Dutch have huge public support but strongly negative attitudes surround immigrant children's bilingualism. Policy makers rejected bilingual education in the Dutch context not because of its linguistic results but because of its implication for separate schooling for immigrant pupils. In a typical anti-bilingual fashion, many Dutch teachers believe that immigrant children are overloaded by dealing with two languages, which lowers their proficiency in Dutch. Apparently, this old-fashioned *separate underlying proficiency* (SUP) model can still find some supporters in the Dutch context. In this subtractive bilingual environment, most immigrant children are reluctant to speak in their first language, which also has implications in their socio-emotional development. In most cases, such children are identified as having language problems. As indicated by Verhoeven and van Balkom (2004: 6), such children 'no longer have an open, uninhibited attitude toward the environment, and they develop a fear of failure with regard to school learning'. As a matter of fact, what is identified as SLI for most immigrant children turns out to be inappropriate schooling and inaccurate assessment of their language skills. In the following sections, after presenting a brief overview of instrument(s) to assess first language skills of Turkish immigrant children, we will present the results of SALT analyses and their implications for use as a diagnostic instrument with bilingual children.

Diagnostic Instruments for First Language Assessment of Bilingual Children Used in the Netherlands

As documented in detail by de Jong *et al.* (Chapter 13, this volume), there are serious difficulties with the screening of Turkish children for language development disorders. The only instrument available is a translated Turkish version of a Dutch tool called the Lexilijst van de Schlichting test. The Lexilijst for Turkish children is used for screening language development at the age of about two years. It aims at measuring productive skills in Turkish (Schlichting, 2006). As covered fully in this volume, a broad range of diagnostic techniques is needed to trace language problems in natural and structured situations. Measuring only speech production might not show the extent and depth of impairment. As pointed out by Verhoeven and van Balkom (2004), such instruments should cover speech production, speech perception, morphosyntactic knowledge, lexical/semantic knowledge and pragmatic skills. Such detailed instruments are not available for Turkish immigrant children in the Netherlands. As a result, Turkish immigrant children are assessed on the basis of their Dutch skills, which certainly turn out to be highly inaccurate. Below, we will present the feasibility of SALT as a diagnostic instrument for use with bilingual Turkish children.

SALT as a diagnostic instrument

SALT (Miller & Chapman, 1993) is a software package developed for English by Miller and colleagues in the late 1980s at the University of Wisconsin in the United States. SALT is a clinical tool for assessing language performance on the basis of language samples. Although standardized tests are the most frequently used methods for assessing language proficiency, there is growing interest in language sample analysis as an additional clinical tool (Acarlar & Johnston, 2006). In language sample analysis, natural interactions between a child and one or more adults are recorded, transcribed and subsequently analyzed. Areas of analysis in SALT are quite rich in scope: phonology, utterance complexity, morphology, discourse and so on. The main advantage of language sample analysis over language tests is that they provide a more valid picture of a child's everyday language abilities (Acarlar & Johnston, 2006). Several studies have shown that methods for language sample analysis correlate significantly with standardized tests (e.g. Bornstein & Haynes, 1998; Ukrainetz & Blomquist, 2002). The kind of information provided by language sample analysis is different, however, and can therefore be used as a useful addition to tests, which usually focus on only a limited set of language abilities. In order for language sample analysis to be not too time and labor intensive, software tools have been developed for transcription and analysis, of which SALT is the most widely used. An important feature of SALT is that it contains data of normally developing reference groups of different ages. Recently, SALT was adapted for Turkish by Acarlar *et al.* (2006). Acarlar and Johnston (2006) describe the nature of the adaptation process in detail.

The Present Study

In this study, we want to find out whether normally developing Turkish-Dutch bilingual children at the age of three differ significantly from monolingual Turkish children in Turkey on language proficiency, as assessed with SALT for Turkish. If so, in what ways do they differ and how can SALT for Turkish be adapted for use in bilingual contexts?

Methods

Informants

The current study compares language samples of seven bilingual children in the Netherlands with reference groups provided by the SALT analysis software. The data from the children in the Netherlands are available in the Van der Heijden bilingual corpus (Van der Heijden, 1999) and in the Nap-Kolhoff bilingual corpus (Nap-Kolhoff, 2009). All bilingual children were born in the Netherlands but are dominant in Turkish. Their backgrounds as well as the setting in which the data collection took place differ considerably. The parents of the four Turkish girls (Selma, Berrin, Filiz and Şükran) in the Van der Heijden corpus were first-generation immigrants. The children were exposed to different amounts of Dutch language input in day-care centers, preschool playgroups, at home and/or in the neighborhood where they were living. The data were collected in the early 1990s. Data for the three boys (Mehmet, Batuhan and Yunus) in the Nap-Kolhoff corpus were collected in the early 2000s. The three boys had one parent who was a second-generation immigrant and fluent in Dutch. The other parent was a first-generation immigrant. All three children had been attending a Dutch preschool playgroup from the time of their second birthdays for about 12 hours per week.

Both corpora contain spontaneous speech data collected longitudinally at 1–3 month intervals. Data for Selma and Berrin were collected in the day-care centers they attended. All speech produced by the informant during a morning or an afternoon in the center was recorded. A bilingual Turkish research assistant was always present and spoke only Turkish to the informants. Data for Filiz and Şükran were collected in their homes, because they did not attend a day-care center. During those recordings, the same research assistant was present. A Dutch researcher, who visited the children in their homes, as well as in the playgroup, collected data for

Mehmet, Batuhan and Yunus. During the recordings at home, the mothers were encouraged to talk Turkish with their children.

Conversion to SALT

From the corpora, two transcripts were selected for each child: one around at age 3;0 and one around age 3;6. Since the data are available in the CHAT format (MacWhinney, 1996), the transcripts had to be converted to the SALT format. From each transcript about 160 utterances were used, as this is the maximum number of utterances available for the reference groups (see below).

Several problems were encountered when converting the transcripts to the SALT format and adding the morpheme codes. First, SALT for Turkish has been developed for monolingual speech data. The data under investigation were, however, bilingual in nature. Children and adults conversed in both Dutch and Turkish and regularly mixed the languages within utterances. As the aim of this study was to investigate the Turkish speech data of the children, only Turkish utterances were extracted from the bilingual data. Mixed utterances were excluded from the present analyses. Each child utterance in the bilingual corpora was coded for language (Turkish, Dutch, mixed or 'undecided'), which made extraction of the Turkish utterances straightforward.[1]

A result of excluding the non-Turkish parts of the child data was that the adult speech data could not be used either. The tools SALT has for analyzing discourse, such as the number of responses to questions, the length of the turns and overlap, therefore could not be used. Finally, some changes had to be made, because of the fact that most of the bilingual children were acquiring a dialect of Turkish, rather than using the standard variety. Morphemes not included in the SALT analyses are -(y)nEn as instrumental (-(y)lE in standard Turkish), -(y)Ek and -(y)Em as optative (-(y)Elİm and -(y)Eyİm in standard Turkish), -gil as a family marker (annemgil 'mother-my-family: my mother's family'), and the informal imperative -sEnE (baksana 'look-sEnE: 'just look'). The former two suffixes were relatively frequent in the data and coded with their form in the standard variety. The latter two suffixes appeared only infrequently and were not further analyzed.

Reference groups

SALT for Turkish contains reference data for 140 children between ages 2;6 and 6;6. In the present study, reference groups were selected for children ranging in age from two months younger to two months older than the bilingual informant. The children in the monolingual reference groups attended preschools in Ankara, Turkey, and were assessed as typically developing (Acarlar & Johnston, 2006). Most of the children were from middle-class families with parents who had completed at least secondary education. The language data were collected in dyads with a researcher

Table 12.1 Data and reference groups (age: +/– 2 months)

	Selma	*Berrin*	*Filiz*	*Şükran*	*Mehmet*	*Batuhan*	*Yunus*
Time 1							
Age	2;10	3;1	3;0	3;0	3;0	3;0	3;0
Size reference group	7	9	8	8	8	8	8
Number of utterances	142	147	143	140	128	82	131
Time 2							
Age	3;6	3;6	3;6	3;6	3;8	3;6	3;6
Size reference group	21	21	21	21	18	21	21
Number of utterances	100	142	71	142	139	150	147

in a room in the preschools or in the children's homes. The conversations typically included activities like book reading and playing with play dough or talking about topics such as holiday and home activities. Differences in the settings in which data were collected are visible in the present analyses and discussed when relevant. An overview of the data used in the present study is given in Table 12.1.

Results

By means of the SALT for Turkish software (Acarlar *et al.*, 2006), so-called Standard Analyses were run with 'Standard Measures', and 'Word lists, Bound morphemes and Utterance distribution'. The scores of the informants were compared with reference groups ranging from two months younger to two months older in age than the individual informants. The scores were assessed as deviating if they differed by more than 1 or 2 standard deviations (SD) from the mean of the reference group.

Intelligibility

Table 12.2 gives an overview of the proportion of utterances without unintelligible parts. It turns out that at both time 1 (around age 3;0) and time 2 (around age 3;6), the bilingual informants are less intelligible than the reference groups. For all children, this difference is of a size of 1 SD or 2 SD at time 1 and/or time 2.

Two aspects of the bilingual data may explain the fact that the bilingual children are less intelligible. First, most of the data was collected in settings

Table 12.2 Intelligibility compared with reference groups (age: +/−2 months)

	Selma	*Berrin*	*Filiz*	*Şükran*	*Mehmet*	*Batuhan*	*Yunus*
Time 1							
% Intelligible utterances	85[‡]	92	91	91	79[‡]	77[‡]	88[†]
+/−SD	−3.26	−0.67	−0.69	−0.76	−4.04	−3.88	−1.64
Time 2							
% Intelligible utterances	93[†]	92[†]	86[‡]	88[‡]	82[‡]	91[†]	95
+/−SD	−1.05	−1.39	−2.91	−2.7	−4.56	−1.39	−0.27

*>1 SD; **>2 SD; †<1 SD; ‡<2 SD.

with at least three participants, and some data even with up to 15 participants, in a day-care center. It is not unlikely that as a result the spontaneous speech data were overall less intelligible. A second aspect may, however, also be the bilingual nature of the data. The children also regularly spoke Dutch during the conversations, which may have led to more doubt among the transcribers about what a child was actually saying.

Word types and tokens

Table 12.3 gives an overview of the total number of words uttered by each child, the number of different word roots and the type/token ratio (TTR).[2] With the exception of Yunus, all bilingual children were almost as talkative as or even more talkative than the children in the reference groups. Only Yunus produced 2.55 SD less word tokens at time 1 and 1.58 SD less at time 2. However, all children but Mehmet produced at least 1 SD less word types than the monolingual reference group at time 1 and/or time 2. Mehmet scored around the average of his reference group at both times. For most children, the TTR was also at least 1 SD lower at time 1 and/or time 2. Exceptions include Selma as well as Yunus. This means that although Yunus was less talkative, the diversity of his words was still similar to the reference group (2).

The fact that the bilingual children use fewer different words may be explained by their bilingualism. Bilingual vocabularies do not usually contain translation equivalents of the words in both languages. Rather, bilinguals tend to use specific words in only one language, other words in the other language as well as words in both languages (known as *doublets*, Oller *et al.*, 2007). As all Dutch words were excluded from the present analyses, it is not surprising to find that the bilingual children use fewer different types of words than their monolingual peers.

Table 12.3 Types, tokens and TTR compared with reference groups (age: +/–2 months)

	Selma	*Berrin*	*Filiz*	*Şükran*	*Mehmet*	*Batuhan*	*Yunus*
Time 1							
Types	95†	87†	111	93†	96	56†	80†
+/–SD	–1.19	–1.59	–0.05	–1.1	–0.48	–1.53	–1.68
Tokens	275	298	338**	282	252	199**	206‡
+/–SD	–0.03	0.21	2.84	0.48	0.32	2.71	–2.55
TTR	0.35	0.29†	0.33†	0.33†	0.38	0.28‡	0.39
+/–SD	–0.93	–1.64	–1.1	–1.16	–0.58	–2.06	–0.48
Time 2							
Types	93	113	65†	110†	131	107†	99†
+/–SD	–0.5	–0.88	–1.38	–1.04	–0.21	–1.43	–1.75
Tokens	209	333	164	365	402	392	253†
+/–SD	–0.55	0.03	0.01	0.61	0.99	0.7	–1.58
TTR	0.44	0.34	0.40†	0.30†	0.33†	0.27†	0.39
+/–SD	0.04	–0.86	–1.41	–1.43	–1.04	–1.74	–0.05

*>1 SD; **>2 SD; †<1 SD; ‡<2 SD.

Mean length of utterance

A standard measure of utterance complexity is the mean length of utterance (MLU; Brown, 1973). Although MLU can be measured both in words and in morphemes, since Turkish is an agglutinating language, morphemes are the most relevant measure.

Table 12.4 gives an overview of MLU for the seven bilingual children. It turns out that most of the children score around the average MLU of the reference groups. There are two children who score at least 1 SD (Selma) or 2 SD (Yunus) below the reference groups.

Bound morphemes

Table 12.5 gives an overview of the number of omitted bound morphemes that were marked as such in the transcripts. Note that a score below the reference groups is 'positive' rather than 'negative' in those analyses (and vice versa). The data show that most children do not omit bound morphemes, which is in most cases similar to the reference groups. At time 2, Berrin and Filiz omit at least 1 SD more morphemes than the reference groups, but because the number of omissions is only one or two, the reliability is not very high.

Table 12.4 MLU in words and morphemes compared with reference groups (age: +/–2 months)

	Selma	*Berrin*	*Filiz*	*Şükran*	*Mehmet*	*Batuhan*	*Yunus*
Time 1							
MLU in morphemes	3.08†	3.1	3.49	3.36	3.19	3.44	2.02‡
+/–SD	–1.03	–0.68	0.73	0.24	–0.24	0.35	–3.75
Time 2							
MLU in morphemes	3.18†	3.51	4.03	3.99	4.32	3.95	2.41‡
+/–SD	–1.29	–0.87	–0.1	–0.19	–0.03	–0.25	–2.42

*>1 SD; **>2 SD; †<1 SD; ‡<2 SD.

Table 12.5 Omitted bound morphemes compared with reference groups (age: +/– 2 months)

	Selma	*Berrin*	*Filiz*	*Şükran*	*Mehmet*	*Batuhan*	*Yunus*
Time 1							
Number of morphemes	0*	0	1	0	0	0	0
+/–SD	–1.07	–0.71	0	–0.84	–0.85	–0.5	–0.88
Time 2							
Number of morphemes	1	2†	1†	0	0	0	0
+/–SD	0.77	1.64	1.15	–0.66	–0.79	–0.66	–0.66

*<1 SD; **<2 SD; †>1 SD; ‡>2 SD.

Case markers

Table 12.6 gives an overview of the case markers produced by the seven bilingual children. In general, the picture is rather diffuse. For almost all case markers, children score both above and below the average of the reference groups, as well as around the average. The only exception is the locative, which all children use as frequently as the reference children or even at least 1 or 2 SD above the average. For all children, it is the case that at a given point in time, they do not produce more than two case markers more than 1 SD lower than the reference groups.

The diffuse picture can probably be explained by the fact that it is largely dependent on the exact context and topics of conversation that

Table 12.6 Production of case markers compared with reference groups (age: +/–2 months)

	Selma	*Berrin*	*Filiz*	*Şükran*	*Mehmet*	*Batuhan*	*Yunus*
Time 1							
Accusative -(y/n)İ	23**	20**	9	7†	8	5	4‡
+/–SD	3.61	2.24	–0.46	–1.06	–0.6	–0.29	–2.07
Dative -(y/n)E	8	10	15	13	14	17**	8
+/–SD	–0.96	–0.27	0.59	0.3	0.74	2.74	–0.6
Locative -DE	20**	8	29**	8	19**	1	3
+/–SD	2.04	0.27	3.99	0.14	2.32	–0.92	–0.74
Ablative -DEn	9**	1	2	0	0	0	0
+/–SD	3.51	–0.78	0.28	–0.82	–0.82	–0.85	–0.82
Genitive -(n)İn	11**	12*	13**	9*	0†	4	2
+/–SD	2.44	1.25	2.08	1.00	–1.36	0.91	–0.82
Instrumental -lE	2	1	2	0†	0†	0	1
+/–SD	–0.31	–0.75	–0.41	–1.22	–1.29	–0.97	–0.84

(Continued)

Table 12.6 *Continued*

	Selma	*Berrin*	*Filiz*	*Şükran*	*Mehmet*	*Batuhan*	*Yunus*
Time 2							
Accusative -(y/n)İ	8	12	14**	19	13	6†	13
+/–SD	–0.72	–0.58	2.16	0.79	–0.54	–1.74	–0.47
Dative -(y/n)E	7†	6†	6	17	21*	9†	11
+/–SD	–1.07	–1.79	–0.87	0.35	1.4	–1.32	–0.88
Locative -DE	14*	9	6	13	13	35**	14
+/–SD	1.89	–0.06	0.34	0.77	0.22	5.12	0.93
Ablative -DEn	1†	8	4	2	7	2	1
+/–SD	–1.01	0.22	0.05	–0.73	0.13	–0.77	–0.91
Genitive -(n)İn	3	16*	2	3	1†	5	0†
+/–SD	–0.65	1.36	–0.45	–0.9	–1.33	–0.62	–1.41
Instrumental -lE	4*	0†	1	4	0†	1	0†
+/–SD	1.64	–1.08	–0.26	0.41	–1.34	–0.71	–1.08

*>1 SD; **>2 SD; †<1 SD; ‡<2 SD.

case markers occur. This explains the differences between time 1 and time 2, as well as the fact that although some case markers are used frequently, others are not. The data show that none of the bilingual children has a serious problem with using case markers.

Plural and possessive markers

An overview of the plural and possessive markers used by the bilingual children is presented in Table 12.7. The data show that at time 1, all bilingual children use fewer plural markers than the reference groups. In all cases but Filiz's, the difference is more than 1 *SD*. At time 2, none of the children uses plural markers, but apparently the reference groups do not produce many plural markers either, as the difference is in none of the cases more than 0.5 SD. It is not clear as to what developments lie behind those difference between age 3;0 and 3;6.

With respect to possessive markers, the picture turns out to be as diffuse as the picture for the case markers presented before. Children tend to score around, below or above the average for all case markers and differently at time 1 and time 2. Presumably, it is the exact situation and topic of conversation that influences the choice of a particular possessive suffix. As none of the children produces more than one of the three suffixes more than 1 SD below the average of the reference groups at a specific point in time, it can be concluded that none of the children has severe problems with possessive markers.

Verb inflections (tense)

The picture that arises from Table 12.8 about the production of verbal tense inflections is different from the diffuse ones discussed for case markers and for plural and possessive markers. What is remarkable in the data for tense inflections is that relatively often the bilingual children score more than 1 SD below the average of the reference groups. For the progressive suffix, the differences are the largest: four children score more than 1 SD below the average at both time 1 and time 2, two children (Mehmet and Batuhan) score at least 1 SD below the average at time 1 and around the average at time 2, and only one child (Şükran) scores around the average during both recording sessions. For the past simple and the evidential, scores at least 1 SD below the averages are found in about half of the cases. At time 2, there are two children (Şükran and Mehmet) who score at least 1 SD above the average. For the aorist, children generally score around the average at time 1 and/or time 2.

In sum, it appears that at least for some bilingual children, the difference with the reference groups with respect to the production of verbal tense suffixes is structural. This is most clearly visible for Selma, who scores at least 1 SD below the average for all suffixes at time 1, and Yunus, who scores below the average for three or four suffixes at both time 1 and time 2.

Table 12.7 Production of plural markers and possessive suffixes compared with reference groups (age: +/−2 months)

	Selma	*Berrin*	*Filiz*	*Şükran*	*Mehmet*	*Batuhan*	*Yunus*
Time 1							
Plural	0†	5†	6	3†	0†	0†	0†
+/−SD	−1.45	−1.02	−0.66	−1.31	−1.8	−1.95	−1.96
Possessive 1.sg	8	3	2	6	5	2	0†
+/−SD	0.62	−0.65	−0.97	0.1	0.04	−0.28	−1.56
Possessive 2.sg	3**	1	2*	1	1	0	0
+/−SD	2.38	0.76	1.98	0.66	0.66	−0.66	−0.66
Possessive 3.sg	7†	6†	7	15	8	2†	5
+/−SD	−1.19	−1.4	−0.69	0.89	−0.27	−1.05	−0.94
Time 2							
Plural	0	0	0	0	0	0	0
+/−SD	−0.38	−0.5	−0.35	−0.35	−0.35	−0.35	−0.35
Possessive 1.sg	5‡	15	11†	13	18	13	4‡
+/−SD	−2.51	−0.72	−1.23	−0.88	0.16	0.83	−2.47
Possessive 2.sg	2	9**	5**	3	13**	3**	1
+/−SD	0.31	5.96	2.14	0.77	8.93	3.31	−0.29
Possessive 3.sg	6**	4**	2	0	1	0	1
+/−SD	2.44	3.46	0.44	−0.98	−0.21	−0.84	−0.27

*>1 SD; **>2 SD; †<1 SD; ‡<2 SD.

Table 12.8 Production of verbal tense markers compared with reference groups (age: +/–2 months)

	Selma	*Berrin*	*Filiz*	*Şükran*	*Mehmet*	*Batuhan*	*Yunus*
Time 1							
Progressive	10‡	19†	12‡	29	17†	9‡	9‡
+/–SD	–2.69	–1.91	–2.89	–0.38	–1.83	–2.09	–3.01
Simple past	11†	13	13†	17	17	5	6‡
+/–SD	–1.04	–0.92	–1.04	–0.22	0.28	–0.39	–2.71
Evidential	3†	4	6	0†	5	0†	4
+/–SD	–1.53	–0.62	–0.43	–1.71	–0.61	–1.64	–0.9
Aorist	0†	1	1	0	0	1	0
+/–SD	–1.01	–0.59	–0.69	–0.99	–0.99	–0.48	–0.99
Time 2							
Progressive	12†	18†	8†	28	25	31	15†
+/–SD	–1.23	–1.16	–1.25	–0.24	–0.53	–0.15	–1.48
Simple past	5†	19	11	9†	5†	24	8†
+/–SD	–1.15	–0.49	–0.2	–1.29	–1.6	–0.21	–1.42
Evidential	5	2†	3	27**	20*	0†	2†
+/–SD	–0.33	–1.23	–0.54	3.02	1.83	–1.58	–1.26
Aorist	0	2	0	4	14*	2	2
+/–SD	–0.95	–0.74	–0.86	–0.46	1.42	–0.76	–0.76

*>1 SD; **>2 SD; †<1 SD; ‡<2 SD.

Verb inflections (aspect/modality)

Table 12.9 gives an overview of the results for aspect or modality marking suffixes on verbs. It appears that most suffixes are rather infrequent in the data of the reference group, and similarly also virtually absent in the bilingual data. Most children produce the negation marker relatively frequently. Sometimes they use it below the average of the reference groups, and sometimes above or around the average. For all children, it is the case that they produce it around the average at time 1, time 2 or both. A similar picture arises for the gerund -(y)İncE. The only exception is Yunus, who produces at least 1 SD lower than the average of the reference groups at both time 1 and time 2. The picture for the optative is also similar. The only exception for this suffix is Batuhan, who produces at least 1 SD more than the average of the reference groups at both time 1 and time 2. In general, however, the picture that arises is again a diffuse one.

Discussion and Conclusion

Language samples of seven bilingual children were analyzed using the software package SALT for Turkish (Acarlar *et al.*, 2006) and compared to the results of monolingual reference groups. A summary of the results is given in Table 12.10.

On the basis of the findings, it can be concluded that using SALT with bilingual children has certain implications. The fact that bilinguals often score lower in comparison to monolingual reference groups in SALT should be taken into account when using SALT as a clinical tool. The deviations from monolingual scores should not be seen as a problem or as an indication of lower skills in the language measured. Secondly, the 'diffuse' patterns observed for the use of some bound morphemes (such as case markers, possessive markers and some verbal suffixes) indicate that there are no structural problems in those areas. Those areas are potentially interesting for diagnosing children with SLI. Thirdly, if SALT is to be used in bilingual contexts, it is recommended that a bilingual standardized version be developed. Because of the bilingual nature of the data, not all analyses (e.g. discourse related ones) could be done. In addition, a bilingual reference group would make the picture complete. On the basis of the approaches presented in this volume, a combination of various techniques and instruments can be utilized for such a comparison. Fourthly, more research is needed to explain why bilingual children score structurally lower on verbal tense markers. Most probably, the difference is related to lower amounts of Turkish input available to immigrant children. Finally, the socio-cultural background of parents may also play a role in these linguistic differences as most of the immigrants come from rural backgrounds compared to the reference group informants. Naturally, the quality of Turkish language input is a lot different from the

Table 12.9 Production of verbal aspect and modality markers compared with reference groups (age: +/−2 months)

	Selma	***Berrin***	***Filiz***	***Şükran***	***Mehmet***	***Batuhan***	***Yunus***
Time 1							
Negation -mE	14*	9	5†	26‡	18**	4	4
+/−SD	1.11	−0.41	−1.03	3.68	2.36	−0.23	−1.01
Gerund -(y)İncE	15*	4	9*	1†	3†	1	1†
+/−SD	2.05	−1	1.02	−1.71	−1.02	−0.91	−1.71
Conditional -sE	0	0	0	0	0	0	0
+/−SD	−0.38	−0.84	−0.54	−0.54	−0.35	−0.35	−0.35
Optative -(y)E	1	6	0†	12**	2	9**	2
+/−SD	−0.87	0.85	−1.12	2.86	−0.47	3	−0.47
Necessitative -mElİ	0	0	0	0	0	0	0
+/−SD	0	0	0	0	0	0	0
Potential -Ebil	0	0	1*	0	0	0	0
+/−SD	−0.8	−0.33	1.62	−0.54	−0.54	−0.35	−0.54
Causative -Dİr	0	0	0	0	0	0	0
+/−SD	−0.38	−0.5	−0.35	−0.35	−0.35	−0.35	−0.35

(Continued)

Table 12.9 *Continued*

	Selma	*Berrin*	*Filiz*	*Şükran*	*Mehmet*	*Batuhan*	*Yunus*
Time 2							
Negation -mE	3	8	3	8	10	5†	5
+/–SD	–0.91	–0.25	–0.17	–0.25	0.01	–1.05	–1.00
Gerund -(y)İncE	7	6	10**	15*	2	4	0†
+/–SD	0.63	–0.21	2.82	1.88	–0.9	–0.81	–1.69
Conditional -sE	0	0	1	0	2	0	0
+/–SD	–0.47	–0.49	0.56	–0.49	0.35	–0.49	–0.49
Optative -(y)E	4	3	3	3	11*	9*	0†
+/–SD	0.38	–0.45	0.96	–0.45	1.97	1.01	–1.28
Necessitative -mElİ	0	0	0	0	0	0	0
+/–SD	–0.22	–0.22	–0.22	–0.22	–0.24	–0.22	–0.22
Potential -Ebil	0	0	0	1	2	3**	0
+/–SD	–0.58	–0.51	–0.51	0.38	0.59	2.17	–0.51
Causative -Dİr	0	0	0	0	0	0	0
+/–SD	–0.32	–0.32	0	–0.32	–0.24	–0.32	–0.32

*>1 SD; **>2 SD; †<1 SD; ‡<2 SD.

Table 12.10 Overview of the results of the comparisons between seven bilingual children in the Netherlands and the monolingual reference groups

Domain	*Bilinguals (compared to monolinguals)*
Intelligibility	Less
Lexical diversity (TTR)	Less
Utterance complexity (MLU)	Similar (some less)
Morphology	
Case markers	Diffuse
Plural markers	Similar or less
Possessive markers	Diffuse
Verbal inflection (tense)	Less
Verbal inflection (aspect/modality)	Diffuse

monolingual Turkish environment. The Dutch context can be characterized as a submersion environment, which is highly counter-productive for bilingual development. On the basis of this chapter, the concluding statement can be as follows: Whether SLI or normally developing, bilingual children are a special population and instruments aiming at assessing their language skills need to be developed for this specific group. Monolingual assessment instruments might not show the nature and extent of the possible language impairment.

Notes

1. For language codes, a so-called dependent tier was used (%lan). On this tier, Turkish utterances were coded with '$Turkish'. The CLAN command used to extract the relevant child utterances is: kwal *filename.cha* +t*chi +t%lan +o@UTF8 +o@* +s$turkish* +d +o@Begin +o@UTF8 +o@Participants +o@Languages +o@End +o@ID | kwal +s* +d +o@Begin +o@Participants +o@Languages +o@End +o@ID +f. The output is now saved as pipeout.kwa.cex, which can be changed with the command: rename pipeout.kwa.cex *filename.salt.cha.*
2. Note, however, that TTR is sensitive to sample size: a smaller sample leads to a TTR (Malvern *et al.*, 2004; Vermeer, 2000). This may explain the pattern found for Yunus.

Chapter 13

Language Impairment in Turkish-Dutch Bilingual Children

JAN DE JONG, NAZİFE ÇAVUŞ and ANNE BAKER

Introduction

Specific language impairment (SLI) is defined on the basis of clear linguistic symptoms in the absence of a clear etiology. The language delay cannot be explained by a primary disorder such as mental retardation, perceptual impairment or obvious neurological dysfunction (Stark & Tallal, 1981). Previous research has highlighted inclusive characteristics of SLI for many languages – they constitute the linguistic symptoms of the disorder. In this chapter, we will focus on the grammatical, primarily morphological, symptoms in a specific population: bilingual – Turkish-Dutch – children with SLI.

Diagnosis of SLI in bilingual children poses a specific challenge. The exclusionary criteria mentioned above, that is intelligence and hearing status, etc., still apply. The inclusionary criteria – the language skills themselves – make it necessary to consider the influence of the child's bilingualism.

Diagnosis of SLI in bilingual children is not always adequate. Genesee *et al.* (2004) make a useful distinction between two – all too common – types of misdiagnosis in bilingual children. One is that of 'missed identity', where a child is language-impaired but is not recognized as such. The other is 'mistaken identity', where a typically developing (TD) child is mistaken for a child with SLI. Yagmur and Nap-Kolhoff (Chapter 12, this volume) highlight the second type of misdiagnosis and suggest some explanations. A main cause is that there is a lack of knowledge about what should be considered normal in bilingual children. Is it normal, for example, for a bilingual child to omit determiners in the second language after two years of exposure? If a particular linguistic behavior is normal in bilinguals, then a similar lack of knowledge can also explain 'missed identity'. After all, if normal development cannot be properly profiled, there is no benchmark for establishing deviance either.

In this chapter we will discuss some assessment tools used in the Netherlands. The main focus, however, will be on the differences between bilingual children with and without SLI. We will argue that the characteristics of bilingual SLI cannot be identified reliably without referring to a *bilingual* control group without SLI. We will substantiate that claim for both the first language (Turkish) and the second language (Dutch). Research on bilingualism and SLI has taken many forms (for a review, see de Jong, 2008). For instance, TD bilinguals have been compared to monolingual children with SLI; bilingual children with SLI have been compared to monolingual children with SLI; and, finally, bilingual children with SLI have been compared to TD controls. The latter comparison will be the prime focus of this chapter, whereas comparison with monolingual (Dutch) children with SLI will serve as an additional point of reference.

SLI across Languages, in Monolinguals and Bilinguals

In this chapter, we will present some of the results from the Amsterdam research project on Turkish-Dutch children with SLI. In this project, both the children's languages are investigated.[1]

Previous research on the typological characteristics of SLI has generated different predictions about the symptoms in the Turkish and Dutch output of the bilingual children. Leonard and his colleagues (for a review, see Leonard, 1998) have conducted a number of studies on SLI as it appears in different languages. They find cross-linguistic similarities as well as differences. In each language studied, SLI children have delayed acquisition of language with the primary symptoms being in grammatical morphology. In that respect, we therefore expect similar phenomena in monolingual Turkish and Dutch children with SLI and in the two languages in a language-impaired bilingual child.

However, Leonard has also shown important differences. First of all, difficulties with grammatical morphology are less severe in languages that have a rich morphological system and are also more visible in languages in which the morphology is sparse, as research on languages such as Italian, Spanish and Hebrew (rich) reveals compared to English (sparse). Following this dichotomy, Turkish would group with Italian, etc., and Dutch with English. Consequently, in Turkish-Dutch bilingual children, we would expect more errors in Dutch than in Turkish. Leonard has also pointed out the role of perceptual saliency in the children's performance. Leonard refers to SLI children's limited processing capacity. A morpheme that is highly salient, that is, syllabic or can be lengthened, is more perceptible and thus it requires less processing effort. A morpheme that consists of a single consonant, on the other hand, is more problematic. This variable correlates with typological differences, partly overlapping with morphological richness: morphemes in languages in which morphology is rich are often also salient. Turkish and Dutch differ in this respect as well – Turkish morphology in general is more salient.

There are differing positions regarding what to expect in a bilingual child. Paradis (2007) discusses two opposing views. The 'representational' theory posits that SLI children's linguistic knowledge is faulty. The grammar itself shows signs of impairment. If this is the case, the same problems should show up in both languages, although their appearance may vary due to typological differences. As Leonard (in his preface to Genesee *et al.*, 2004) puts it: 'the same child with SLI will show two different grammatical profiles depending on the language being spoken' (Genesee *et al.*, 2004: xvi). Following this theory, our bilingual children should have the symptoms of Dutch monolinguals with SLI in their Dutch as well as those of Turkish monolinguals with SLI in their Turkish. Their bilingual status should have no influence. Crucially, the severity of the problem should not exceed the profile of monolingual SLI in either language. The alternative view posits that children with SLI need more time to process the linguistic information needed. Once a child is faced with input in two languages, this process is slowed down even further. The child 'would have twice as much linguistic information to deal with in the same amount of exposure time as monolinguals' (Paradis, 2007: 553). This should lead to a delay compared to monolingual children with SLI in both languages, though not necessarily to different symptoms. This position is described as a 'processing' account: the innate linguistic knowledge itself is presumed to be intact. In this chapter, we will also compare our findings with the predictions based on these two positions.

The Amsterdam Study on Bilingualism and SLI

Subjects

We compared four groups, each consisting of 20 children: monolingual (Dutch) children with SLI and two groups of Turkish-Dutch children: with and without language impairment. The children were between six and eight years old. Both languages were studied. In addition, we included a group of TD younger children whose first language is Dutch. One group that is conspicuously missing here is a group of Turkish monolinguals with SLI. Such a group was not available, and, importantly, not much is yet known of the grammatical symptoms of SLI in Turkish (for more information, though, see other chapters in this volume). We cannot therefore fully verify whether the outcomes on SLI in Turkish are also valid for monolingual SLI children.

The findings for both languages will be discussed in turn and are followed by a cross-linguistic comparison.

Turkish

Variables

As mentioned above, there has been very little research on the symptoms of SLI in Turkish. A recent explorative study by Acarlar and Johnston (2006) reported on the verbal output of a small number of impaired Turkish monolingual children. These children, it should be noticed, were not *specifically* language-impaired. They were described as having a pervasive developmental disorder or a general delay. However, since the language of children with non-specific delay tends to share vulnerable domains with the language of children with SLI (see Rice & Warren, 2004), Acarlar and Johnston's study might offer a window on the symptoms of SLI in Turkish. An important observation in their study is that nominal morphology appears to be more vulnerable than verbal morphology. This finding echoes what is known about typical language acquisition in Turkish, where verbal morphology is acquired quickly (Küntay & Slobin, 1999). This is different from what is known about SLI in, for instance, Germanic languages. Acarlar and Johnston specifically single out errors in the genitive–possessive construction, in which one suffix has to agree in grammatical person with another suffix (Göksel & Kerslake, 2005). This agreement relationship is, in their findings, more severely affected than subject–verb agreement. Another aspect of the nominal domain that can be argued to be vulnerable is case marking. Data on other languages that have case marking on nouns suggest that case is impaired in SLI, as for example in Hungarian (see the $n = 1$ study by Vinkler and Pléh (1995)). Consequently, for the present study, accusative marking and possessive marking were included among the research variables.

Studies on normal acquisition show early mastery of subject–verb agreement in Turkish (Aksu-Koç, 1997). Nevertheless, given the fact that verb agreement has been shown to be affected in SLI in many languages, albeit to different extents, it was also included in this study. In addition, it allowed us to compare the children's specific performance cross-linguistically since this domain was also investigated for Dutch.

Data

All variables were addressed in grammatical closure tasks, in which the child had to complete a sentence and, in so doing, supply the relevant morphological marker. Additional data came from narratives that were elicited using the Frog Story (Berman & Slobin, 1994; Mayer, 1969). Our findings, for obvious reasons, concern the two bilingual groups only: Turkish-Dutch children with and without language impairment.

Results

Subject–verb agreement was measured in past-perfect forms – after the morpheme – *DI* or one of its allomorphs. Within this inflectional paradigm, one form, the third person singular, does not have an overt agreement marker.

Agreement marking was faultless in the TD bilingual children. This is possibly not surprising in 6–8-year-old children since forms marked for agreement in Turkish are mastered around age 2 in monolingual children (Aksu-Koç, 1997). The bilingual children with SLI, on the other hand, did produce errors, although the groupwise percentage of correct forms in obligatory contexts (89%) was close to the conventional 90% criterion for acquisition of a morpheme; only six children failed to fulfill that criterion. The group difference was significant. In only a few cases was the zero-morpheme associated with the third person singular substituted for an overt morpheme; this might be called an omission. Most errors involved the substitution by an overt marker. An example of a substitution of a second person form by a first person form by a language-impaired boy (age 7.5) is given in Example (1) below. Remember that cloze procedures were used so that the child's contribution is indicated in brackets.

(1) *Afferin oğlu-m, sen güzel bir çiçek . . . (kes-ti-m).*
Well done son-POSS.1SG, you beautiful a flower. . (cut-PST-1SG)
'Well done, my son, you have cut a beautiful flower'

Substitutions are common in SLI in languages with a rich morphology. Chilla and Babur (Chapter 16, this volume), in slightly younger children with SLI, also found bare forms: forms in which not only the agreement marker but also the tense–aspect–modality morphemes were omitted. These errors were also found in a case study of a TD monolingual Turkish child by Aksu-Koç and Nihan Ketrez (2003) during what they called the 'premorphological stage'. No such errors were found in the present study.

Case marking was measured in two contexts in which the direct object in the sentence must have an accusative marker: where the object is immediately preverbal, but definite, and where an object is not immediately preverbal (Göksel & Kerslake, 2005). A significant group difference was found for the task in which the word order created the obligatory context, that is when the word order was not object–verb, but not for the definite condition.

In Example (2), a girl with SLI (age 7:.10) omits an accusative marker.

(2) *küçük (bardak-Ø adam tutuyor)*
small glass- Ø man hold-DUR-3SG
Correct form:
küçük (bardağ-i adam tut-uyor)
small glass-ACC man hold-DUR-3SG
'The man holds a small glass'.

The word order in this example is object–subject–verb. Since the direct object does not immediately precede the verb, it must be marked for the accusative case.

The word-order task was designed to elicit several possible word orders, precisely because some word orders necessitate the accusative marker.

However, there is a strong preference in Turkish for the SOV order (Batman-Ratyosyan & Stromswold, 1999). The children in our study also reflected this preference: they often changed the target sentences to fit the canonical word order. As a consequence, the number of analyzable responses in the word-order condition decreased. To further investigate the children's awareness of the correlation between word order and case marking, a grammatical judgment task was used. On this task the children with SLI performed significantly worse than the bilingual TD group. This finding confirms the impression that case marking is weak in the SLI group.

A first analysis of a sample of Frog stories (five bilingual SLI children and five bilingual TD matched for age) showed a higher frequency of case marking errors in the SLI subjects. In addition, a lower frequency of case markers was found in the impaired children. This concerned not only the accusative case, but also the genitive and the dative. This observation mirrors findings for younger Turkish-German children (Chilla & Babur, Chapter 16, this volume). In the study of Turkish language impaired children by Acarlar and Johnston, it was found that '(1) noun suffix errors occurred three times as often as verb suffix errors, and (2) the frequency of use for most noun inflections was well below the normal range' (Acarlar & Johnston, 2006: 91). Given the performance of the SLI group in the verb agreement and case marking tasks (89% versus 56%),[2] we can confirm the dissociation between verbal and nominal morphology; the initial findings from the Frog story show a similar picture. The significant difference between the two research groups, at least for one accusative context, suggests that case marking is a candidate for a clinical marker of SLI in Turkish.

The *genitive–possessive construction* is interesting in that it represents an agreement relation beyond the verbal domain. It is a composite noun phrase constructed of two noun phrases marked as follows: (noun phrase + genitive) + (noun phrase + possessive) (Göksel & Kerslake, 2005). The possessive marker must agree with the first noun phrase for person. In our study, there was no significant difference between the SLI group (52%) and the bilingual TD children (69%). The percentage in the latter group, and thus the frequency with which these children omit the possessive marker, is intriguing: it is well below the level at which the marker can be said to be mastered. Out of 20 TD children, only eight reached 90% realization in obligatory contexts. Since the application of the rule by these TD children is not consistent and since there is no difference between the two groups, the morpheme cannot serve as a marker of SLI. In contrast, the pilot study on the Frog story data revealed a different picture: the TD children supplied the correct possessive morpheme in 97% of the contexts in these narrative data; the SLI children in only 64% of the contexts.

The data from the elicitation task may prompt the hypothesis that the use of this particular morpheme is undergoing change in Turkish as spoken in the Netherlands and the performance of the bilingual TD children may be the reflection of this. However, no conclusive evidence is yet available about this aspect of language change in the host country. On the other hand, Yagmur and Nap-Kolhoff (this volume), in their exploration of possessive marking in seven TD Turkish-Dutch children, found *no* difference between their bilingual children and Acarlar *et al.*'s monolingual normative SALT data.[3] Summarizing the suggestion by Acarlar and Johnston (2006) that the genitive–possessive construction is a vulnerable domain in SLI was not confirmed in our study. The discrepancy with studies on Turkish in the country of origin warrants further investigation of the source of this difference.

In conclusion, the three domains investigated present three perspectives on SLI in Turkish as well as on bilingualism. Problems with subject–verb agreement are less severe than in, for instance, Germanic languages. This finding resembles what is known about other languages with a rich morphology. Case marking is a domain that has been little researched and, as Acarlar and Johnston (2006) suggest, it may be a more vulnerable area for SLI in Turkish than verb morphology. Finally, possessive marking shows that what is known about Turkish in the country of origin may be different in the host country and, consequently, in the first language that bilingual children are acquiring. If this is the case, it adds to the need to create bilingual language norms.

Dutch

Variables

For the Dutch part of the study, two linguistic domains were selected. Subject–verb agreement was chosen because it is a key area of difficulty in Dutch children with SLI (de Jong, 1999). The other domain selected is that of gender marking on articles and adjectival morphology, two interrelated phenomena. This particular domain presents persistent problems to learners of Dutch as a second language and has not been studied sufficiently in SLI children. By jointly addressing variables that characterize language impairment and normal second language learning, we aim to shed light on the relative impact of both factors on bilingual SLI.

Dutch, like German, is a verb-second language. Key features of these languages are thus similar. An important similarity concerns the correlation of verb form and verb position: finite forms appear in second position; non-finite forms are sentence-final. Chilla and Babur (Chapter 16, this volume) observe that German monolingual children with SLI produce 'sentences with finite or non-finite verbs in verb-final position' (Chilla & Babur, this volume: Chapter 16). This observation does not hold for Dutch, where the correlation that is found in monolingual TD children is also strong for children with SLI: finite forms are seldom found in utterance-final position. Inflection itself, on the other hand, is significantly impaired in these children (de Jong, 1999).

Dutch has two definite articles: the article *het* for (singular) neuter nouns and *de* before common nouns. There is only one indefinite article, *een*. Adjectives in Dutch are inflected when they are used attributively, that is, before a noun. Here, the gender distinction becomes important. The inflectional marker is – *e*, except for one particular context. If the noun phrase is indefinite, singular and neuter, the adjective has zero-marking. So the gender distinction that is not visible in the indefinite article has to be reflected in the adjective. This is illustrated in Example (3).

(3) a. *een grote* (groot-**e**) *tafel*
'a large table'
b. *een groot* (groot- **Ø**) *huis*
'a large house'

The 'exceptional case' (3b) is the one that is difficult for learners of Dutch as a second language and, to a lesser extent, for native learners of Dutch.

Data

Data for both domains were elicited in a sentence completion task. For the verb inflection task, agreement marking was targeted, not verb placement. This meant that the verb was elicited in the second position, where the verb must be finite. To ensure that the verb position was unambiguous, transitive verbs were used, since with intransitive verbs, the second and final positions cannot be distinguished.

For Dutch, an additional group of children could be used for comparison: monolingual children with SLI. This makes it possible to test the hypothesis that bilingual children with SLI show the symptoms of monolingual children with SLI, as predicted by the representational-deficit hypothesis. This hypothesis could not be tested for Turkish. As described in the section 'SLI across Languages, in Monolinguals and Bilinguals', the processing hypothesis predicts the opposite result. Bilingualism should put an additional demand on the resources that the impaired child has at its disposal and thus lead to an additive or cumulative effect of impairment and bilingual status.

Results

Verb morphology: Table 13.1 presents the percentages of correct agreement marking for all groups. First of all, there was a difference between

Table 13.1 Subject–verb agreement: Percentage of realization of morphemes in the obligatory context; means

	TD bilingual children	*Bilingual children with SLI*	*Monolingual children with SLI*
Subject–verb agreement	88	77	81

the monolingual children with SLI and the TD bilingual children. This finding contradicts previous research in which similarities were observed between language impairment and normal bilingualism (Håkansson & Nettelbladt, 1996). Paradis (2005) argued that this similarity might make it even more difficult to identify SLI in bilingual children. In our comparison, there were two important findings that complement this evidence. Bilingual children with SLI differed from bilingual TD children but not from monolingual children with SLI. Apparently, in this linguistic domain, the effect of SLI can be isolated from the effect of bilingualism.

How do these findings compare to the hypotheses discussed in the section 'SLI across Languages, in Monolinguals and Bilinguals'? The prediction, based on a processing explanation, that there is a difference in severity between the monolingual and bilingual SLI group is not confirmed. One observation should be added here. In adult learners of Dutch as an L2, a specific kind of substitution is often found: the use of the marker – *en*, which can express both plural as well as non-finiteness, with the verb in the second position (Blom *et al.*, 2006). This error was, however, rarely found in the children. In this respect, the error *types* of monolingual and bilingual children with SLI, as well as of monolingual and bilingual TD children, were similar.

As mentioned above, adjectival agreement is a domain which is quite challenging for learners of Dutch as a second language. Errors made here tend to be persistent. The description of the 'exceptional case' above illustrated the complexity of the rule that has to be learned.[4] In the same groups of subjects that participated in the verb agreement task, significant differences were found between TD groups of monolingual and bilingual children (Orgassa, 2009; Orgassa & Weerman, 2008). This was also the same for the comparison between bilingual and monolingual children with SLI. In addition, there was a difference between TD children and children with SLI. Consequently, for verb agreement the effects of bilingualism and SLI cannot be disentangled: they are both at work here.

To return to the hypotheses in the section 'SLI across Languages, in Monolinguals and Bilinguals': the results are mixed. For one of our domains (verb agreement), no additive effect is found; for adjectival agreement, there is evidence for such an effect (see Table 13.2).

Table 13.2 Adjectival inflection: Percentage of correct (zero) marking in the 'exceptional case'

	TD bilingual children	*Bilingual children with SLI*	*Monolingual children with SLI*
Indefinite neuter gender	39	14	31

In conclusion, a comparison between the Turkish and Dutch findings

The error patterns in the Dutch and Turkish output of the children with SLI should reflect the typological differences that Leonard and his colleagues have identified (Leonard, 1998, 2000). Here this prediction could be tested in one domain only, subject–verb agreement. Bilingual children with SLI indeed produced more errors in Dutch than in Turkish. Since these languages differ in morphological richness, the direction of the difference is correctly predicted by Leonard's hypothesis. The percentage of use in Turkish (89%) cannot be said to be within a 'clinical range' and thus must be dismissed as a clinical marker, at least in this age range.

The other variables that were investigated do not allow for a cross-linguistic comparison but they can inform us about the characteristics of SLI in these bilingual children.

For Turkish, evidence was found that case marking, in particular, is affected in bilingual SLI when word order creates an obligatory context. Evidence that this is also true for monolingual Turkish children with SLI is sparse. A study by Topbaş (2006c) of 15 language impaired children (mean age 6;2) revealed '[n]ot many errors in noun or verb inflections'. Acarlar and Johnston (2006) found more errors in noun morphology than in verb morphology, but they pointed out possessive marking specifically. As explained above, the possessive morpheme cannot be considered an SLI marker in Turkish, at least in the Netherlands, due to its low frequency in the TD bilingual group.

In the Dutch findings, in one domain (adjectives), the bilingual children with SLI show the influence of impairment as well as of second language learning, and in another (verbs), the SLI effect is predominant. This is relevant for diagnostic practice. There are no errors that are exclusive to bilingual children with SLI; neither are there any that resemble errors made by adult learners of Dutch as an L2. As in the monolingual population, the SLI group is primarily characterized by its error *frequency*.

These findings have a dual implication. On the one hand, when SLI and bilingualism cannot be separated, criteria for SLI in bilinguals are needed. These can only be defined by creating a normative database of bilingual learners of Dutch. On the other hand, when an SLI effect can be isolated, a monolingual (Dutch) assessment tool may be able to identify bilingual children with SLI.

Bilingualism and Diagnosis of Language Impairment in the Netherlands

In the introduction to this chapter, we referred to two types of misdiagnosis, leading to instances of mistaken identity and missed identity (Genesee *et al.*, 2004), respectively. This current study had implications for clinical practice. We will first give a brief survey of the tools currently available for diagnosing bilingual children in the Netherlands. In conclusion, we will revisit the results of our study and question the adequacy of the assessment tools in the light of our findings.

In the Netherlands, children with SLI are cared for in a number of ways. Initially, they are referred to a speech therapist. If the impairment is significant, the child may be referred to a diagnostic team. If the language impairment turns out to be SLI, the child can either go to a special school for children with language difficulties or receive peripatetic treatment, a service usually provided by professionals from the special schools. The choice between these two options lies with the parents.

The number of children attending special schools amounts to almost 4% of Dutch primary school children. The *percentage* of children with a non-Dutch language background who visit these special schools is higher than among children who are native speakers of Dutch.[5] Non-native speakers constitute 14% of the mainstream school population, but 19% of special schools. At the special schools for children with speech and/or language difficulties, the percentage of children who are not native speakers of Dutch is around 24%. Of course, if there were no misdiagnosis, the percentage of children identified with language impairment should be identical in monolinguals and bilinguals. The ratio suggests that there is still a certain measure of misdiagnosis. It is probably not the application of exclusionary criteria that leads to misdiagnosis. Rather, the language assessment itself seems to be inadequate.

The numbers presented above are at odds with some findings in the literature. Salameh (2006), describing the situation in Sweden, discusses two factors that may *prevent* bilingual children from being referred for treatment. First, diagnostic assessment and referral to a special school are refused more often by parents of non-native children. Another observation, echoed by Crutchley (1999) for the United Kingdom, is that the selection of bilingual children who are referred may be skewed. Bilingual children who are referred have more severe problems than the monolingual children referred. They also have a more even profile in that more language levels are affected. The implication is that bilingual children with a less severe problem, but who are still in need of care, are overlooked. As Crutchley stresses, this pattern may be an artifact of late – and more reluctant – referral. Diagnosticians may have more 'patience' with these children. With bilinguals, they may be more willing to think that the children will catch up.

As in Germany (Chilla & Babur, Chapter 16, this volume), children in the Netherlands are commonly assessed in their second language only. No Turkish language tests are available and, in addition, administration of such a test would require a Turkish-speaking diagnostician. There is, however, a vocabulary screening test for Turkish (Schlichting, 2002), based on the Language Development Survey (Rescorla, 1989) and a test for bilinguals (Verhoeven *et al.*, 1995) that includes items for Turkish. In addition, questionnaires that include items about the language history of the child necessarily include information on the first language that the parents supply. In order to acquire more information about the first language, some interpreters are trained to specifically gather information about language (Blumenthal & Julien, 2000).

For assessment of the proficiency in the second language, there is a widely used test battery, the (TAK) the Taaltoets Alle Kinderen ('Language Test for All Children'[6]) (Verhoeven & Vermeer, 2006) that aims to broaden the scope to monolinguals *and* bilinguals ('all children'). The route chosen is the establishment of separate norms for native speakers of Dutch and for bilingual children. One of the norm groups selected consists of bilingual children. The resulting test score can be translated into one of three levels of performance – high, average and low. A low score on the TAK plays a role in a child's referral to special education. It will be clear that a task that allows only for three 'scores' runs the risk of creating a 'mistaken identity' (Genesee *et al.*, 2004). After all, not all children who perform at the level 'low' on the test will turn out to be language-impaired. This does not subtract from the value of this particular enterprise, but it stresses the fact that one should not rely on this or any single test.

Concluding Remarks

Our research has some implications for diagnostic practice. In previous research, it has sometimes been claimed that monolingual SLI and typical bilingualism have many characteristics in common. This finding is discouraging for the identification of SLI in bilinguals, at least based on their second language (Paradis, 2005). However, the diagnostic confound can be solved in a straightforward way, by including a third group in the comparison. After all, the only valid benchmark for bilingual children with SLI is the performance of TD *bilingual* children. Diagnostic markers of SLI in bilingual children should derive from comparisons with that group, for their first language as well as for their second language. In this chapter we have suggested some domains in which SLI may be apparent. In the first language, Turkish, noun morphology may be a useful index – more so than verb morphology, at least for the age range we have addressed here. In the second language, Dutch, the SLI group differs from the bilingual TD children in verb morphology as well as in adjectival morphology.

The remaining clinical challenge is twofold. First, we should agree on what constitutes markers for SLI in the first and second languages – that is the variables that are clinically sensitive. Second, as a point of reference, we should create bilingual norm groups that enable us to measure SLI children's performance in the linguistic domains in the L2 that are vulnerable.

Given the fact that information on performance in the L1, arguably a litmus test of SLI, is obviously needed but often not available, these L2 norms may fill a diagnostic gap.

Notes

1. The research was undertaken at the University of Amsterdam and funded by the Dutch Research Council NWO (NWO Research grant 254-70-010). Besides the authors, Antje Orgassa and Fred-Weerman participated in the project. The Dutch data to be presented here are part of Antje Orgassa's dissertation (Orgassa, 2009).
2. For accusative marking in the word-order condition, in the definiteness condition, the percentage was 63%. Mean percentages for the TD group were 90% and 86%, respectively. The error percentages in the SLI group exceed those found by Chilla and Babur (Chapter 16, this volume).
3. Of course, these data are not readily comparable to ours, since use of a morpheme in an obligatory context differs from the spontaneous production of the same morpheme. Nevertheless, the similarity, for this variable, between Yagmur and Nap-Kolhoff's subjects and the children in the Turkish Systematic Analysis of Language Transcripts (TSALT) normative database does not support the interpretation that the use of the possessive morphemes decreases in Dutch-Turkish.
4. We will only discuss this condition, because the other conditions show quite high percentages of realization. Again, while all child groups behave alike – using the *e*-marker as a default form – adult learners of L2 also use zero markers instead of – *e*.
5. It should be noted that the category applied here is named 'cultural minority' in the Netherlands and does not include, for instance, children whose first language is English. If a school includes members of a 'cultural minority', this grants access to additional funding in education. All numbers are taken from the website of the Centraal Bureau voor de Statistiek (*Statistics Netherlands*) – www.cbs.nl. For additional information, we thank Marja Vollaard, of *Siméa*, the association of schools for children with language difficulties.
6. A previous version was named *Taaltoets Anderstalige Kinderen, anderstalig* meaning 'with another (first) language'. In that version, separate norms were given for children with Turkish as their L1.

Chapter 14

Measuring the Language Abilities of Turkish-English Bilingual Children Using TELD-3: Turkish

THEODOROS MARINIS and DUYGU ÖZGE

Introduction

A large number of primary school children in the United Kingdom speak a language other than English at home, and some do not start learning English systematically until they begin school. According to a report from the Department for Education and Skills (DfES), in 2005, 18% of the primary school children in England were classified as belonging to an ethnic minority and 10% spoke English as a second language (L2) (DfES, 2005). The number of children with English as an L2 in London is even higher, reaching approximately 30% of the school children (Baker & Eversley, 2000).

Research on the language abilities of successive bilingual children has revealed that at an early stage of development, they show transfer effects from their first (L1) to their second (L2) language (Gavruseva, 1998; Haznedar, 1997; Unsworth, 2005; Whong-Barr & Schwartz, 2002) and their language profile in their L2 seems to resemble the profile of monolingual children with specific language impairment (SLI). For example, studies comparing language development in children acquiring Swedish as L2 to Swedish children with SLI revealed that both groups of children make similar errors of word order that are not attested in monolingual Swedish children (Håkansson & Nettelbladt, 1993, 1996). English children acquiring French as L2 show similar morpho-syntactic errors (finiteness and tense marking, subject–verb agreement and use of clitics) to those of French children with SLI (Paradis & Crago, 2000, 2003). Children acquiring English as L2 show a high rate of omission of grammatical morphemes relating to tense marking (Paradis, 2005) that have been argued to be clinical markers of SLI in English (Rice & Wexler, 1996).

Speech and language therapists and teachers in multilingual settings have long identified the difficulty in discriminating between successive bilingual children, whose abilities in their L2 lag behind those of L1 children due to lack of sufficient exposure to the L2, and L2 children who have a language impairment and need clinical intervention to successfully acquire both their L2 and their L1 (Crutchley *et al.*, 1997; Cummins, 1984; Genesee *et al.*, 2004; Gutierrez-Clellen, 2000; Pert, 2003). This can lead to problems of 'mistaken identity' or 'missed identity' (Genesee *et al.*, 2004; Paradis, 2005). The problem of 'mistaken identity' arises when L2 children without language impairment are inappropriately diagnosed as language impaired and receive unnecessary services. Conversely, the problem of 'missed identity' occurs when language impaired L2 children remain undiagnosed and do not receive appropriate treatment because their observed language deficits are attributed to their L2 background.

To avoid these types of misdiagnosis, it is important to assess both languages spoken by the children (Mahon *et al.*, 2003; SIG in Bilingualism, 2007). This is based on the assumption that language impairment should manifest itself in all languages spoken by the child. However, most studies on successive bilingual children have focused on their L2 language. It is unclear whether or not their L1 develops in the same way and at the same rate as monolingual children, and whether monolingual norms for the L1 are valid for successive bilingual children. For example, Yagmur and Nap-Kolhoff (this volume: Chapter 12) show that many Turkish-Dutch successive bilingual children have lower scores on the Turkish Systematic Analysis of Language Transcripts (SALT) (Acarlar & Johnston, 2006) compared with monolingual norms. This has important implications for the use of the Turkish SALT as a diagnostic tool with successive bilingual children. Yagmur and Nap-Kolhoff recommend the development of standard scores on SALT for successive bilingual children. In a similar vein, de Jong *et al.* (this volume: Chapter 13) report that in an elicitation task, Turkish-Dutch Typically Developing (TD) children omit the genitive possessive marker at a similar level as children with SLI and suggest that the use of the genitive possessive may be undergoing change in the Turkish spoken in the Netherlands. This would make the use of monolingual norms inappropriate for Turkish-Dutch children. Similar to Yagmur and Nap-Kolhoff, de Jong *et al.* suggest that bilingual norms are necessary for both the L2 and the L1 of successive bilingual children.

The present study addresses the issue of the development of bilingual norms by investigating the performance of Turkish-English successive bilingual children in their L1 using the Turkish Test of Early Language Development (TELD-3:T) (Topbaş & Güven, 2007). TELD-3:T is a recently developed Turkish assessment that is currently being normed in Turkey with monolingual typically developing children and children with SLI (Topbaş, this volume: Chapter 7; Topbaş & Güven, 2007). The results of the present study are a first step toward developing bilingual norms for TELD-3:T for Turkish-English successive bilingual children in the United Kingdom.

The Turkish-Speaking Community in the United Kingdom

According to the Turkish Consulate in London, the number of Turkish-speaking individuals in the United Kingdom is around 150,000. The largest Turkish-speaking communities in the United Kingdom are based in the greater London area in the Boroughs of Hackney, Haringey and Enfield, but smaller communities are also present in the Midlands and Scotland. A large number of members of the Turkish-speaking community in London own or work in small businesses. Turkish is largely preserved as a language for communication among this population as it is used not only as a language of socialization but also as a minority language for which service is available in public sectors such as hospitals, libraries and community centers (Wright & Kurtoğlu-Hooton, 2006). Despite this unifying aspect, the Turkish-speaking community in the United Kingdom is far from being a culturally and linguistically homogeneous group. It is mainly composed of Turkish and Kurdish immigrants from mainland Turkey and Turkish immigrants from Cyprus.

Turkish spoken in the Turkish-Cypriot community should be distinguished from Turkish in the Turkish and Kurdish communities from mainland Turkey because of differences in the time of the migration and linguistic differences between Turkish-Cypriot and mainstream Turkish (Tözün, 2005). In terms of migration waves, migration from Cyprus dates back to 1878 when Cyprus became a British colony. On the other hand, migration from Turkey started in the late 1950s as part of a general migration to Europe, but gained speed only after 1980 (Tözün, 2005). Therefore, the Turkish-Cypriot community in London has adapted to the English language and the British culture to a greater extent than the Turkish and Kurdish communities from Turkey. In addition, the Turkish-Cypriot dialect differs from mainstream Turkish at the level of syntax, vocabulary and phonology (Creese *et al.*, 2007).

Due to the outlined differences between Turkish-Cypriot and mainstream Turkish, the present study only includes children of migrant families from Turkey that have settled in London in the late 1990s.

The Present Study

The present study is part of the project 'Real-time processing of syntactic information in children with English as a Second Language and children with SLI' funded by the Economic and Social Research Council. The primary objective of this project is to investigate how Turkish-English successive bilingual children with typical and atypical language development process sentences. A secondary objective of this project is to investigate how Turkish-English children perform in a wide range of assessments normed with monolingual children. The present chapter falls within this objective by investigating how Turkish-English children perform in TELD-3:T (Topbaş, this volume: Chapter 7; Topbaş & Güven, 2007).

TELD-3:T is an adaptation of the English assessment TELD-3 (Hresko *et al.*, 1999) that assesses receptive and expressive language in children between the ages 2;0 and 7;11. Both tests have two forms (Form A and Form B), each of which has a receptive language and an expressive language subtest. Each subtest and each form of TELD-3:T includes items assessing morpho-syntax and semantics.

TELD-3:T is in the process of standardization. The pilot study has been finished with 335 monolingual typically developing children, 35 monolingual language impaired children and six children with mental retardation. The normative sample was collected in 14 cities in five different regions of Turkey. Details about the reliability and validity of TELD-3:T are provided in Topbaş (this volume: Chapter 7).

In the present study, we used only the receptive subtest of TELD-3:T. This subtest is composed of the following task types: following basic and complex oral instructions, word–picture matching task, sentence–picture matching task, understanding meaning relations in words, detecting ungrammaticalities and sentence repetition. Because the standardization process has not yet been completed, both Form A and Form B were used with each child.

The present chapter addresses the following research questions:

(1) Is there a difference in the scores of the bilingual and monolingual children between Form A and Form B?
(2) Is there a difference between the scores of bilingual and monolingual children in the receptive part of TELD-3:T?
(3) Do the scores of the bilingual and monolingual children differ from the scores of the norming sample?
(4) How do the bilingual children score in each item and do they perform better in items tapping morpho-syntax or in items tapping semantics?

Method

Participants

Ten children (five females and five males) participated in this study. The children had a mean age of 5;11 (SD = 8.9 months; range = 4;10–6;11) and had no history of a neurological or psychological condition, hearing impairment, language delay or language impairment. All children were born to Turkish-speaking families in the United Kingdom and the language spoken at home was Turkish since most of the mothers had poor English skills and preferred using Turkish, although they were also competent in

Kurdish. All mothers of the children were housewives and attended English courses provided by community centers in London. Although the children lived in the United Kingdom and had some exposure to English from birth, consistent input and communication in English started at around the age of 3;5 when they attended English nursery school. At the time of testing, the children had between 1 and 3 years of exposure to English. English was the language spoken at school, and in the informal interviews with the children and their parents revealed that at the age of testing, the primary language for socialization of the children seemed to be English. Children commented that they prefer to communicate in English with their siblings and their English or Turkish friends inside and outside school and that they use Turkish only when they communicate with people who are not competent in English.

The Turkish-English children were matched to 10 monolingual children from the standardization sample of TELD-3:T on the basis of age and socioeconomic background. Matching on the basis of age was one-to-one and each pair of children had the same age in years and months ($t(18) = 0.000$, $p > 0.1$).

Procedure

Each child was tested individually in a silent room in their school or in the DAYMER Turkish community center, which provides supplementary education for Turkish-speaking children in the Borough of Hackney. Children were told that they would do a fun task related to their Turkish. Instructions were given orally and it was made sure that the children understood the instructions. TELD-3:T is administered in the following way. Testing begins at the entry point for each child, which is based on their age. To specify their basal point in the test, children are expected to answer three consecutive items correctly. If a child does not succeed in three items in a row, testing continues backwards until this is met. The ceiling is determined when the child makes three mistakes in a row.

Results

Tables 14.1 and 14.2 present the overall scores for the bilingual and monolingual children for Form A and Form B separately and also the basal and ceiling point for each child.

To investigate the first research question, which is whether the children performed differently in the two forms, we analyzed the scores of each group in Form A separately from Form B. This showed that bilingual children had in Form A a mean score of 27.2 (range = 11–21; SD = 3.9) and in Form B a mean score of 28.6 (range = 10–22; SD = 3.4). A paired-samples t-test revealed no significant difference between the two forms ($t(9) = -1.769$, $p > 0.1$). Monolingual children had in Form A a mean score of 31.2

Table 14.1 Performance on the bilingual children in TELD-3:T

ID	Age (years; months)	Form A: Basal (item/ age)	Form A: Ceiling (item/ age)	Form A: Score	Form B: Basal (item/ age)	Form B: Ceiling (item/ age)	Form B: Score
PZ	4;10	31/7	34/7	31	30/7	35/7	31
NR	4;11	21/5	29/7	23	30/7	33/7	30
LG	5;6	19/4	27/6	21	22/5	25/6	22
NA	5;8	31/7	34/7	31	29/7	37/7	32
NS	5;9	21/5	32/7	25	22/5	31/7	25
SE	5;10	20/5	33/7	24	21/5	32/7	25
YB	6;4	24/5	33/7	26	29/7	34/7	30
ND	6;6	31/7	36/7	32	30/7	36/7	32
IA	6;11	28/7	36/7	31	25/6	36/7	29
NH	6;11	25/6	37/7	28	27/6	36/7	30

Table 14.2 Performance on the monolingual children in TELD-3:T

ID	Age (years; months)	Form A: Basal (item/ age)	Form A: Ceiling (item/ age)	Form A: Score	Form B: Basal (item/ age)	Form B: Ceiling (item/ age)	Form B: Score
119	4; 10	24/5	27/6	24	25/6	28/7	25
86	4; 11	18/4	28/7	22	24/5	27/6	24
144	5; 6	26/6	34/7	29	23/5	26/6	23
155	5; 8	31/7	–	34	34/7	–	35
291	5; 9	33/7	36/7	33	25/6	34/7	28
185	5; 10	30/7	–	33	30/7	33/7	30
261	6; 4	31/7	34/7	31	31/7	37/7	32
211	6; 6	31/7	–	33	31/7	34/7	31
225	6; 11	37/7	–	37	31/7	–	34
321	6; 11	34/7	–	36	36/7	–	36

(range = 15 – 22; SD = 4.9) and in Form B a mean score of 29.8 (range = 13–23; SD = 4.7). Similarly to the bilingual children, a paired-samples *t*-test revealed no significant difference between the two forms ($t(9) = 1.583$, $p > 0.1$). Finally, a Pearson correlation showed a strong positive correlation between the scores from Form A and Form B ($r(18) = 0.79$, $p < 0.001$). This provides evidence for reliability of the two parallel forms.

To address the second research question and find out whether or not there is a difference between the scores of bilingual and monolingual children, we calculated the raw scores of each group in each form, as shown in Figure 14.1. Overall, bilingual children were slightly less accurate than monolingual children. To address whether this difference was reliable for each one of the two forms and for the two forms combined, we conducted independent samples *t*-tests for each form separately and for the two forms combined. These revealed a trend for a significant difference between the two groups in Form A ($t(18) = 2.013$, $p = 0.059$), but the difference between the two groups in Form B was not significant ($t(18) = 0.657$, $p > 0.1$). The difference between the two groups was also not significant when we combined the scores of the two forms ($t(18) = 1.434$, $p > 0.1$).

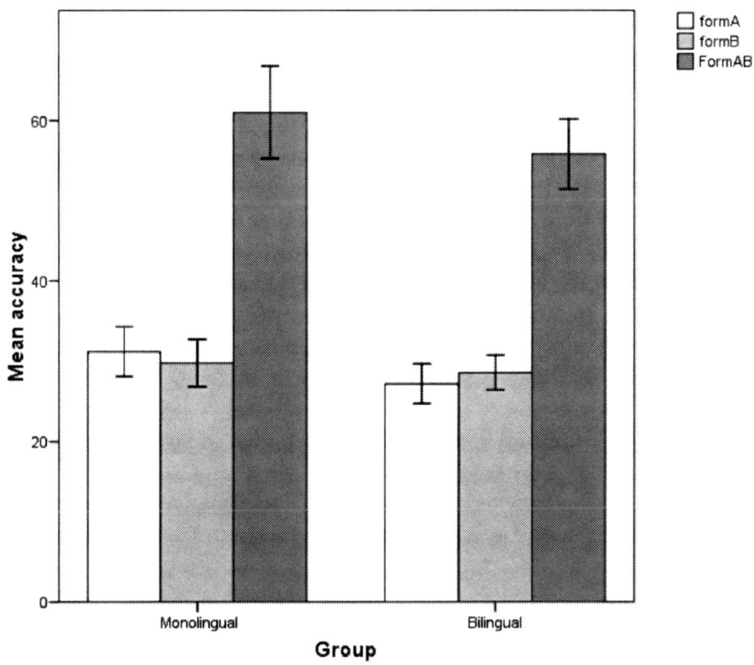

Figure 14.1 Performance of the bilingual and monolingual children in the two forms

Table 14.3 Mean score of the TELD-3:T Receptive Test based on the norming sample

Age (in months)	*Form A*	*Form B*
78–83	31.73	31.04
72–77	32.08	31.02
66–71	26.65	28.80
57–59	27.50	26.45

To tackle the third research question addressing whether or not the bilingual and monolingual children's scores differ from the scores of the norming sample, we compared the scores of the bilingual and monolingual children in Form A and Form B per age band to the mean scores of the children from the norming sample, as shown in Table 14.3.

Five bilingual children (NH, YB, SE, NS and LG) and two monolingual children (119 and 86) performed slightly lower than the means of the norming sample in both forms and two bilingual (IA and NP) and two monolingual children (144 and 261) performed slightly lower than the means of the norming sample in one of the two forms. To ascertain whether there was a significant difference between the scores of the two groups and the norming sample, we conducted one-sample t-tests for each group per age band for each form separately. These showed that despite the small differences mentioned above, bilingual and monolingual children did not perform below the mean of the norming sample for any of the two forms (all p values > 0.05). In contrast, the scores of the four 5;6–5;10 years old monolingual children in Form A ($M = 32.25$) were significantly higher than the mean of the norming sample in the same age band ($M = 26.65$) ($t(3) = 5.051$, $p = 0.015$), and there was a trend for a significantly higher scores of the two 4;10–4;11 years old bilingual children in Form B ($M = 30.5$) compared to the mean of the norming sample ($M = 26.45$) ($t(1) = 8.100$, $p = 0.078$). It should be mentioned that these two children have attended the aforementioned Turkish community center and received extra support in Turkish.

To address the bilingual children's performance in Form A compared to Form B per item and to find out whether they perform better in items tapping morpho-syntax or in items tapping semantics, we first analyzed the data per item for each one of the two lists, as shown in Figures 14.2 and 14.3.

Paired-samples t-tests showed no significant difference between the scores per item in Form A ($M = 7.5$, SD = 3.44, range = 0–10) and Form B ($M = 6.9$, SD = 3.6, range = 0–10) ($t(9) = 0.732$, $p > 0.1$). Finally, comparisons between the bilingual children's performance in morpho-syntax versus their performance in semantics reveal that they performed better in items tapping morpho-syntax (51.7%) than in items tapping semantics (35.3%).

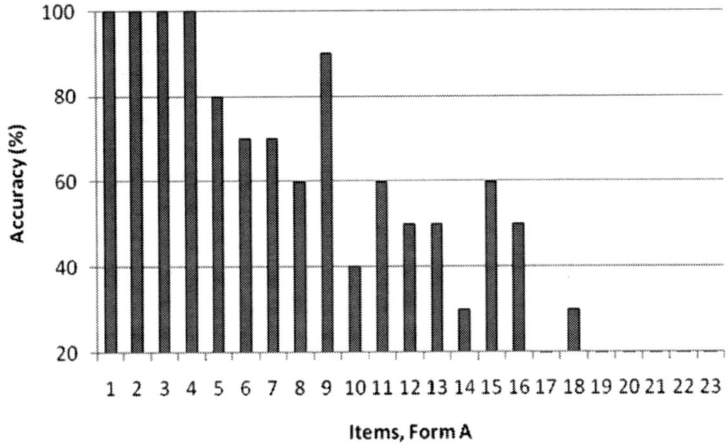

Figure 14.2 Bilingual children's accuracy per item in Form A

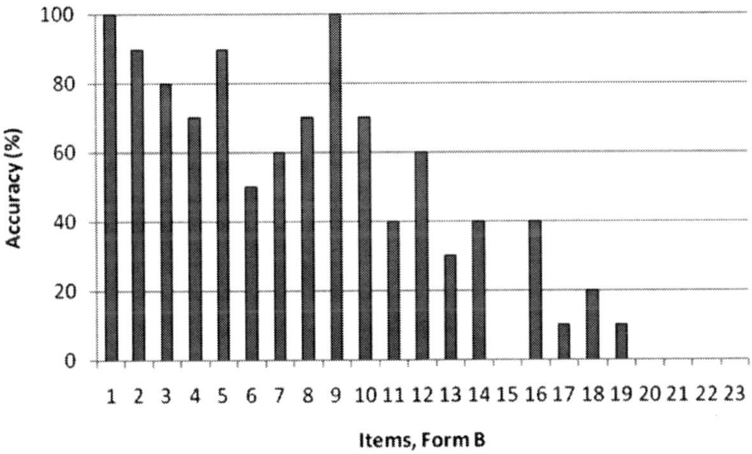

Figure 14.3 Bilingual children's accuracy per item in Form B

Discussion

The primary aim of this study was to investigate whether or not norms from monolingual Turkish children are valid for successive bilingual Turkish-English children in the United Kingdom. This was motivated by the fact that most studies on successive bilingual children have focused on the children's L2 and very little research has investigated the children's L1. Therefore, there is a lack of norms for successive bilingual children and it is unclear whether or not monolingual norms are valid for the L1 of successive bilingual children. Research on the language abilities of successive bilingual children in the Netherlands has revealed that TD successive bilingual children have lower scores in SALT than TD monolingual Turkish children (Yagmur & Nap-Kolhoff, this volume: Chapter 12). In addition, de Jong *et al.* (this volume: Chapter 13) have shown that TD successive bilingual children in the Netherlands make similar errors of omission in the use of the genitive possessive to those of children with SLI and have pointed out that Turkish spoken in the Netherlands may be undergoing change. This discrepancy between the performance of monolingual and successive bilingual children may cause a misdiagnosis of TD successive bilingual children as language impaired because their performance in both their L2 and L1 may be below monolingual norms. Against this background, we investigated the performance of a group of 10 Turkish-English children from the Turkish community in London in the receptive subtest of TELD-3:T compared to 10 monolingual Turkish children growing up in Turkey and the test's norming sample. A secondary aim of the study was to test the reliability of the two parallel forms of the receptive subtest of TELD-3:T that is currently being standardized with monolingual Turkish TD children and children with SLI.

The results of the study can be summarized as follows. Comparison of the results in the two parallel forms for each group of children separately showed no significant differences in the performance of the children in Form A versus Form B and a strong correlation was found between the scores of the children in the two forms. This provides evidence for reliability of the two parallel forms of TELD-3:T.

Comparison between the scores of monolingual and bilingual children revealed that bilingual children were slightly less accurate than monolingual children, especially in Form A, but when we combined the scores of the two forms, the numerical difference was not statistically significant. This shows that the two groups performed equally well despite the numerical advantage of the monolingual children. Comparison between the scores of the monolingual and bilingual children against the norming sample showed that despite some small numerical differences, monolingual and bilingual children did not perform below the mean of the norming sample for any of the two forms. In contrast, four 5;6–5;10 years old monolingual children performed in Form A significantly better than the norming sample, and two 4;10–4;11 years old bilingual children who attended a Turkish community center performed in Form B significantly better than the norming sample. Finally, analysis per items revealed that the bilingual children performed better in items tapping morpho-syntax than in items tapping semantics.

Taken together, these results are promising regarding their usefulness of the norms of the receptive section of TELD-3:T for the population of successive bilingual Turkish-English children in the United Kingdom. The discrepancy between our findings and the findings of Yagmur and

Nap-Kolhoff (this volume: Chapter 12) and de Jong *et al.* (this volume: Chapter 13) may be due to the different modality tested in these studies. Yagmur and Nap-Kolhoff and de Jong *et al.* tested production, whereas we tested comprehension. Alternatively, this could be due to differences in the Turkish spoken in the Netherlands versus that in the United Kingdom. As mentioned in the de Jong *et al.* study, the Turkish spoken in the Netherlands seems to be undergoing change, but to date such an effect has not been discussed for the Turkish spoken in the United Kingdom. In addition, the nature of the tasks used in the present study, compared to the Yagmur and Nap-Kolhoff and de Jong *et al.* studies, was different. Yagmur and Nap-Kolhoff (this volume: Chapter 12) used SALT and showed differences between TD monolingual and successive bilingual children in terms of intelligibility, lexical diversity, Mean Length of Utterance (MLU) and the use of grammatical morphology. de Jong *et al.* (this volume: Chapter 13) showed an asymmetry in the performance of successive bilingual children between different phenomena involving grammatical morphology. TD bilingual children were more accurate than bilingual children with SLI in subject–verb agreement and case marking, but not in the use of the genitive–possessive construction. In contrast to those two studies, we did not use a production, but a comprehension task, the receptive section of TELD-3:T. This task includes a variety of items tapping mainly vocabulary and semantics, as well as grammar, although it does not include items tapping the genitive–possessive construction that was proven to be vulnerable in Turkish-Dutch TD children.

However, our results have to be interpreted with caution because of the small sample size of the present study and the narrow age range. Future research should include a larger number of both unimpaired and impaired children in a wider age range. This could provide more conclusive evidence as to whether or not monolingual Turkish norms of TELD-3:T are valid for the population of successive Turkish-English children in the United Kingdom.

One last point we would like to make is that given the lack of norms of bilingual children and the large heterogeneity relating to differences in the age of onset, years of exposure, quantity and quality of input, it is important to use more than one modality and more than one assessment tool. This can provide a wider picture of the strengths and weaknesses of successive bilingual children and avoid the problems of 'mistaken' and 'missed identity'.

Acknowledgments

This research was supported by the Economic and Social Research Council research grant 'Real-time processing of syntactic information in children with English as a Second Language & children with Specific Language Impairment' awarded to Theo Marinis (RES-061-23-0137).

Chapter 15

Aspects of Language Acquisition and Disorders in Turkish-French Bilingual Children

MEHMET ALI AKINCI and NATHALIE DECOOL-MERCIER

Introduction

In the past 40 years, a large influx of immigrant families in the industrialized European countries has modified the demography of these nations and generated contexts of language contact. These contacts have raised a significant number of important social and linguistic debates, especially with a bearing on school difficulties in children from immigrant families whose background cultures and languages differ from those of the mainstream school system (Extra & Verhoeven, 1999; Extra & Yagmur, 2004). In reality, language practices of immigrant families evolve as they settle in the host country and as their children grow up (Deprez, 1994). Often parents may adapt themselves to this new situation, and this raises many questions as far as the maintenance of home language and cultural practices is concerned (Yagmur & Akıncı, 2003).

Numerous studies on the language of children from immigration backgrounds in European countries have yielded conflicting results. Some researchers suggest a 'language deficit' to explain why immigrant children do not attain the same levels at school as their native-speaking peers (Ammerlaan *et al.*, 2001). Others suggest that their language difficulties may be due to quite narrowly defined areas of literacy-related activities rather than to general language use (Akıncı *et al.*, 2001). Still others associate difficulties with child-specific factors such as home and/or host language, individual personalities and socio-cultural identities rather than with background literacy or school-based activities (Gregory & Williams, 2000; Wong-Fillmore, 1991). In addition, many educationally oriented studies (Billiez, 1990; Deprez, 1994; Grosjean, 1982; Hélot, 2007; Lüdi, 2001; Lüdi & Py, 2003) stressed that, in practice in France and elsewhere in Europe, minorities are not given the chance to fully develop their bilingualism. These studies also point out the paradoxical policies that restrict bilingualism when it concerns migrants' children, but encourage it for the 'elite' by supporting early second-language learning. They also assert that differences in school performance may reflect negative teacher attitudes concerning the academic abilities of children from ethnic minority groups (Billiez, 1990; Gadet & Varro, 2006; Hélot, 2007; Lüdi, 2001). They propose the idea that difficulties may be due to inferior institutional and instructional facilities available to such populations. Another suggestion is that children from such backgrounds represent highly heterogeneous populations that show considerable inter-group diversity, and so they cannot automatically be identified as 'poor achievers', whether in language or in other domains. Lüdi and Py agree with this position, affirming that 'the more balanced the use of two languages is, the higher will be the increase in value of the home language on the language market, which is to say that bilinguals are capable of accomplishing cognitively demanding and de-contextualized tasks in their two languages, both orally and in writing. Consequently the problem of bi-literacy, the competence to read and write in both languages, arises' (Lüdi & Py, 2003: 186). Furthermore, school constitutes the primary place of acquiring the language of the host country and hence literacy. According to Dabène and Billiez (1987), school is not the only place where this occurs, but for the first time, it brings the child stemming from immigration into contact with the standard variety of this language.

The aim of this chapter is to outline aspects of language acquisition, development and disorders in Turkish-French bilingual children born in France. In order to do this, we will first briefly present French language policies concerning linguistic minorities and bilingualism in children from immigration backgrounds. Then, we will introduce the Turkish immigrant community in France. Next, we will focus on two aspects: the acquisition and development of language in Turkish children before and during their first years of schooling; and on the studies carried out on language impairments in Turkish. After having presented our methodology in a third part, the main body of the text analyzes two phenomena of language abilities of Turkish bilingual children and adolescents from Turkish immigration backgrounds in France: connectives in Turkish and French corpora and anaphors in French data. We will conclude with implications for speech and language pathologists (henceforth SLP) working with Turkish clients in France, focusing on the SLP process in French for Turkish people and assessment tools used for Turkish children with language disorders in context.

French Language Policies and Bilingualism in Children from Immigration Backgrounds

Compared to other West European countries, French policies concerning ethnic minorities differ in many respects. However, like many other

West European countries, nation-state ideology and maintenance of nationhood rooted in a commonly shared notion of cultural unity underlies French language policies (Archibald, 2002; Gadet & Varro, 2006). Rather than promote linguistic and cultural pluralism, French policies explicitly prefer integration and linguistic assimilation of immigrants. For the purpose of facilitating the transformation of immigrants into French nationals, a commission on nationality was set up in 1987. The commission took a number of measures to set up the legal framework for assimilating immigrants into the mainstream society (Zirotti, 2006). Along with many other factors, mastery of French was seen to be the most fundamental aspect of the acculturation process because language is considered to be of overarching importance in achieving social cohesion and national unity in France.

When one talks about children from an immigration background in French schools, the common perception seems to be that the variable 'child stemming from immigration' is a factor in school failure. Yet Deprez (1994) speaks positively about 'family bilingualism' in the context of immigrant families, since the children who were born and raised in France introduce the language of schooling into the home environment.

In the last three decades, one of the most influential theories in the field of language contact was doubtless the ethnolinguistic vitality theory developed by Giles and his colleagues (Giles *et al.*, 1977). According to this theory, the language and culture of origin tend to undergo changes in situations of contact, and their maintenance is conditioned by several factors. The factors involved are generally divided into two categories: those affecting a speech community and those affecting individuals within a speech community (Kipp *et al.*, 1995). However, it is not always easy to draw the line between individual and societal factors as there is an ongoing interaction between an individual and the speech community. In the majority of cases, these factors are interdependent.

Since the first studies of Skutnabb-Kangas and Toukomaa (1976) showed that there was a direct relation between a child's competence in his first language and his or her competence in the second language, numerous investigations have been carried out to confirm these findings. Many studies referring to Cummins' interdependence hypothesis (Cummins, 1979) showed that poor development of skills in the first language hinders progress in the second language, both in quantity and in quality. Thus, one will put at risk the cultural identity and linguistic development of migrant children who are schooled by 'immersion' in the language of the host country and are urged to give up their home language following the principles of assimilation policies (Cummins, 1991; Hamers & Blanc, 1983). As discussed by Skutnabb-Kangas and Toukomaa (1976) and Haugen (1977), some theories on bilingualism do not hesitate to classify children from an immigration background as semilinguals who not only confuse and mix both languages but also, like second-language learners, have unstable skills, as indicated by restricted vocabulary, faulty grammar, hesitation in production and difficulties in expression in both languages. The study conducted by Gonzo and Saltarelli (1983) concerning immigrant families advances the idea that linguistic and cultural attrition can take years with first-generation immigrants, while children belonging to the second generation acquire a weakened language and culture of origin. These languages and cultures are in their turn transmitted in an even weaker form to a third generation. Influenced by a follow-up effect, authors such as Thomason and Kaufman (1988) and Lüdi and Py (2003) affirm that in three or four generations, the languages and cultures of migrant children who are in contact with the language and culture of the environment will become extinct.

Turkish immigrants in France

The immigration history of the Turkish community in France is shorter compared to other immigrant communities. The Turkish population arrived in France mainly in the seventies, 'coming from a country having not a historical background related to colonization, neither knowledge of France' (Petek-Salom, 2001: 98). In most cases, Turks came to France by default, because they could not go to Germany, the main destination at the time for the vast majority of Turkish economic immigrants.

Shortly after World War II, only 7770 Turks lived in France. This number declined to 5273 in 1954 and increased slightly to 7628 in 1968. The first bilateral immigration agreement between France and Turkey was signed in 1965, but large-scale Turkish migration only started at the beginning of the 1970s and continued in the 1980s. Between 1968 and 1972, the Turkish population increased to 50,860; between 1972 and 1982, it rose further to 123,540. The increase is due not only to labor migration, but also due to family reunification for those immigrants whose families had remained in the home country. In the 1982 census, the consequences of family reunification were already apparent. It revealed a sharp rise in the number of both women and young people (between 10 and 34 years). By the year 1990, there were 202,000 Turks in France. They were then the fourth largest immigrant community in the country. In 1990, for half of the Turkish population, the average age was below 20. Thus, as opposed to less educated first-generation Turkish immigrants, the young generations have been through the French school system and their educational and vocational profiles are much better than the previous generations. This modifies the general profile and outlook of the Turkish population in France. Many Turkish families have now settled in France and maintain contacts with the homeland. These families may end up staying in France indefinitely, whereas at first they intended their stay to be only temporary. Today, the Turkish population in France is estimated to be 400,000, of which around 15,000 Turks have acquired French nationality (the number is very low due to the French language proficiency condition for the applicants). According to Kastoryano (2003), 47% of the Turks in France have the nationality of their home country.

The majority of Turkish immigrants in France are blue-collar workers. According to Echardour and Maurin (1993), 43.7% of Turks are working in production, 28.5% in construction and 23.5% in services. Although, following the study of Brabant (1992), there has been a slight shift in the occupational structure from blue-collar (89.9% in 1982 and 80% in 1989) to white-collar jobs and self-employment (both were 6.6% in 1982 and 18.5% in 1989), the majority of the working Turkish population can still be identified as blue-collar.

Today, the largest proportion of the Turkish population can be found in the region of Île de France (27% of all the Turks live in this region; Manço, 2004). The second region is Rhône-Alpes (17%) with 38,185 individuals. Alsace comes next with 15% (Villanova, 1997).

As in other major immigration contexts (Germany and The Netherlands), in-group marriage tendencies are very strong. According to INSEE (National Institute of Statistics and Economic Studies) (1997), 98% of girls and 92% of boys marry a person from Turkey, so that the migration process renews itself continuously. Young immigrants born in Turkey arriving in France through family reunification contribute also to language maintenance. The population structure of Turkish immigrants in France is very young, which is the same pattern observed in other immigration contexts as well. According to INSEE, 90% of immigrants are less than 55 years old and 40% are less than 25 years old. Women represent nearly half of their members (46%). If we consider that 57.2% of the children are now born in France, nonetheless 82% of the couples are composed of two persons of Turkish nationality or origin. According to the education attaché in The Turkish Consulate, the number of pupils of Turkish origin, from nursery school to university, is 71,321 in France. While the level of education is rising with the second generation, which could be considered as perfectly French-speaking, among the first generation, about 100% of the women and 75% of the men hardly speak any French or do not speak any French at all. According to INSEE, in Turkish families, 17% of fathers and 3% of mothers speak to their children in French (as compared to 69% and 52% of Algerians).

As in other immigration contexts (such as Germany and The Netherlands), Turkish immigrants in France are able to visit their homeland at least once every year. The Turkish-language media is readily accessible to Turkish immigrants in France. Most of the major Turkish newspapers have rather high-circulation European editions. There are weekly magazines and journals coming from Turkey as well. Turkish bookshops provide a wide range of Turkish-medium books in major areas of Turkish concentration. On a regular basis, Turkish-language plays are performed by actors from Turkish state theaters and private theaters, as well as by local immigrant Turkish theater groups. Movies, concerts and exhibitions by Turkish artists are also very common all over Western Europe. In the main centers of Turkish concentration, there are rich collections of Turkish books in public libraries. These libraries also organize panels during which novelists from Turkey meet Turkish immigrants and interested mainstream community members. Along with print media, major Turkish TV channels can be received by cable or satellite dish. Members of the receiving societies are mostly critical of satellite dishes, arguing that they delay 'integration' of immigrants. Some marginal groups even support the idea of a ban on satellite dishes. Nevertheless, there is a growing demand for Turkish-medium broadcasting, and Turkish immigrants who have satellite dishes can receive all Turkish-medium channels. Additionally, in the age of the internet, immigrants are able to access a rich variety of first-language medium resources on the web. These support factors presumably contribute to maintenance of the Turkish language and provide a wide (and rich) social network for Turkish immigrants.

Finally, the learning and teaching of Turkish contribute considerably to the maintenance of first-language skills among younger generations. On the basis of a bilateral cultural agreement, the French and Turkish governments agreed to provide mother tongue education for Turkish children in French schools. In line with the practice in many other European countries, the Turkish government sends teachers from Turkey to teach Turkish language, history and geography in French schools (Akıncı, 2009).

The use of Turkish remains very active in many families, as demonstrated above. Turkish mothers, whose French skills are often very limited, are the guaranteed source of language transmission and maintenance. Thus, during early childhood and until the beginning of nursery school, the child develops his language in an exclusively Turkish linguistic environment. The entry to school marks a break in language learning. In what follows, we will present briefly the characteristics of language development in Turkish children in France before and during their schooling.

Turkish children acquiring and developing languages before and during schooling

Before describing the acquisition of language by Turkish children, it is necessary to distinguish the several types of such children that exist:

- those born in France;
- those who arrived in France before the age of 6; and
- those who arrived after the age of 6.

In these last two types, children arrived in France within the framework of family reunification. In all cases, parents may share the same nationality and speak only Turkish; the couple may be mixed and use only one language, often French, or they may use both languages. One parent may have been born and raised in France and will therefore use French with his or her child. All these children could be subject to language pathology or not. Our study concerns only children born in France of first- or second-generation parents.

Generally, a child born in France of Turkish migrant parents first begins learning to speak in Turkish. The language spoken around the children in the majority of Turkish families is only Turkish. Surrounding family, neighbors and parents speak to them in Turkish. Even though the children are living in France, they will thus develop their Turkish-language capacities. Their first babbling, sounds and words are in Turkish. The lexicon develops according to parental interaction with the child, and also according to the cultural and linguistic environment. To our knowledge, up to now, no studies have been carried out on babies born following Turkish immigration to France.

The children born in France thus develop their language and their linguistic abilities in an exclusively Turkish-speaking environment. The first contact with French language for these children will be done only with the entry to nursery school around the age of two-and-a-half or three. However, young children have obviously already heard French around them in the neighborhood, at supermarkets, on television, without needing to adopt French as a means of communication.

The entry to nursery school is a major turning point in several respects: children leave the safe environment of their family to enter a new space where they will first need to find their ways around. They find themselves in an unknown environment with peers and adults who do not speak the same language as them and with whom they will spend long hours during school days. This new situation will represent for them a rupture in the language learning process. In an ordinary and monolingual situation, the school should constitute the place where the child increases his knowledge of the language. As for children with a Turkish background, since the linguistic continuity of Turkish is not ensured by the school, they will then be confronted with a new situation in which they have to speak French. Language development thus occurs on two levels, in two different areas. In her study, Tinelli (2004: 49) reports what a seven-year-old Turkish girl answered when asked whether she liked French: 'not too much because when I was baby, I could speak a little bit Turkish. Then I went to nursery school, and after I learned French. Then for me, my head speaks in Turkish', she continued, 'I spoke with nobody at school, I understood nothing, nobody played with me'.

Parents' motivation and a child's personality play an important role in how to deal with this new environment and language, and determine the speed of progression in French and the child's integration into the class. As our purpose is not to describe in a theoretical perspective the acquisition and learning styles of French (see Bates *et al.*, 1988) or the various adaptation phases the Turkish-speaking child goes through in nursery school (Tabors & Snow, 1994),[1] we do not go into details of these processes that are already described elsewhere.

In our previous studies (e.g. Akıncı, 2001), we showed that for Turkish children, French very quickly becomes their dominant language by the age of five or six, which matches with the beginning of primary school. Even if their Turkish continues to develop, their mother tongue becomes their weak language. Then, there exists two types of Turkish children: those who are beginning to learn academic Turkish in the second year of the French primary school (within the framework of mother tongue education) and those who do not have the chance to learn Turkish and are satisfied with what their parents can transmit to them. For the first group, Turkish will continue to develop, whereas for the second group, we can speak about fossilization of the language of origin. However, for both groups with French schooling, the effect is that they have better control of French than Turkish and feel more comfortable speaking French. According to our previous studies (Akıncı, 1996; see also Akıncı, 2008), 68% of Turkish children would use only French with each other, 23% use both languages and 9% use only Turkish. In addition, we also showed that Turkish children mostly speak only Turkish with their parents. There are very few who interact only in French. These results are supported by findings of previous research carried out in France (Akıncı *et al.*, 2004; Gautier-Kızılyürek 2007; Irtis-Dabbagh, 2003; Yagmur & Akıncı, 2003), in which children from Turkish immigrant families and adolescents in France report that they almost exclusively communicate in Turkish with their parents but mostly in French with their siblings.

As has been described in many studies, with schooling, the language of school enters homes and, as described above, children use this language with each other and sometimes with parents.

According to the observations of many people involved with parents and children from migrant families (Steib, 2006; Tinelli, 2004), and also of teachers with whom we have done training on bilingualism in schools, Turkish parents fear that their children will give up their mother tongue and culture.[2] According to our own experience of Turkish parents in France, this is not true for all cities where Turks are living. In some places, French is seen as a utility language without emotional load.

Schooling of Turkish children in France therefore raises problems not only for teachers in nursery schools but also for those in primary schools who underestimate the Turkish community and as a result the children to whom they teach French. One day, I received a phone call from a nursery school teacher who found my work on the internet. She complained about Turkish children in her class who have considerable difficulty learning

French, contrary to other children with immigration origins, such as Maghrebi or Portuguese children. Then, she asked me if their difficulties might not be linked to their genetic heritage. One can imagine my distress and anger about such unfounded thoughts. But does the fault lie with the teacher who repeated what she knew or that of the national policy that did not provide sufficient teacher training?

The following section summarizes, to our knowledge, the very few existing background studies of language impairments in Turkish children in France.

Background Studies of Language Impairments in Turkish

France is a country with a strong monolingual culture. The acknowledgment of regional languages is recent; this is even truer for languages of immigration (see in particular the Cerquiglini report – April 1999, published in 2003). For a major part of the population, including the majority of those working in education and health, bilingualism is still regarded as a marginal phenomenon, monolingualism being standard. However, the census of 1999 showed that 26% of adults living in Metropolitan France had had parents usually speaking to them in a language other than French, and from this census 400 languages were identified (Deprez *et al.*, 2002).

Attitudes and behavior toward bilingualism vary according to the languages involved: for some languages, bilingualism will be encouraged, while for others – and in particular a number of languages of immigration – the use of the mother tongue could be stigmatized. This is also the case for Turkish. Not very long ago, it was recommended that parents refrain from using Turkish with children at home.

In this context, studies relating to speech difficulties of immigrants are poorly developed. There are no studies to our knowledge concerning speech difficulties in Turkish. Some rare studies are concerned with speech therapy for young Turkish patients and difficulties encountered in French by children from Turkish immigrant families. These studies concern especially Turkish children in the Alsace region where, as we said above, 15% of the Turkish community lives; indeed, this region has a well-established Turkish population. For the moment, no statistical studies relating to linguistic disorders of Turkish children exist. The two studies presented below consist of case studies by two speech-therapy students in Strasbourg (the capital of Alsace).

Fanny Steib (2006) bases her analysis in particular on an interview with one speech therapist of Strasbourg.[3] About 30% of this speech therapist's patients are of Turkish origin. According to her, 'one can observe the same speech difficulties in Turkish-speaking children as in working-class French children; and the disorders are roughly similar' (Steib, 2006: 87, authors' translation).

The second study conducted by Alexia Tinelli (2004) relates to children from Turkish communities living in and around Strasbourg. Twenty speech therapists answered her inquiries, having followed 100 Turkish background children during two years preceding the investigation. She concludes, from answers to the questionnaire, that Turkish children present specific difficulties in oral and written language.

In spoken language, these difficulties are as follows (Tinelli, 2004: 109–111):

Difficulties due to linguistic differences between Turkish and French: Pronunciation, articulation (some sounds are pronounced differently in Turkish), gender of nouns (no gender in Turkish), disorders of syntactic structuring (the structure of Turkish sentences is different).

Difficulties due to the introduction of the French language: Some Turkish children lack the desire and need to learn French, as this language is less spoken within Turkish families.

Disorders of communication: Speech therapists observed that some Turkish children speak little, almost do not communicate and are sometimes selectively silent. Disorders of comprehension, a poor and approximate lexical stock and phonological disorders are common.

In written language, speech therapists note

Orthographical consequences of speech difficulties: Children are often confronted with agreement errors; they are also unable to notice word relations, segmentation of words, and show lack of vocabulary, and spelling disturbances.

Disorders of comprehension: As their vocabulary is reduced in French, written sentences are not understood.

Instrumental disorders: The prerequisites for writing have not yet been established (i.e. spatio-temporal orientation, handedness, audio-verbal structuring, and visuo-spatial perception).

Difficulties with starting to read: In the beginning, reading is often difficult. Some speech therapists suspect word blindness; access to books is not commonly available in Turkish families.

Late arrival in rehabilitation for the written language is observed.

Except difficulties possibly due to linguistic differences between Turkish and French, other disorders mentioned can however not be regarded as specific to Turkish children: the question was indeed the following one: 'According to you, what are the most frequent difficulties presented by Turkish children coming for oral language difficulties; for children coming for written language difficulties?' This study thus gives an indication of perceived reasons for the referral of Turkish children, of some types of interference, but does not permit any specific conclusions. Santelli (2007: 228) notes the same problem concerning migrants coming from the Maghreb: 'assessment tools do not exist that are devised to detect possible specific difficulties and consequently, standard tools are used. Such a report is much more detrimental than knowledge, even superficial, of the mother tongue or language of origin which could make it possible, on the other hand, to understand certain linguistic constructions and, consequently, to deal in a more effective way with the difficulties encountered by these children' (authors' translation).

We think that other studies using protocols allowing a comparison of Turkish and French language levels of children who consult for speech therapy would be necessary to support our knowledge of Turkish children's speech difficulties. The following is an attempt to fill this gap providing baseline research on children without SLI.

Biliteracy Competences of Turkish-Speaking Children and Adolescents in France

In order to characterize the Turkish and French acquired by Turkish-French bilingual children and adolescents in France, we investigate here, in the following paragraphs, two types of syntactic phenomena: the use of connectives and the use of anaphors in written texts in both languages. For *connectives*, we will first measure differences between clauses containing coordination and those containing subordination, then we will look for types of semantic link (temporal, additive, causal and adversative). Recent studies (Akıncı, 2006; Blanche-Benveniste, 1995; Gayraud *et al.*, 2001; Verhoeven *et al.*, 2002) show that the use of subordinate clauses is more frequent in written texts of adults than in those of young pupils, while the use of juxtaposition is more frequent in spoken discourse. The quantity and the type of syntactic connectivity constitute a good index of language development.

Anaphors are traditionally defined as any repetition of a previous element in a text (Riegel *et al.*, 1994: 610). An anaphoric relation can be defined as the relation between two elements, where the interpretation of one element (the anaphor) depends in some way on the interpretation of the other (the antecedent). Two types of anaphors can be distinguished: sentence-internal and discourse anaphors. The first type of anaphor refers to an antecedent within the same sentence, while in the second type the antecedent must be sought in another sentence. Finding the antecedent of a discourse anaphor is much more difficult because that depends not only on syntactic, but also on pragmatic and semantic aspects (Aarssen, 1996: 30).

Methodology

In our study, participants in three age groups (11-, 13- and 16-year-olds) were asked to produce two types of text (personal narration and expository) in two modalities (spoken and written).[4] The texts were elicited in two successive sessions. In Session I, participants were asked to tell and write a

Table 15.1 Order of presentation across the tasks and groups

Session	*I*	*II*
Order A	Narrative spoken/Narrative written	Expository spoken/ Expository written
Order B	Narrative written/Narrative spoken	Expository written/ Expository spoken

story about an incident of interpersonal conflict that they had experienced personally. In the following session, expository discussions were gathered, where participants were asked to give a talk as if they were in front of their class, or write an essay or composition discussing the issue of interpersonal conflict. All subjects produced both the narrative and expository texts in two modalities of speech and writing. The mode of presentation was balanced across the tasks, so that half of the subjects performed the spoken task first, and then produced a written text, while the other half started with the written text and continued with the spoken task. The sessions and the texts elicited in these sessions are depicted in Table 15.1.

In the remaining part of this paper all of the analyses will be based on written texts of monolingual and bilingual children.

The research groups of bilingual and monolingual subjects were organized according to their school-grade level. The texts were elicited from one group of primary school children, one group of secondary school children and one group of high school students. Each group consisted of at least 20 subjects. Table 15.2 illustrates the information about number and age of the bilingual informants in each group.

Table 15.2 Age, number, mean age and range of ages of bilingual and monolingual informants

School type	*Primary*		*Secondary*		*High*	
Group	A	B	A	B	A	B
Population	**Turkish-French bilingual**					
Number of subjects	11	13	12	12	9	13
Mean age	11;00		13;01		16;01	
Population	**French monolingual**					
Number of subjects	11	12	11	11	11	12
Mean age	11;01		13;04		16;03	
Population	**Turkish monolingual**					
Number of subjects	11	12	10	12	10	10
Mean age	11;00		12;09		15;06	

The bilingual informants for this study were selected from the Turkish immigrant community living in Rouen and Grenoble. In order to control the gender factor, we included equal numbers of males and females. They are sons and daughters of first-generation immigrants to France all of whom were born in France. The French monolinguals were raised and educated in French with low educational and socio-economic family backgrounds. They attend the same schools and live in the same neighborhoods as the immigrant children mentioned above. Data from Turkish monolinguals were collected in 2003 in Denizli (in western Anatolia) that matched the place of origin of the parents of the bilingual informants. In terms of socio-economic status, these monolingual groups can be compared to our bilingual group.

The fathers of all of the bilingual informants, except one, are unskilled workers and freelance building workers. Compared to the parents of monolingual informants, they are under-represented in the categories of farmer or in very qualified jobs such as technician, trade or office workers. The French monolinguals' fathers belong much more often to the middle-class professions, or are qualified technicians, or trade or office workers. The Turkish monolinguals' fathers are often farmers, craftsmen, storekeepers or teachers, or are retired.

As far as the mothers' occupation is concerned, we observed that mothers of bilinguals and Turkish monolinguals are much more often housewives than those of French monolinguals. This situation concerns respectively 72% and 73% of the bilingual and Turkish monolinguals' mothers. In contrast, the mothers of French monolinguals are represented in almost all occupations. They most often work as managers or as cleaning ladies.

Like other children whose native language is not French, the children in our study acquired their home language, in this case Turkish, exclusively within the family up to the age of seven. From that age on, some of these children have the possibility of attending the HLI classes (Home Language Instruction) in France until the end of secondary school. In HLI classes, the children are given the possibility of reading and writing in Turkish. Children also learn Turkish history and geography in these classes. All of our subjects attend HLI classes.

Before the data -collection phase began, the background information of our subjects was collected with a literacy questionnaire filled in by the child. With the help of that questionnaire, we tried to get information about the demographic variables and the literacy-related activities in and outside the subjects' homes. All subjects in France and in Turkey were given similar motivational instructions.

Connectives in Turkish and French written texts

This part of our paper aims to characterize the developmental profile of connective use in written texts of Turkish-French bilingual children and teenagers. In a linear sequence of oral and written texts, connectives contribute to the structure by marking semantic relations between clauses or sequences (Halliday & Hasan, 1976). From a cognitive viewpoint, it is necessary for a speaker or a writer to analyze beforehand the event as an association of two or several components and to perceive that two situations can be built as belonging to only one event (Fayol, 1997). That is why acquiring competence in combining clauses in order to produce oral texts and coherent writing is a sign of development that extends well beyond childhood (Jisa, 1987; Verhoeven *et al.*, 2002).

Authors have different views concerning the role of connectives. For some, a relation expressed by a connective (i.e. a marked relation) is an equivalent variant of a relation expressed without a connective (unmarked). This is the case, for example, in 'I get up, I wash, I get dressed', where a simple juxtaposition is sufficient for both the speaker and the listener, unless stated otherwise, to consider that the events occur in succession. For other authors, marked and unmarked relations are not equivalent (for a detailed presentation of the various viewpoints, see Rossari, 2000; Segal *et al.*, 1991). As noted by McCabe and Peterson (1991), in comparison with other types of text, narratives have a very high density of these markers of discourse cohesion, even if, for example, it is unnecessary for inter-propositional temporal links to be present for the narrative to be understood.

Our previous studies on connectives used by 5-, 7-, 10-, 12- and 14–17-year-old bilingual Turkish-French children and adolescents in France (Akıncı, 2006; Akıncı & Jisa, 2000)[5] showed that for Turkish texts, overall, about 50% of all connections are simple juxtaposed sentences. If the subjects mark the connection with syntactic means, they mainly use coordination. Significant differences between all groups concerned deictic expressions (5- and 17-year-olds use more deictic forms than others) and subordination (adolescents use more subordinate sentences than the younger children). Temporal deixis is used to ground the story in a temporal framework by the majority of high school students. The development of complex means (subordination) appears to stagnate until the age of 12, but after this age, there is a real development.

In both languages, the majority of subjects use juxtaposition to connect sentences. When they connect with syntactic means, coordination is the preferred means. Statistical tests[6] reveal significant differences between the younger and older groups only for subordination. The 5- and 7-year-old children show a much lower proportion of subordination in comparison to students of other ages.

This study allowed us to conclude that the Turkish texts produced by the bilingual French-Turkish children were sometimes weaker in terms of clause linkage. Until the age of 10, in Turkish texts children employed more juxtaposition and coordination than subordination, whereas for French texts, the percentage of subordination was higher and this began at a very young age and developed rapidly at the age of 10.

In our new study, each occurrence was assigned a two-part code. The first indicated the type of connectivity: coordination or subordination (Kornfilt, 1997; Topbaş & Özcan, 1995). The second indicated the type of semantic link; these types are as follows (Vion & Colas, 2005: 48):

(1) *Additive*: Two simultaneous or consecutive elements, objects, events or states, often enumerations. Each element is semantically independent, and the meaning is the same when the two are combined or taken separately.
(2) *Temporal or chronological*: Two elements related by temporal succession.
(3) *Causal*: Relations of cause, consequence or effect. The cause is a sufficient cause of the consequence. One proposition refers to a planned or current action or state, and the other gives a reason or a result.
(4) *Adversative*: A relation of contrast between two events and/or states. The expected outcome of what is described in the first proposition is not what is described in the second. The relation between the propositions is opposition, where one proposition refutes or opposes the other, or one proposition qualifies or restricts the other.
(5) *Others*: Includes other semantic functions such as results, manner, condition and alternation.

Examples given in Turkish (1) and in French (2) illustrate encoded connectives; the categories are shown in Tables 15.3 and 15.4.

(1) Ben eve gidecektim **çünkü** saat beş bucuğa geliyordu. İki gün **sonra** bir Cumartesi günü, bir daha yüzmeye gittim, **o anda** (o kızı) gördüm benlen arkadaşlık yapan kızı gördüm. **Ama** onlan oynamayaya git**tiğimde** beni (boğuyordu) **yani** benlen oynamıyordu. Şimdi o kızdan nefret ediyorum.

I'll go to home ***because*** *it was around half past five. Two days* ***after*** *one Saturday, I went to swim again,* ***at this moment*** *I saw (this girl) I saw the girl who was friends with me.* ***But when*** *I went to play with her (she was choking) me* ***that is to say*** *she was not playing with me. Now I hate this girl* (TB-S07B-WN).[7]

(2) **Quand** j'étais en vacance dans un Camping je me promener une fille est arrivée elle commencer a parler sur moi a ces copains **alors** j'ai était là voir **et** je les prevenue que si elles recommencer à parler sur moi je la defoncerer **après** elle commencer a me traiter **Donc** j'ai était la voir **et** on ces battu.

When *I was on holiday at a Campsite I was walking a girl came and started to talk about me to her friends* ***then*** *I went to see her* ***and*** *I warned them that if they began again to talk about me I would smash her* ***after*** *she started to call me names* ***So*** *I went to see her* ***and*** *we fought.* (FM-S09B-WN).

Tables 15.3 and 15.4 summarize all connective forms observed in our data according to their semantic meaning in Turkish (Table 15.3) and French (Table 15.4).

Table 15.3 List of the conjunctions according to their meaning in Turkish

	Additive	*Temporal*	*Causal*	*Adversative*	*Others*
Most frequent	ve (*and*) da (*and, and then*) {-Ip} (*and*)	sonra (*after*) ondan sonra (*and then*) {-dIğIndE} (*when*) {-IncE} (*when, as soon as, although*) {-kEn} (*as, when, while, although after which*)	çünkü (*because*) için (*so*) bunun/onun için (*so that*)	ama (*but*)	- Result: Diye (for, *so that, in order to*) - Condition: {-sA} (*if*) - Alternative: yani (*that is to say*)
Less used		daha sonra (*after then*) {-dIktEn sonra} (*after, subsequent to*) {-dIğI zaman} ilk önce o zaman o sırada (*meanwhile*) birden bire/birden {-mEdEn+önce} (*before*) {-E değin/-E dek, -E kadar} (*until*) {-dIkçE}(*as, as long as, whenever*)	{-E göre} bu yüzden (*because of, due to*) {-dEn dolayı} (*because of, due to*) {-dIğIndEn} (*because of…*) {-dIğI için} (as, *because, whereas*) {-mEk için} (*because of, due to*)	fakat (*but, though*) ancak (*but, except*), {-E rağmen}	- Result: ki (*that, as, though …*) {-sIn diye} (*lest*) - Manner: {-ErEk} ((*in, by*) *-ing*) {-E … -E} - Condition: {-sA bile} (*even if*) - Alternative: veya (*or*), ya da (*either … or*) öyle (*so, that*) Böylece Örneğin Mesela

Note: List taken from Akıncı & Jisa, 2000; Slobin, 1995; Topbaş & Özcan, 1995; Vion & Colas, 2005

Table 15.4 List of the conjunctions according to their meaning in French

	Additive	*Temporal*	*Causal*	*Adversative*	*Others*
Most frequent	et (*and*)	puis (*after*) alors (*then*) quand (*when*) après (*then*) et puis et après et alors (*and then*)	parce que (*because*) car (*because*) donc (*so*)	mais (*but*)	si (*if*) ou (*or*)
Less used	pendant que (*while*) lorsque (*when*) depuis que (*since*) dès que (*as soon as*) avant que (*before that*)	puisque (*since*) peut-être que (*perhaps that*) à cause de (*because of*) pour que (*so that*)	au lieu que (*isntead, but*) mais sinon (but if not) mais dès fois (*but sometime*)	même si (*even if*) en fait (*in fact*) et que (*and that*) aussi que (*also that*) tant que (*as long as*) déjà que (*already that*)	pendant que (*while*) lorsque (*when*) depuis que (*since*) dès que (*as soon as*) avant que (before that)

Results for connectives in Turkish

Before presenting the results concerning connectives across language groups (bilingual versus monolingual) and across school grades, the length of the texts produced will be discussed. In this study, the unit of analysis is 'the clause', which is defined by Berman and Slobin (1994) as a unified predicate describing a single situation (an activity, event or state). Table 15.5 gives the length with total number of clauses and mean number of clauses per subject for each group and the range of clauses.

Table 15.5 shows that monolingual subjects produced longer texts than the bilingual group. The differences in terms of text lengths are statistically significant for all groups except for the narratives of primary school children. We can also observe that for bilinguals, the only students that produce longer texts than the others are high school children. When we look at the range of clauses produced by both populations, again, interpersonal differences become important. For example, in the expository texts of the last group, one student produced 32 clauses out of 115. These results show that monolinguals produced longer texts than bilinguals and there is a continuing development in text production abilities in Turkish monolinguals. However, such a development is not observed until high school among bilinguals.

Length is not necessarily a sign of development. As was found in earlier research (e.g. Akıncı, 2001; Berman & Slobin, 1994), young children generally give elaborate descriptions of single pictures, without creating cohesive and coherent texts. Older children develop the skills to analyze situations into components and, hence, to relate events into a narrative. They are able to encode these events into multiclausal constructions, creating compact, and thus shorter, stories.

Table 15.5 Total text lengths in Turkish written texts

Text type	*Narration*			*Expository*		
School type	*Primary*	*Secondary*	*High*	*Primary*	*Secondary*	*High*
Population	**Turkish-French bilingual**					
Total clauses	180	238	415	184	174	332
Mean clause/ subject	7.2	11.9	20.7	7.3	8.7	16.6
Range clauses	2–15	2–24	8–46	3–20	3–27	5–32
Population	**Turkish monolingual**					
Total clauses	234	458	651	376	478	775
Mean clause/ subject	14	20.8	32.5	16.3	21.7	37.7
Range clauses	4–31	10–40	12–56	6–38	4–48	22–69

Table 15.6 presents the total number of connectives as well as the percentage of coordination and subordination in Turkish written texts of bilingual and monolingual informants.

First, the comparison of the total number of connectives for both populations shows similar use for both types of texts. Differences are not significant for any group except for expository texts of high school students.[8] As compared to high school students for both populations, primary and secondary school children show lower total numbers of connectives. However, a developmental schema can be observed with age: both in narratives and in expository texts, the mean of connectives increases from 4 (primary school pupils) to 13 (high school students).

Secondly, in an analysis of the types of connectors, despite a significant increase in the use of subordination with age, coordination dominates bilinguals' texts, regardless of group or type of text; for monolinguals, results show differences depending on type of text: if coordination is more common for narratives, use of subordination is clearly high in expository ones.

As far as the semantic link expressed by connectives in narratives is concerned, Table 15.7 shows that bilinguals use more additive relations. Monolinguals, however, prefer also temporal conjunctions for this type of text. We do not observe any big differences for causal and adversative relations. Expository texts' results show the contrary: monolinguals use more additive links than bilinguals, who use more causal ones. Even

Table 15.6 Total number of connectives and percentage of coordination and subordination in Turkish written texts

Text type	*Narration*			*Expository*		
School type	*Primary*	*Secondary*	*High*	*Primary*	*Secondary*	*High*
Population	**Turkish-French bilingual**					
Total connectives	112	154	311	109	118	271*
Mean/subject	4.4	7.7	13.5	4.3	5.9	13.5
Coordination	77	77	63	62.5	63	57.5
Subordination	23	23	37	37.5	37	42.5
Population	**Turkish monolingual**					
Total connectives	117	179	262	114	157	354*
Mean/subject	5	8.1	13.1	4.9	7.1	17.7
Coordination	55.5	62.5	57.5	52	51	52.5
Subordination	44.5	37.5	42.5	48	49	47.5

*Significant difference: $F(1,41) = 7.42$, $p < 0.009$.

Table 15.7 Percentage distribution of marker occurrences by semantic link in Turkish written texts

Text type	*Narration*			*Expository*		
School type	*Primary*	*Secondary*	*High*	*Primary*	*Secondary*	*High*
Population	**Turkish-French bilingual**					
Additive	47.5	51	47.5	38.5	30.5	27.5*
Temporal	29.5	27	25	24	7.5	14.5
Causal	3.5	6	8.5	16.5	22	17.5
Adversative	8	9	10	6.5	6	8.5
Others	11.5	7	9	14.5	34	32
Population	**Turkish monolingual**					
Additive	39.5	44.5	38	42	39	43*
Temporal	36.5	39.5	35.5	22	27.5	18.5
Causal	5	4.5	10.5	9	9	7.5
Adversative	12	8.5	9.5	6	8	5.5
Others	7	3	6.5	21	16.5	25.5

*Significant difference: $F(1,41) = 11.92$, $p < 0.01$.

though bilinguals differ from monolinguals for causal links in percentage terms, the differences are not significant.

Results for connectives in French

Table 15.8 gives the lengths of written texts for French. It shows that both populations produce texts of nearly the same lengths. When we look closely, the texts of young bilingual are often longer than those of monolinguals. Statistical analyses showed significant differences for bilingual secondary school subjects for narratives and bilingual primary school subjects for expository texts: in these cases, bilinguals produce longer texts than monolinguals. There is a continuous development in text production capacities in French for all, since for narratives, for instance, the mean clause per subject increases from seven (primary school bilingual children) to 18 (high school students); we see the same developmental pattern for French monolinguals: from 8.3 to 21.1.

Table 15.9 presents the total number of connectives as well as the percentage of coordination and subordination in French written texts.

Comparison of groups by age for the total number of connectives shows significant differences for narratives of secondary school children and for expository texts of primary school children. In both of these groups, bilingual subjects use more connectives than monolinguals.

Table 15.8 Total text lengths in French written texts

Text type	*Narration*			*Expository*		
School type	*Primary*	*Secondary*	*High*	*Primary*	*Secondary*	*High*
Population	**Turkish-French bilingual**					
Total clauses	170	353*	398	258*	242	285
Mean clause/ subject	7	14.1	18	10.7	9.7	13
Range clauses	2–15	6–24	3–34	4–42	3–29	5–25
Population	**French monolingual**					
Total clauses	192	192*	486	126*	188	365
Mean clause/ subject	8.3	8.3	21.1	5.4	8.1	15.8
Range clauses	3–22	1–17	8–53	2–12	3–15	5–37

*ANOVA test is statistically significant.

Table 15.9 Total number of connectives and mean per subject and percentage of coordination and subordination in French written texts

Text type	*Narration*			*Expository*		
School type	*Primary*	*Secondary*	*High*	*Primary*	*Secondary*	*High*
Population	**Turkish-French bilingual**					
Total connectives	98	192*	234	173*	161	175
Mean/subject	3.9	7.7	10.6	6.9	6.4	8
Coordination	80.5	65.5	48	35	43	35.5
Subordination	19.5	34.5	52	65	57	64.5
Population	**French monolingual**					
Total connectives	100	112*	290	87*	108	204
Mean/subject	4.3	5.1	12.6	3.8	4.9	8.9
Coordination	70	66	47	43.5	42.5	41
Subordination	30	34	53	56.5	57.5	59

*Significant difference: $F(1,45) = 7.83, p < 0.007$; $F(1,46) = 9.15, p < 0.004$.

Table 15.10 Percentage distribution of marker occurrences by semantic link in French written texts

Text type	*Narration*			*Expository*		
School type	*Primary*	*Secondary*	*High*	*Primary*	*Secondary*	*High*
Population	**Turkish-French bilingual**					
Additive	55.5	46	45	29	36	35
Temporal	32	33	28	20	7	9
Causal	4*	9	14.5	37*	24.5	28.5
Adversative	6	10	9	2	7	15
Others	1	2	3.5	12	25.5	10
Population	**French monolingual**					
Additive	55.5	52.5	45	41.5	40.5	38
Temporal	19	25.5	20	18.5	11	14.5
Causal	16.5*	9	11.5	23.5*	25	16
Adversative	7	6	14.5	10	9.5	14.5
Others	2	7	9	6.5	14	17

*Significant difference: $F(1,45) = 6.15, p < 0.01$; $F(1,45) = 7.67, p < 0.008$.

As for type of text and type of connectives, coordination is used more often in narrative texts than in expository texts for all age groups and both populations, except for both bilingual and monolingual high school subjects who prefer subordination in narratives. However, for expository texts, subordination is clearly the form that all groups use predominantly. Nevertheless, this preference for subordination over coordination in expository texts is stronger in all bilingual groups than in the French monolinguals.

As shown in Table 15.10, comparing the use of categories by semantic role of the conjunctions, bilinguals and monolinguals shows similar results. The only statistical difference concerns the use of causal connectives by primary school children: for both types of text, bilinguals use more than French monolinguals.

To summarize, whatever the population (bilingual or monolingual), age (primary, secondary or high school informants) and type of text (narratives or expository texts), using connectives in Turkish and French written texts follows the same path. If we have to make a distinction, this should be between young subjects (primary and secondary students) and the older ones (high school students). Indeed, the former use more coordination, while the latter use more subordination. This does not mean in any way that the young subjects do not have full control of subordination. In

French expository texts, we find subordination occurs three times more frequently than in narratives.

Anaphors in written texts in French

In order to succeed in school, children must master different types of texts. These texts have to be cohesive and coherent. One important indicator of mastering cohesion and coherence is anaphoric reference.

Discursive functions of languages, implying command of the reference system at various levels of coherence and cohesion, appear late, around seven years old, and continue to evolve up to 10 years and older (Hickmann, 2004). In the field of reference maintenance, non-anaphoric repetitions are prevalent at a young age, while anaphoric repetitions increase until the age of 8 or 9, with stabilization from a quantitative point of view at the age of 9–10 years, the age at which almost all repetitions have an anaphoric status.

In this context, our purpose is to answer the following question: do 10-year-old Turkish-French bilingual children differ quantitatively and/or qualitatively in their use of anaphoric units compared to their monolingual French peers? Following De Weck's (1991) classification of anaphors, we propose to study anaphoric density units and to analyze distribution of anaphors on both the quantitative and qualitative levels.[9]

Pronominal anaphora

(1) Third-person pronouns

(3) Je me suis batut avec sésbastien quart **il** mernever
I fought with Sebastian because he irritated me (FM-P04A-WN)

(2) Demonstrative pronouns (simple and compound)

(4) **ca** sert à rien
It is not useful for anything (TB-P01A, WE)

(3) Third-person possessive pronouns and adjectives

(5) Ma mère devait partir en Turquie pour **son** père qui était malade
My mother had to go to Turkey for her father who was sick (TB-P09B-WN)

(4) First- and second-person possessive pronouns and adjectives

(6) **Mon** ami a dit qu'il n'en avait pas
My friend said that he did not have any (TB-P02A-WN)

(5) Relative pronouns

(7) Il y en avait **qui** comme Thibault et Sacha me supportait pour que je la tape
There were [some people] such as Thibault and Sacha who defended me because I beat her (FM-P01B-WN)

(6) Indefinite pronouns

(8) Si **l'autre** fait une erreur
If the other one makes an error (TB-P04A-WE)

Anaphoric nominal processes

(7) Repetition

(9) Moi je pense que **la violence** ce n'est pas une chose très bien car: les problèmes ne se règle jamais avec **la violence**
Me, I think that violence is not a good thing because: problems never fix themselves with violence (TB-P08B-WE)

(8) Definitivization

(10) **un grand** à demander ... et après **le grand** a dit ...
An older one asked ... and then the older one said (TB-P02A-WN)

(9) Textual exophoric reference

(11) **Ma** grave **maladie** (...) j'avais 6 ans quand j'ai eu **cette maladie**
My serious illness (...) I was 6 years old when I had this disease (FM-P11B-WN)

(10) Lexical substitution

(12) j'ai reçus dais coup de pied par **un garçon** (...) je l'ai dit au maître et il a puni **l'élève**
I got kicked by a boy (...) I told the teacher and he punished the pupil (FM-P06B-WN)

(11) Nominalization

(13) Etant petite, chez **mon tonton, mon grand frère** jouait à la pétanque, **tout le monde** disait de pas passer derrière eux
When I was young, with my uncle, my elder brother played games of bowls, everyone said not to pass behind them (FM-P10A-WN)

Others

(12) Mainly adverbs of place

(14) A l'école et **dehors**, les choses bien et pas bien
At the school and outside, good things and not good ones (TB-P11A-WE)

In order to classify anaphoric occurrences in one of the categories illustrated above, we have taken as a starting point the first mention of a referent. Calculation of anaphoric density makes it possible to obtain an evaluation of its ratio according to the type of text and the modality, by neutralizing the length of texts. This calculation will be applied to (1) all kinds of anaphors to get total density; (2) pronouns; (3) nominal anaphors; and (4) the category of 'others'. We will then study types of anaphors used in texts and try to describe the specificities of each type of text on both the quantitative and qualitative levels.

Analyses of anaphors

Before presenting the results on the number of anaphors in texts, Table 15.11 gives text length in terms of number of words for the primary school

Table 15.11 Text lengths based on number of words in French written texts for primary school children

Type of text	*Narratives*		*Expository texts*	
Population	***Bilingual***	***Monolingual***	***Bilingual***	***Monolingual***
Text lengths (word number)	1149	1303	1792	866

children in French. Table 15.8 illustrated differences in French text lengths in clauses; however, here we have chosen to display text lengths in words.

For French monolinguals narratives are longer than expository texts, while the quantitative relation is reversed for Turkish-French bilingual children. Moreover, the number of words in expository texts provided by bilinguals is higher than that of their monolingual peers. A qualitative analysis of written expository texts shows differences in terms of content. Whereas monolingual children produced expository texts on the topic of violence in schools or between people, as we expected, Turkish-French bilingual children relied more on support from videos we showed them before data collection. Many bilingual children's expository texts thus contain references to episodes showed on video, instead of discussing the issue of interpersonal problems.

We then calculated anaphoric density according to two parameters: (1) population (monolingual versus bilingual) and (2) type of texts (narratives versus expository texts).

We expect to find higher anaphoric density in narratives than in expository texts, whatever be the population. Indeed, anaphoric operation is mastered earlier for narratives than for discursive text types, which are mastered at around 14 years (De Weck, 1991). We also think that bilingual children will achieve similar anaphoric density as concerns the comparison according to type of texts (narrative versus expository). Table 15.12 shows anaphoric density in French written texts provided by the 10-year-old primary school children of both populations.

For both populations, these results demonstrate the strong correlation between text length and anaphoric density. With respect to French monolinguals, anaphoric density is quite a bit higher in narratives compared to expository texts. As for bilingual children, we get the opposite

Table 15.12 Anaphoric density[a] (in %) in written texts of monolingual and bilingual children

Type of text	*Narratives*		*Expository texts*	
Population	***Bilingual***	***Monolingual***	***Bilingual***	***Monolingual***
Anaphoric density	12.1	11.44	11.94	6.81

[a]This calculation consists of a ratio of number of anaphors to number of words in text.

result: expository texts contain more anaphors than narratives. We can therefore wonder how relevant the differences in anaphoric density are. Although differences are in favor of bilingual children, their anaphoric density is at least equivalent to that of monolinguals.

In a second stage, we studied the distribution of types of anaphors for both types of texts and both populations. Our hypotheses for this were

Hypothesis 1: For narratives, we will find more pronominal anaphors than noun phrases. Indeed, because of disjunction related to referent and autonomous discursive mode, we should find more third personal pronouns, possessive pronouns and adjectives and relatives. Concerning expository texts, we expect more pronominal anaphors, followed by nominal ones and then others.

Hypothesis 2: We expect no differences in use of anaphors between Turkish-French bilingual children and French monolinguals.

Table 15.13 presents the percentages obtained for each category of anaphor.

In both types of text, pronominal anaphors are strongly represented. As we predicted in our second hypothesis, percentages are very close between both populations, with, however, a small advantage for bilinguals concerning the use of nominal anaphors. The category 'others' is hardly used by either population. Concerning pronominal anaphors, we observe a small percentage difference between narratives and expository texts. We need a deeper analysis of types of anaphor in order to explain the different uses with types of texts. Indeed, pronominal anaphors comprise six types of anaphors. The total percentage of pronominal anaphors can thus hide differences in types of pronominal anaphors between narratives and expository texts. Nominal anaphors are slightly more common in expository texts, whatever the population. In this case, it will also be necessary to perform qualitative analysis of type of nominal anaphors in order to understand the mechanisms involved.

As we already stressed, bilingual children from an immigration background are often stigmatized and bilingualism is considered to

Table 15.13 Percentage of types of anaphors in French written texts of primary school children

Type of text	*Narratives*		*Expository texts*	
Population	***Bilingual***	***Monolingual***	***Bilingual***	***Monolingual***
Pronominal anaphors	78.5	86	89.5	90
Nominal anaphors	21.5	13.5	10	8.5
Others	0	0.5	0.5	1.5

be responsible for school failure. School success requires control of particular linguistic competences, both in written and oral language; abilities are often related to de-contextualized situations and require a high cognitive level in the standard language. Anaphors appear to be a good indicator of linguistic control levels compatible with school requirements.

Previous studies of anaphors primarily involved narratives. However, texts produced within the school framework at primary school level are expository or argumentative texts as often as narratives. It thus appeared judicious for us to compare the use of anaphors in these two types of texts. Our first results linking anaphoric density to text type show that Turkish-French bilingual subjects' results for narratives are equivalent to those of monolinguals. Anaphoric density also appears higher in expository texts from bilingual children. We must relate this finding to the characteristics of expository texts written by bilinguals. Comparison of each type of anaphor (pronominal, nominal and other anaphors) leads us to conclude that bilingual and monolingual children use the same amount of anaphors. This result should obviously be supplemented by detailed and qualitative analyses of anaphors in writings. Also, comparing oral versus written modalities of texts should enable us to validate these conclusions.

Implications for SLPs Working with Turkish Clients in a Clinical Setting

The SLP process in a French multilingual setting for Turkish people

Speech therapy as a profession was legally recognized in France by the law of July 10, 1964, which instituted a national diploma: the Certificate of Competence of Speech-therapy (Certificat de Capacité d'Orthophoniste).

Speech therapists are medical auxiliaries, which mean that they intervene on medical prescription. The first step in the SLP process is the speech assessment, which is divided into two parts: the anamnesis (or preliminary case history) and the assessment itself.

During anamnesis, speech therapist asks parents about the reason for seeking services, symptoms, and medical and academic history of their child. Parents are questioned about the language spoken with the child, the child's language development (age of first words, which language is used by the child, with whom and so forth) and any history of language impairment in the family. At this stage, speech therapists may be confronted with the problem of the language spoken by the parents. There will be no problem if the parents speak French, or if the speech therapist speaks Turkish. However, if the parents speak only Turkish or Turkish with low levels of French and the speech therapist cannot speak Turkish, anamnesis will be difficult to conduct. In this case, parents often come with an interpreter (a family member or a neighbor who speaks French). In some cases, one of their older children acts as an interpreter. However, when there is an interpreter, the anamnesis may be more difficult because parents may feel uncomfortable answering certain private questions in the presence of the interpreter. Speech therapists who answered the questionnaire established by Tinelli (2004: 107–109) mentioned four types of difficulties encountered:

(1) *The linguistic barrier*: Many Turkish families are not fluent enough in French and rely on the help of siblings who will act as interpreters.
(2) *A lack of understanding about speech therapy*: Speech therapy is not often understood by Turkish families. Not knowing about speech therapy, the parents imagine it as support with school work. The parents are not very motivated because they are not aware of the child's difficulties and, in a sense, they do not understand the point of long-term monitoring.
(3) *A difficulty in accessing the history of the pathology*: During the anamnesis, it is often difficult to recapture the child's medical or language history.
(4) *A cultural barrier*: Cultural references, religion and traditions are factors that can appear complicated to anyone who does not belong to the community. Speech therapists misread the cultural references of families, and families often do not necessarily understand the job of the speech therapist.

It is necessary to have these difficulties in mind in order to try to prevent them. Concerning the first point, the linguistic barrier, the only answer, apart from turning to an interpreter, is to find a bilingual speech therapist, which may be difficult. Indeed, we do not have at our disposal any index of bilingual speech therapists. Nevertheless, some solutions might be taken into consideration. As for the second point above, it is necessary to take time to explain what speech therapy consists of. Through developing bilingual questionnaires and gathering documentation on the cultural environment of Turkish families, the speech therapist will be able to reduce these barriers. Speech therapists working with bilingual patients have to integrate the patient's family as a real partner in the therapy, even if it seems difficult because of linguistic and cultural barriers.

After anamnesis, the speech therapist proceeds to an assessment. Its clinical modalities depend on medical prescription, age of the child and his or her level of participation. A speech therapist has at his or her disposal the following:

- Many assessment tools: standardized tests that make it possible to get quantitative results in terms of age (lexical age for example) or of standard deviation in reference to a statistical standard.
- Clinical experience that allows a qualitative analysis of a child's production and behavior.

However, as Chevrie-Muller (2007: 95) points out, 'beyond the modular approach it is essential that the child has to be considered as a whole'.

Assessment tools used for language disordered Turkish children in context

In France, there are no specific assessment tools used for language disordered Turkish children. The Turkish child will be asked to take tests in French. If the speech therapist speaks Turkish, he or she will be able to conduct a qualitative analysis of the child's Turkish language, but no standardized tests in Turkish are published in France. If the speech therapist does not speak Turkish, the only way to approach the specificities of the child's Turkish will be to ask parents or the interpreter, keeping in mind the problems noted above.

Calbour (2006) uses a table that allows analyzing the particular linguistic situation of the child who comes in for consultation (see Table 15.14). It is a useful aid to help adapt the therapy for the particular client and to measure linguistic development during therapy.

As for the French language, many assessment tools can be used, according to age and language components. We present in Table 15.15 a non-exhaustive list of the existing materials divided into three categories: tools for oral language, those for written language and those for both.

These assessment tools are only a small part of those used by speech therapists in France. Furthermore, as we saw before, the most important aspect of the assessment is the meeting between the child, their family and a speech therapist.

After the anamnesis, which involves similar questions for all children, assessment must be age appropriate. Three age ranges can be considered:

- before starting schooling (i.e. before the age of three years),
- between the start of schooling and the entry into primary education, and
- after entering primary education (usually after the age of six years).

The assessment is adapted to the age and capacities of the child; for example, the use of standardized tests is restricted to children of school age.

(1) Before schooling: It is rare that children consult speech therapists, except for children with specific handicaps, or in the case of a child without language who also presents behavioral problems. In these cases, consultation is often done on the advice of a 'Maternal and Infantile Protection' physician (PMI) or of a pediatrician. This is unfortunate as, at this age, preventive intervention can be most effective, especially for children with bilingualism resulting from immigration.

Table 15.14 Bilingualism typology of the child

	Mother				*Child*					
					Early linguistic development		*Mastery of the language*			
	Mother tongue		*Second language*		*Mother tongue*	*Second language*	*Mother tongue*		*Second language*	
	Compre-hension	*Produc-tion*	*Compre-hension*	*Produc-tion*			*Compre-hension*	*Produc-tion*	*Compre-hension*	*Produc-tion*
Oral language										
Written language										

Bilingualism typology of the child
According to the linguistic abilities of the mother and the child (Calbour, 2006).

Table 15.15 Some assessment tools classified according to oral or written modality (details of these tests are presented in the appendix)

Oral Language	***Written language***	***Oral and written language***
Batterie d'évaluation psycholinguistique (BEPL-A, BEPL-B), Chevrie-Muller *et al.* (1985a, 1985b)	*Epreuve d'évaluation de la compétence en lecture Lecture de mots et compréhension – Révisée (LMC-R)*, Khomsi (1999)	*Batterie « Langage oral et écrit, mémoire – attention » (L2MA)*, Chevrie-Muller *et al.* (1997)
Nouvelles épreuves pour l'examen du langage (N-EEL), Chevrie-Muller and Plaza (2001)	*Bilan de lecture informatisé (BLI)*, Khomsi (2002)	*Une batterie cognitive d'examen du langage oral et écrit (EXALANG 5–8)*, Helloin *et al.* (2002)
Epreuves verbales d'aptitudes cognitives (EVAC), Flessas and Lussier (2003)	Alouette-R, Lefavrais (2005)	*Une épreuve de compréhension syntaxico-sémantique (E.CO.S.SE)*, Lecocq (1996)
Evaluation du langage oral (ELO), Khomsi (2001)	*Analyse du savoir lire de 8 ans à l'âge adulte (ANALEC)*, Inizan (1998)	*Batterie prédictive de l'apprentissage de la lecture (BP/BL)*, Inizan (2000)
Epreuve d'évaluation des stratégies de compréhension en situation orale (O-52), Khomsi (1987)	*Vol du PC*, Boutard *et al.* (1997)	*Outil de dépistage des dyslexies – version 2 (ODEDYS – version 2)*, Zorman and Jacquier-Roux (2005)
Test de Langage Oral Complexe pour collégiens (TLOCC), Maurin (2006)	*Test de Compréhension Syntaxique (T.C.S.)*, Maeder (2006)	
Sacré Nestor, Crunelle *et al.* (2004)		
Test de vocabulaire en images (VOCIM), Légé and Dague (1976)		
Protocole d'évaluation rapide (P.E.R. 2000), Ferrand (2000)		
Une batterie cognitive d'examen du langage oral (EXALANG 3–6), Helloin *et al.* (2006)		

In the case of children below the age of three years, speech therapists will primarily center their assessment on

- Observations by parents of the language used by their child in daily life. In French, there is the IFDC (French inventories of communicative development) adapted from the MacArthur-Bates communicative development inventories by Kern (2003, 2004) and the French Association of Ambulatory Pediatry (http://www.afpa.org). Parents fill out analysis charts, which are distributed by the pediatrician during a consultation or by a speech therapist. These inventories have the advantage of being calibrated but are difficult to use with bilinguals since they are available only in French. The Standing Liaison Committee of EU Speech and Language Therapists and Logopedists propose analysis charts dealing with 18-, 30- and 54-month-old children. These charts are less elaborate, but they have the advantage of being translated into several languages including French and Turkish.
- An observation of the child when playing freely.
- Use of standardized tests such as the Batterie d'évaluation psycholinguistique (BEPL-A, BEPL-B) of Chevrie-Muller *et al.* (1985a, 1985b) for children of at least 2;9.

The major difficulty at this age lies in the fact that before schooling, children of Turkish origin are only exposed to the Turkish language: the standardized tests in French will be thus difficult or even impossible to use with them and speech therapists who do not speak Turkish have to rely on the observation of non-verbal communication and on the assistance of parents or interpreters. This assessment, therefore, will not necessarily lead to a therapeutic intervention plan, but advice and support could be suggested in order to allow favorable development of language.

(2) Between the beginning of schooling and the entry into primary education (usually from three to six years): It is often at this age, as we saw, that a child will start a prolonged contact with the French language. It is also often at this period that an assessment is required for children of Turkish immigrant families. The referral often comes from a PMI physician, the school physician and/or the teacher. Parents do not always consult a speech therapist at this stage: the second author often met children for whom a referral had been made at this age but whose parents, for cultural reasons, came for a consultation only when an older sibling encountered great difficulties in written language.

Between three and six years, the assessment of oral language will comprise

- An observation of the child in a play situation and of its behavior throughout the assessment (the desire for communication, nonverbal communication, communication strategies).

- Standardized tests: Standardized tests are numerous and make it possible to explore wide-ranging competences, in particular articulation, phonology, both lexical expression and comprehension, semantics and syntax, pragmatics, attention and memory.

Among test batteries concerning this age range, speech therapists have at their disposal

- *Batterie d'évaluation psycholinguistique (BEPL-A, BEPL-B)*, Chevrie-Muller *et al.* (1985a, 1985b)
- *Protocole d'évaluation rapide (P.E.R. 2000)*, Ferrand (2000)
- *Nouvelles épreuves pour l'examen du langage (N-EEL)*, Chevrie-Muller and Plaza (2001)
- *Evaluation du langage oral (ELO)*, Khomsi (2001)
- *Epreuve d'évaluation des stratégies de compréhension en situation orale (O-52)*, Khomsi (1987)
- *Test de vocabulaire en images (VOCIM)*, Légé and Dague (1976)
- *Une batterie cognitive d'examen du langage oral (EXALANG 3–6)*, Helloin *et al.* (2006)

With these tests, speech therapists can build up an inventory of competences and difficulties in the French language of the child. In comparison with this profile in French, it will be advisable to get as precise information as possible about the child's competences and difficulties in the mother tongue by questioning parents or the interpreter. Interpretation of French tests should balance both quantitative and qualitative analyses; it must also be remembered that norms obtained from these different tests are those for monolingual children and not for bilingual ones. That is why tests should be used cautiously. Qualitative analysis will allow speech therapists who assess the mother tongue of the child to differentiate interference from pathology.

(3) After entry into primary education (usually after six years old): As we saw, at this age, the French language becomes dominant for Turkish children. At this age, children learn to read and write in French. Some of them will, furthermore, benefit from supplementary mother tongue education.

Children who have difficulties are identified by teachers. They refer for speech and/or writing difficulties and physicians will specify the type of assessment needed.

Assessment of oral language

The same competences as previous described are examined by means of tests appropriate to the age and capacities of the child:

- *Nouvelles épreuves pour l'examen du langage (N-EEL)*, Chevrie-Muller and Plaza (2001)

- *Evaluation du langage oral (ELO)*, Khomsi (2001)
- *Epreuve d'évaluation des stratégies de compréhension en situation orale (O-52)*, Khomsi (1987)
- *Test de vocabulaire en images (VOCIM)*, Légé and Dague (1976)
- *Epreuves verbales d'aptitudes cognitives (EVAC)*, Flessas and Lussier (2003)
- *Sacré Nestor*, Crunelle *et al.* (2004)
- *Test de Langage Oral Complexe pour collégiens (TLOCC)*, Maurin (2006)

Assessment of written language

The aim is to test the following competences (some or all of them according to the age of the child):

- knowledge of letters and graphemes,
- speed and quality of reading aloud,
- quality of lexical addressing and phonological assembly in reading,
- reading comprehension,
- lexical and syntactic spelling (under dictation and in spontaneous production) and
- text competences.

Some of the tests used for both oral and written language of children over six years old are listed in Table 15.15 and detailed in the appendix.

It would also be interesting to ask children about their use of written Turkish. As for oral language, we do not have at our disposal specific Turkish-French bilingual tests.

Therapeutic implications

In France, we have only recently begun to take into account the variable of bilingualism. Lack of information and specific assessment tools leads many speech therapists to unsatisfactory classification of clients. Because of this, they often seek advice from professional forums about bilingualism on the internet, trying to get information from each other. There is still a long way to go, but studying bilingual children's language development may be the first step in helping speech therapists in their work with this population.

In this study about Turkish-French bilingualism, some elements should help us to understand the Turkish-French bilinguals' language development. One very important discovery is that at the age of 10, their abilities in French are similar to those of monolingual French children. Speech therapists should bear this in mind when they carry out an assessment of the language of a Turkish-French bilingual child.

Another implication concerns prevention. The provision of informative materials about language for Turkish families may help these families to manage their particular language situation, with benefits for their children. Such documents have begun to be developed, notably by the CPLOL (Standing Liaison Committee of Speech and Language Therapists/ Logopedists in the European Union, 1988–1998).

In any case, as Calbour (2006) points out, 'As it is impossible for a speech therapist to learn all the native languages and cultures with which he is confronted, he must integrate the family in the therapeutic process with its linguistic, cultural and social referents, specific to its original ethnic group. He acts with coherence and efficacy when he respects the child's linguistic roots'. More than any other case, speech therapy with a Turkish child requires cooperation with the family. Rosenbaum's work in Switzerland (1997) gives some interesting ideas of what form this cooperation should have. She proposes the realization of a 'genogram': it begins by drawing, with the help of the child's family, a family tree of three generations. The location of different family members (in our case in France or in Turkey), comparison of first names and different information about each member (age, dead or alive) are discussed with the child. This work should help children to write their own history and to situate themselves.

General Discussion and Conclusion

While for some children the two languages develop independently and simultaneously, leading to early almost balanced bilingualism, our previous results have shown the status of strong and weak language changes for Turkish-French bilinguals in their development. While children show Turkish as a dominant language in early childhood, their mother tongue stagnates or fossilizes until the age of 10 and it becomes close to the language used by Turkish monolinguals at the age of 14 (Akıncı, 2001). Our previous research also showed that French becomes dominant at the age of six. However, bilingual children's abilities in French are not similar to those of monolingual French children until the age of 10. Figure 15.1 shows the development of the two languages for Turkish-French bilingual children in France.

Usually, nursery school is an emotional shock for a child, and each child adopts strategies corresponding to his or her personality to manage this new situation. The first months are a sensitive period, because teachers with little awareness of the processes involved put pressure on bilingual children, judging them negatively. We believe that it is essential to allow the child a period of silence without engaging in false interpretations such as 'language delay' or 'refuses to speak'. Some children with a Turkish background probably do need speech therapy, but in any case we should not generalize this practice.

Recent studies (see Backus, 2004, for reviews of this work) on the language of Turkish bilingual children in European countries point to the fact that these children face important problems in learning the language of the country in which they live. Our results show, however, that text

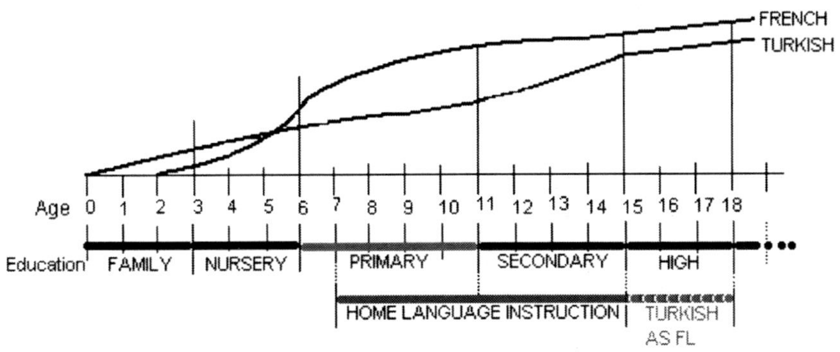

Figure 15.1 Acquisition and development of French and Turkish by Turkish second-generation children and adolescents in France with schooling and age

production abilities in Turkish and French continue to develop through high school in Turkish-French bilingual children and adolescents. If methodological precautions are taken, both bilingual and monolingual populations behave the same, despite myths circulating about lower competencies in the mother tongue and in French, that contribute to school failure. These myths, which are often due to a widespread bilingualism deficit approach in the educational framework, influence the educational relationship and the expectations regarding the performance of pupils.

'The most important thing is not to teach a child to speak a new language differing from his usual one well, but to create for him the desire to explore and learn a new language in interaction with his environment. (…) Taking into account the specificity of the environment is especially even more important for a child from a migrant background since he is often rejected by the environment into which some people want to integrate him and since the only language feeding his roots is the one of his parents' (Calbour, 2006: 6; authors' translation).

Acknowledgments

This research was supported by ACI Young Researchers Programs (French Ministry of Research; Project No. 02-2-0241) and French-Turkish PHC Bosphorus programs (French Ministry of Foreign Office and The Scientific and Technological Research Council of Turkey-TÜBITAK). We wish to thank our colleague C. Pfaff (Freie Universität Berlin, Germany) for her assistance with English corrections.

Notes

1. Tabors and Snow (1994) have identified four stages of sequential acquisition of a new language. The stages describe the learning process for children after the

age of three, whose first language is partly established and who are now in a setting where the second language is predominantly in use.
2. Even if by the age of 5/6 years, French becomes the dominant language for children, attachment to mother tongue remains a strong marker of identity for those families. Confronted with acculturation, migrants feel threatened in their identity; there are values that they try to perpetuate such as language, religion or culture. Besides, it is not rare for some Turkish parents to impose French as the language of the home in the belief that this will somehow improve their children's chances at school.
3. In order to learn more about Turkish families who have a child who is being monitored for speech language disorders, Steib (2006) also conducted interviews with four Turkish mothers in the same city. She asked them their views on a number of issues concerning the Turkish community in France, concepts such as language abilities, their contact with books and school, speech therapy, religion, transmission of traditions, marriage and, finally, television.
4. The conceptual and methodological basis for this study is derived from a crosslinguistic research project on the development of text production abilities as a critical indicator of literacy across and beyond school ages (Berman & Verhoeven, 2002).
5. The data of concern here are spoken stories based upon the picture book '*Frog Where Are You?*' (Mayer, 1969) coded following the procedures outlined in Berman and Slobin (1994) (for details, see Akıncı, 2001).
6. The dataset was subjected to Analysis of Variance (ANOVA) tests: the values of these tests were accepted as significant for $p < 0.05$.
7. Each subject was assigned a code. The first letters indicate the group: TB = Turkish-French bilingual and FM = French monolingual. The letter following the group code indicates the child's school level: P = primary school. The number codes the student individually in a school group, and A or B after the number indicates the presentation group in each school level. The final letters code modalities (W = written texts and S = spoken texts) and types (N = narrative texts and E = expository texts).
8. The values of these tests were accepted as significant for $p < 0.05$.
9. This study is part of the work done by N. Decool-Mercier toward her master's degree thesis (Decool-Mercier, 2008).

Appendix: Details of Assessments

Oral language

Batterie d'évaluation psycholinguistique (BEPL-A, BEPL-B), Chevrie-Muller *et al.* (1985a, 1985b)

The BEPL is a module made up of 23 different subtests for Part A, and observation of the child's play for Part B. It provides standardized scores. This test can be used with children aged from two years, nine months to four years, three months. Part A evaluates oro-facial motility, articulation, visuo-spatial organization, immediate verbal retention and phonological, lexical, semantic and syntactic capacities (expression and comprehension). Part B is a situation where the child is playing: the speech therapist observes spontaneous linguistic expression through which the richness of the vocabulary, the morphosyntax and the psycholinguistic and pragmatic aspects can be studied.

Protocole d'évaluation rapide (P.E.R. 2000), Ferrand (2000)

This test allows for quick evaluation of the linguistic capacities of a child between 3;5 and 5;6. The 'P.E.R. 2000' includes several tests that explore the child's abilities in the following fields: hearing, reproduction of rhythmic structures, instrumental abilities (except language), auditory–perceptive aptitudes, articulation of phonemes, speech and oral language (comprehension, syntactic complexity of the speech).

Nouvelles épreuves pour l'examen du langage (N-EEL), Chevrie-Muller and Plaza (2001)

This test has two forms: the P-form intended for younger children (aged 3;7–6;6) and the G-form for older children (aged 6;6–8;7). Some tests are common to both forms, while others are specific to one or the other of the two forms. The various components evaluated are phonology, expression (lexicon – morphosyntax), comprehension (lexicon – morphosyntax), memory and cognitive capacities.

Epreuves verbales d'aptitudes cognitives (EVAC), Flessas and Lussier (2003)

This test evaluates the mental strategy and the linguistic abilities used in the school context for children aged from 8 to 13 years.

Evaluation du langage oral (ELO), Khomsi (2001)

This test evaluates different aspects of oral language of 3–10-year-old children: lexicon in reception (LexR), lexicon in production (LexP), repetition of words (RépM), comprehension (C), utterance production (ProdE) and utterance repetition (RépE).

Epreuve d'évaluation des stratégies de compréhension en situation orale (O-52), Khomsi (1987)

This test of picture recognition is used with 3–7-year-old children. It allows for the evaluation of syntactic comprehension strategies in oral situations.

Sacré Nestor, Crunelle *et al.* (2000)

This test evaluates detailed oral comprehension. After hearing a story, children aged from 7 to 10;11 years have to retell the story, answer some detailed questions and place pictures in the correct order of the story.

Test de vocabulaire en images (VOCIM), Légé and Dague (1976)

This test examines receptive vocabulary. It can be used with children aged from three to nine years. The child is asked to point to one of the four pictures to identify which illustrates the word that was presented.

Une batterie cognitive d'examen du langage oral (EXALANG 3–6), Helloin *et al.* (2006)

This computerized battery is for children aged from 2;8 to 5;10 years. It evaluates lexical competences (expression and reception), morpho-syntactic competences (expression and reception), non-verbal competences, phonology, attention and memory.

Test de Langage Oral Complexe pour collégiens (TLOCC), Maurin (2006)

This test is a clinical tool that evaluates the complex oral language level of school children: vocabulary (comprehension and expression) and sentences (morphology and meaning).

Written language

Epreuve d'évaluation de la compétence en lecture. Lecture de mots et compréhension – Révisée (LMC-R), Khomsi (1999)

This test, for children from first year infants' class to third grade form, is composed of three parts: reading in one minute, word identification and reading comprehension.

Bilan de lecture informatisé (BLI), Khomsi (2002)

This computerized test is modeled after LMC-R. It is designed for children from the second year to the fifth year of primary school and measures reaction times.

Alouette-R, Lefavrais (2005)

This is a test of text reading speed for 6–16-year-old children. Its objective is to provide indications of performances in a situation of reading texts aloud. It contains elements on the speed and the correctness of the reading.

Analyse du savoir lire de 8 ans à l'âge adulte (ANALEC), Inizan (1998)

This is a set of tests on reading and writing abilities for eight-year-old children to adults: silent reading (speed and comprehension), reading aloud (speed and correctness), spelling with aural input (dictation) and spelling with visual input, analysis and synthesis.

Vol du PC, Boutard *et al.* (1997)

This test provides a functional evaluation of the reading of subjects from 11 to 18 years, by measuring text reading speed, analyzing types of errors (there are some nonsense words in the text) and comprehension.

Test de Compréhension Syntaxique (T.C.S.), Maeder (2006)

The T.C.S. is a test designed for children and teenagers aged from 8;6 to 15;5 years. The purpose is to evaluate morpho-syntactic comprehension on the level of written utterances in isolation.

Oral and written language

Batterie prédictive de l'apprentissage de la lecture (BP/BL),
Inizan (2000)

The predictive set of tests determines if the child is ready to begin learning to read, and it predicts in addition the time necessary to conduct this training. The reading battery used with children in their first and second year of primary school measures their reading ability.

Outil de dépistage des dyslexies – Version 2 (ODEDYS – version 2),
Zorman and Jacquier-Roux (2005)

ODEDYS is a tool for the detection of dyslexia, which concerns children from the second year of primary school to second year of secondary school. The tests are l'Alouette, word reading, word dictation, sentence dictation, repetition of words and nonsense words, fast denomination, metaphonology, memory and visual tests.

Batterie 'Langage oral et écrit, mémoire – attention' (L2MA),
Chevrie-Muller *et al.* (1997)

This test concerns children aged from 8;6 to 11;6 years. It tests oral and written language, memory, attention and visuo-motor aptitudes.

Une épreuve de compréhension syntaxico-sémantique (E.CO.S.SE),
Lecocq (1996)

This test can be used with 4–12-year-old children in oral and/or written modalities. It allows for the measurement of syntactic and semantic comprehension.

Une batterie cognitive d'examen du langage oral et écrit (EXALANG 5–8), Helloin *et al.* (2002)

This computerized test is designed for children aged from five to eight years. It evaluates oral language, metaphonology, memory and written language.

Chapter 16

Specific Language Impairment in Turkish-German Bilingual Children: Aspects of Assessment and Outcome

SOLVEIG CHILLA and EZEL BABUR

Introduction

The linguistic description and the assessment of language impairments in Turkish children is a relatively new research area (Babur *et al.*, 2007; Rothweiler *et al.*, 2007; Topbaş, 2006c). Although many studies focus on the normal acquisition of Turkish (e.g. Aksu-Koç & Slobin, 1985), very little is known about the outcome of a delayed or disordered language acquisition process in general. Recently, several authors have focused on different forms of language impairments in monolingual Turkish children (Topbaş, Chapters 1 and 7, this volume), and phonological disorders have been extensively studied (Topbaş, 1997, 1999, 2007a).

Considering a special form of language impairment, namely specific language impairment (SLI), the lack of linguistic descriptions and assessment tools for Turkish monolinguals leads to a diagnostic dilemma for the clinical assessment of bilingual children in migration settings. About 3–10% of all children are affected by SLI, and authors such as Choudhury and Benasich (2003) or the SLI-Consortium (MonacoAP, SLIC, 2007) assume that the disorder is genetically based. Following this assumption, it is obvious that the disorder must show up in multilingual children as well. About 25% of all children in Germany are bilingual, with Turkish-speaking children being the largest group among them. If the prevalence rate could be confirmed for bilingual children (see, e.g. Goldstein, 2004), approximately 1.25% of all children in Germany would be bilingual children with SLI, and many of them would speak Turkish as their home language. An explicit definition of

SLI, however, is still missing; hence, speech and language therapists have to rely merely on exclusionary criteria. In this sense, SLI children show language acquisition deficits that are not affiliated with hearing loss, mental or social deprivation, or evident neurological damage. A delayed onset of language acquisition and difficulties both in the production and in the comprehension of language have been reported (Leonard, 1998). If the language development of SLI children is compared to a baseline of unimpaired acquisition, their language acquisition process may be characterized as delayed or deviant. Mostly, for these children, the acquisition of grammatical specificities is problematic. The verbal domain seems to be predominantly affected, as studies on SLI in English (e.g. Wexler, 1994, 1996), German (e.g. Clahsen, 1991), Greek (e.g. Tsimpli & Mastropavlou, 2004) or Cantonese (Fletcher *et al.*, 2005) reveal.

These facts on bilingual acquisition and SLI have confronted researchers as well as speech and language therapists with the following problems:

(1) How can it be possible to diagnose bilingual Turkish-speaking children with SLI in their first language, if only a few studies on the outcome of SLI in Turkish monolinguals can be referred to?
(2) Does the acquisition of Turkish as a first language in migration settings (for instance, Turkish-German children acquiring Turkish in Germany) have an impact on the language acquisition process in general? Moreover, to what extent do varieties of Turkish in an immigrant setting like Germany and the outcome of SLI in Turkish affect similar grammatical domains and thus complicate the assessment of SLI in bilingual children?
(3) Do inter-language stages in the acquisition of the L2 grammar pattern with the deviant structures of SLI in German, so that professionals are confronted with the risk of misdiagnosis?

In the following, we will briefly discuss the setting of language acquisition for Turkish-German children, before presenting deliberations on the assessment of language impairments in bilinguals. The second section will refer to the possibility of assessing SLI in Turkish-German children in a non-specific way, and, finally, some recent findings of the Hamburg Project on normal and impaired bilingual language acquisition[1] and on the outcome of SLI in these children will be discussed.

Bilingual Language Development in Migration Settings

The term 'bilingual children' refers in fact to a heterogeneous group of children who acquire their two languages under distinct circumstances. In general, at least four subgroups have linguistically been defined to model different forms of two-language acquisition: simultaneous bilingual children (2L1), successive bilingual children (sL), child second language learners (cL2) and adult second language learners (aL2) (for an overview, see Genesee *et al.*, 2004; Hyltenstam & Abrahamsson, 2003; Rothweiler, 2007). Simultaneous bilinguals acquire both their languages early, for example from birth or in their early preschool years. Ronjat (1913) prescribed the ideal constellation for 2L1 children as the 'one person-one language' principle. The two languages may be acquired as two first languages, leading to the assumption that 2L1 children may develop a first language competence in both. Several studies on grammar acquisition (cf. Meisel, 2004, for an overview) confirm this hypothesis, and show that 2L2 follow the same steps in their acquisition of grammar as do monolinguals of both languages. Unlike 2L1 children, aL2 acquire a second language after puberty or in adulthood, often in migration settings. The aL2 acquisition process is notably more heterogeneous than that of 2L1. Whether or not aL2 or (2)L1 follow the same patterns in acquisition is still under discussion for different language areas. Most studies, however, claim that there are fundamental differences between the two groups (e.g. Bley-Vroman, 1990; Clahsen & Muysken, 1986; Meisel, 1997) in the acquisition of grammar.

The systematic study of child second language acquisition is a relatively new research field. The question in focus is: do successive bilinguals or child L2 learners either acquire their L2 as a second first language, namely as (2)L1 or does their developmental process in language acquisition follow the same pattern as aL2 (e.g. Meisel, 2007; Schwartz, 2004)? Several authors (e.g. Hyltenstam & Abrahamsson, 2003; Lenneberg, 1967; see also Unsworth, 2005, for an overview) assume sensitive periods or critical phases in grammar development, which have an impact both on the developmental process and/or on the achievable competence levels. Henceforth, there has been a discussion over what is the oldest, or latest, age of onset (AO) at which children are able to acquire their second language as a second first language and thus show milestones in acquisition comparable to those known for L1. Lenneberg (1967) sets the cut-off point around puberty, whereas recent work by Meisel (2007) and Rothweiler (2007), for example, assume that the critical phase(s) for grammar development slowly fade out between the ages of three and four years. Some studies strengthen the hypothesis that the development of sentence structure in children acquiring their second language from age 2–3 onwards is to a vast extent indeed comparable to (2)L1 (Prévost, 2003; Rothweiler, 2006; Thoma & Tracy, 2006; but see also Haznedar, 2003). This developmental process has thus been characterized as successive bilingual acquisition (sL), and it is assumed that native competence in both languages, at least for some grammatical domains, may be achieved. The term child L2 comprises an AO of 4–8. If the second language learning starts within this period, the developmental process seems more likely to share commonalities with aL2 (Genesee *et al.*, 2004; Kroffke, 2006; Meisel, 2007; Unsworth, 2005).

The development of Turkish in migration settings

Besides the range of these linguistic models for first and second language acquisition, other aspects such as social and input factors, or the migration setting itself, may influence the language acquisition process both in L1 and L2. Considering the situation of Turkish children in Germany, modeling of bilingual acquisition may not cover all different aspects of the input situation. Especially for children from the second and third generation of immigrants, several variations to these models may be identified. Only some of the bilingual children are 2L1 children in the sense of Ronjat (1913), but most of them speak Turkish at home and acquire German in kindergarten or primary school. Their process of acquisition may thus be characterized either as sL or as cL2, depending on the AO in the second language. But the status of the first language may not be completely captured by linguistic models of bilingual acquisition. Even if different families are comparable with respect to the language spoken at home, the input situation for the Turkish first language varies from family to family. Some parents have been raised in Germany, others have been raised in Turkey and some speak German to their children. As a consequence, the input situation for Turkish children in Germany is only slightly comparable to those in Turkey.

Moreover, the Turkish language in European migration settings has been exposed to several changes for more than 40 years. Several issues with respect to the development of the Turkish language in 'contact' with other languages (such as German, English, Dutch, Danish and recently also French and Norwegian) are discussed by a number of linguistic researchers. Since the 1990s, the specific phenomena observed in the written and oral productions of Turkish-German bilingual speakers have been considered as a result of the influence of German on Turkish. These changes have been characterized by Johanson (1988) as a 'new variety of Turkish'. Rehbein and colleagues specified the idea of a 'European contact-Turkish' (Rehbein, 2001), and finally the term 'Immigrant Turkish' has been established to characterize the new variety (cf. Backus, 2004, for an overview).

The specifics of this new variety were documented in the language practice of several groups of Turkish immigrants, independent of the speaker's age. As an outline, they may be summarized as follows:

(1) The Turkish language has been merely practiced as 'a language of oral communication' that is linked to the immigrant's social life in certain contexts (Rehbein, 2001). Simultaneously, some dialectal phenomena may prevail in the bilingual context more than in the

standard Turkish in monolingual contexts (Backus & Boeschoten, 1998; Boeschoten, 2000; Boeschoten & Broeder, 1999), as can be seen from the omission of the so-called 'question particle (mI)' in yes–no questions in Turkish or from the deviant use of some connectors.

(2) Linguistic phenomena, such as code-switching and code-mixing, have to be considered as valuable resources provided to bilinguals by their languages instead of expressing language deficit in the sense of 'semilingualism' (Hansegård, 1968) or as an outcome of language impairments in bilinguals.

(3) Turkish-German bilingual speakers never were and still are not a homogeneous group of bilinguals. Rather, different groups of Turkish speakers with diverse language backgrounds are found in Germany. Therefore, different aspects of language choice, language maintenance and language shift can be observed within the Turkish community at the same time (Backus, 2004: 694).

Grammatical deviations in the acquisition of Turkish in migration settings

Besides the overall changes in Immigrant Turkish, some specific changes in the Turkish language in migration settings may be at a risk of being interpreted as an expression of language impairments. These structures differ from standard Turkish and should be seen as characteristics of the bilingual children's language use.

A number of substandard forms of the Turkish language found in certain dialects and ethnolects can be observed in the language of Turkish-German bilingual children. Boeschoten (1990: 138) discovered in the data of Turkish-Dutch bilingual children that certain patterns of spoken Turkish became characteristic of the children's language 'independently of the regions [of Turkey] where the children's parents came from', whereas these patterns were not found in the monolingual database of the study. An overuse of ablative forms in locative contexts (e.g. Backus & Boeschoten, 1998) or an omission of interrogative particles in yes–no questions (Hess-Gabriel, 1979) may be an expression of an ethnolect input, for example from the southeast of Turkey. If these overgeneralizations are found in the child's language, they should not be interpreted as a sign of language impairment. Similarly, an interchange of dative and accusative forms in dative and accusative contexts may be due to the fact that the child is exposed to a Turkish variety from Western Anatolia.

In general, Turkish-German bilinguals and monolingual children in Turkey follow the same developmental stages up to the age of six. The milestones in the acquisition of Turkish morphosyntax, such as inflectional marking for case, person and number, and most tense and modality markings, are acquired equally by bilinguals and monolinguals (e.g. Pfaff, 1994; for Turkish in the Netherlands: e.g. Van der Heijden, 1999).

With respect to the more advanced stages in L1 acquisition, deviations between the Turkish in Turkey and the 'Immigrant Turkish' occur especially in the avoidance of using the so-called 'complex structures' of Turkish grammar. The migration setting's influence can particularly be seen in the acquisition of both complement and relative clauses and of participial constructions. Monolingual Turkish children acquire these at an age of approximately five years and older (Aksu-Koç, 1994). Herkenrath and Karakoç (2002) point at the fact that Turkish-German bilingual children at the age of 4–9 prefer finite clauses instead of subordination. These children use suffixes such as -mA, -yAn and -DIK less frequently than their monolingual peers. Further study about interrogative elements as subordinators in the data of bilingual Turkish-German children confirmed these changes in the bilingual Turkish (Herkenrath *et al.*, 2003). They have been interpreted as '[...] making use of a linguistic potential [...] already offered by the Turkish language as such' (Rehbein, 2001: 16).

Another deviation from the Turkish standard language has been observed in narratives of bilingual Turkish-German children. As Pfaff (1994: 91) has already pointed out, bilingual Turkish-German children extensively substitute the evidential form -mIş. Even if bilingual children are forced to produce the evidential forms by means of questions containing the form itself and thus constructing an obvious context (Rehbein & Karakoç, 2004), they tend to substitute.

As soon as Turkish children attend German institutions, for example kindergarten or preschool, the L1 input becomes limited. Adolescents vary in their opportunities for Turkish language use, such as written language/literacy in L1, or print- and audiovisual media in L1. Backus (2004: 700) concludes for later stages in L1 development that, although the acquisition of Turkish in bilingual children may be delayed, bilinguals catch up with their monolingual peers in school-related abilities. He also points at the fact that 12-year-old bilinguals are able to comprehend and produce Turkish morphosyntax almost as completely as age-matched monolinguals. Authors like Dirim and Auer (2004) focus on bilingual language practice in Turkish-German bilingual adolescents and young adults and refer to the development of new ethnolects in bilingual groups with several first languages. Bilingual and monolingual speakers take advantage of linguistic deviants as an expression of their special form of lifestyle in Turkish- and German-speaking environments (Keim, 2007). Cindark and Arslan (2004), however, point out that if the deviations in L1 language production of the young Turkish speakers investigated by Keim (2007) are compared to their monolingual peers, they remain between 2% and 9 % in certain grammatical areas. This small frequency of grammatical deviations seems to be sufficient enough to identify Turkish adults as bilingual speakers ('Deutschtürken'/'Almancı').

As the overall picture reveals, the variety of Turkish spoken in Germany is subject to certain changes, both grammatically and phonologically. Even though these deviations might be identified as characteristics of language impairments in Turkish monolinguals in future studies, they should be excluded as possible criteria for SLI in Turkish-German bilinguals, for they are specific characteristics of 'Immigrant Turkish' itself.

SLI in Bilingual Turkish-German Children in Migration Settings: Assessment and Outcome

In accordance with most researchers focusing on Immigrant Turkish, Babur *et al.* (2007) claim that Turkish-German bilingual children are exposed to the new variety of Turkish mentioned above, and thus we cannot always adapt models or assessment tools for L1 Turkish. A tool for the assessment of language impairments in bilingual children should take into account the possibility that the Turkish spoken in Germany has changed and should therefore consider these variations as a contact-induced language change rather than score the deviant patterns as an indication of language disorders. Both the aspects related to the conditions of an L1 acquisition of Turkish in Germany and the qualitative and quantitative changes of the Immigrant Turkish should be considered. The comparative baseline has to be a bilingual one, and it is conceivable that specific changes of Turkish in the migration setting might share similarities with the outcome of SLI on the surface.

Considering the fact that SLI is a genuine disorder, it has to influence both of the bilingual's languages. A poor language performance in just one of the languages therefore cannot be diagnosed as SLI. Recent studies comparing the language development of monolingual SLI children and that of child L2 learners of Dutch, German or Swedish (e.g. Håkansson & Nettelbladt, 1993; Schöler *et al.*, 1998; Steenge, 2006) reveal similarities in patterns in language acquisition between child L2 and SLI children. It is thus highly problematic that the monolingual German speech and language therapist is unable to assess their subject's Turkish development properly. For example, as Kroffke (2006) points out, both child L2 (AO 6) and SLI children show difficulties in the acquisition of the German subject–verb agreement (SVA). If only German is assessed, the slow Turkish-German cL2 learner may be misdiagnosed as SLI on the one hand, and the successive bilingual SLI child may be incorrectly identified as a slow child L2 learner on the other (Paradis, 2005; Rothweiler, 2007).

How is it, then, possible to discriminate SLI in both languages of Turkish-German bilinguals and to differentiate its conspicuity in grammar from language variations that may follow from the fact that the first and second language acquisition processes are influenced by the migration setting? As long as specific assessment tools for multilingual children are still lacking, the non-specific diagnosis of language impairment in both languages may be a first step toward the identification of SLI multilingual children.

The assessment of (specific) language impairments in successive bilingual children

The first steps toward the identification of SLI in successive bilinguals (and in monolinguals) should include all possible sources of information about language development. The non-specific assessment has to be performed as an interdisciplinary process. At first, all data for anamnesis with respect to the SLI exclusionary criteria, including hearing performance and intelligence, are important. It has to be kept in mind, though, that IQ testing requiring instructions in the second language may not reflect the child's abilities correctly. In some cases, even for the so-called non-verbal IQ testing, the instructions should therefore be given in the L1.

Kindergarten teachers should be asked for their impression of the child's general development. The child's language progression in both languages is of special interest (Rothweiler *et al.*, 2007). In most cases, the kindergarten teachers are monolingual German, of course, but more and more Turkish-German bilinguals are being employed in preschool education and may thus inform about the child's development in Turkish. Educational professionals generally have a very detailed notion about normal or deviant language development of bilingual children in their group and thus often reveal indications of a slow or unexpected language development in the second language. In addition to their impressions, an interview with the parents allows deeper access to the early first and second language development of bilingual children.

Reconstruction of (home) language development as a window to SLI

A reconstruction of the home language development offers an opportunity to distinguish impaired language development from the characteristics either of slow second language learning or of the Turkish spoken in Germany. The parental interview should be carefully planned. It should be designed more as an informal conversation than as a diagnostic questionnaire. If the family language is only Turkish, the monolingual German speech and language therapist may use interpreters. They ought to be trained for their special function in the diagnostic process, for the interpreter has to translate both the questions of the speech and language therapist and the answers/comments of the parents properly. Reports of any illnesses that the child may have had or general remarks about the child's development, especially on late-talker criteria or familial aggregation of difficulties in language acquisition and/or production, should be translated carefully and without additional interpretations (see Kroffke & Meyer, 2007). This information allows for a deeper understanding of the developmental processes. Special questions should be prepared by the interpreter and the therapist beforehand and should be asked with sensitivity. The therapist should research home-language examples in order to examine the syntactical, morphological and phonetic–phonological development of the child and refer to these instead of referring to a list of samples from the second language. In an ideal case, the interpreter may also report to the speech and language therapist any dialectal specificity s/he observes in the parent's variety of Turkish. Phonological changes or non-standard grammatical sentences in the child's speech may therefore be interpreted as characteristics of the input that the child has been exposed to, instead of as an outcome of the disorder. Details on the family language behavior and language preferences of the child are important as well. Changes in the home language preferences could have an impact on the first language development and on the expectations regarding first language competence. A poor development of Turkish in the child may, for example, be an instance of family language attrition instead of being that of SLI.

Following these clues, further and more detailed investigations by a team of experts may allow the phenomena that are typical of the monolingual speech of normally developing children at a certain age to be distinguished from the phenomena related to deficits in the L1 acquisition. Finally, this information on language development should be combined with an evaluation of the child's language development in both Turkish and German. If its findings are compared with studies on first and second language acquisition of Turkish children in Germany, the language profile may be seen as an important part of the first and second language assessment in bilinguals.

Evaluation of typical and deviant language development in L1 and L2

As has been pointed out, an evaluation of deviant language development may be seen as lying between the poles of bilingual acquisition and the outcome of SLI. If the background information allows the interpretation that a bilingual child is acquiring his or her languages as 2L1 or as sL, an evaluation could compare the bilingual's first and second language development to the L1 development of both languages. The sL acquisition may be comparable to L1 and similar milestones in the process of acquisition may be detected. Following the assumption that SLI is language specific, the outcome of SLI in bilinguals may therefore also share similarities with German SLI. But as long as the question of whether sL or cL2 are indeed comparable to L1 or aL2 and therefore share characteristics with one or both processes remains unclear, bilingual SLI children should also be compared to bilingual peers. An 'adult target standard language norm' seems not to be the appropriate measure to evaluate bilingual language acquisition at a certain age. Considering the interpretation of deviant structures in bilingual language acquisition, such a standard might be misleading (Dirim & Auer, 2004: 18ff), especially if intermediate stages like phonological processes or milestones in grammar acquisition are not taken into consideration. The advantage of such in-group comparisons is that bilinguals with and without SLI share the same background situations. Language deviations in SLI children are therefore attributed to the language impairment rather than to the bilingual situation, if the diagnostic process excludes both the exclusionary criteria for SLI and the influence factors named above. The assessment should also take into account spontaneous speech samples instead of assessment tools for the standard language. Experience has shown that the analysis and the interpretation of spontaneous speech data in both languages are sensible instruments for the assessment of deviations in the acquisition of sentence structure and for some aspects of morphology. In the following, we will present findings from the Hamburg study on unimpaired and impaired acquisition of Turkish and German by bilingual children.

SLI in Turkish

The first assessment of the SLI children in the Hamburg study was based on the non-specific diagnosis described above. Most of the SLI children could be characterized as *late talkers*, their first Turkish words were produced between two and three years of age and all requirements of the exclusionary SLI criteria were fulfilled.

In addition to the interdisciplinary steps toward the diagnosis, an assessment of SLI in bilingual children should also be based on language acquisition profiles from unimpaired children. An evaluation of deviant or delayed language acquisition may be facilitated by the use of databases comprising the speech data of monolingual children of both languages. The profiling tool Turkish Systematic Analysis of Language Transcripts (SALT) (Acarlar *et al.*, 2006) offers such a database. Furthermore, the adapted version of the TELD-3 (Test of Early Language Development – 3rd Edition) for Turkish will provide a screening of receptive and expressive language abilities in monolinguals (cf. Topbaş, this volume, Chapter 7). If the influential factors in bilingual acquisition of Turkish already discussed are carefully examined, such assessment tools may enable linguists, speech and language therapists and other Turkish-speaking professionals to compare the speech data of an individual child with an age-matched monolingual group. By using SALT for Turkish, we were able to show that the Turkish-German normally developing sL children (L2–ND) from the Hamburg Project, aged 2.5–6;2, show no difference in their L1 language production compared to age-matched monolingual Turkish children. We conclude that this finding may be due to intensive L1 language use up to the age of 3. Furthermore, our study provides evidence for SLI in bilingual children. As can be interpreted from the language profiles of the bilingual SLI children, a clear difference in the characteristics of language use can be found between the bilingual SLI children on the one hand, and the monolingual L1 and the bilingual normally developing (ND) children on the other (Babur & Chilla, 2008).

Turkish speech samples from one unimpaired monolingual (L1, age 2;5), three unimpaired bilinguals (L2–ND, age range 3;1–6;2) and four bilingual children with SLI (L2–SLI, age range 4;0–6;5) were investigated in more detail (Babur, 2007; Babur *et al.*, 2007; Rothweiler *et al.*, 2007, 2010). A comparison of the groups with respect to the production of Mean Length of Utterance in Morphemes (MLUm) reveals that the L2–ND children reach a MLUm score of 4 or above at the age of approximately 3, whereas the L2–SLI children are more heterogeneous. One of them attains a MLUm score of 2 at the age of 6;5, whereas others are comparable to the ND children.

Furthermore, we were able to detect evidence for SLI in the production of case morphology, as well as in verbal inflections (Babur, 2007; Babur *et al.*, 2007; Rothweiler *et al.*, 2007, 2010). If compared to normally developing monolinguals or to L2–ND children, the acquisition of case morphology in L2–SLI children is delayed. As a MLUm comparison reveals, the overall productivity (i.e. the number of case morphemes as measured by the number of utterances) is individually different so that, for example, one of the children produces case morphemes far less than all other children in the study. Moreover, L2–SLI children do use case morphemes correctly most of the time, but their errors remain at about 10%, even at the age of 6;5 (Babur *et al.*, 2007). If we consider the differences qualitatively, L2–SLI children produce individual errors types. In contrast to younger L2–ND children, they are more likely to omit or replace obligatory case morphemes. Consider, for example, the following sentences from two L2–SLI children at age 6;5 (cf. (1)) and 5;5 (2–3)).

(1)	**Dimmi**	**ben**	**bu**	**gada.**	L2_SLI-Fer, 6;5
	now	I	this	attach-A	
TR:	Şimdi	ben	bunu	tak(ıyorum).	
			this-acc		

'I attach(?) this there'.

(2) **O** **Katze** **bakıyo** **onu.** L2_SLI_Dev, 5;5
this cat look-continous-3.ps. sg. he-acc
TR: 'O Kedi bakıyo ona.'
he-dat
'The cat looks (at) him'.

(3) **Katze** **onu** **dinletmedi,** **kuşu**. L2_SLI-Dev, 5;5
cat he-acc listen-caus.-neg.-perfect-3.ps. sg. bird-acc
TR: Katze ona dinletmedi, kuşa.
he-dat bird-dat
'The cat does not allow the bird to listen'.

These findings were confirmed by the data of a Turkish monolingual girl with language impairments presented by Topbaş (2007b). The girl extensively omits case morphemes in her spontaneous speech. Furthermore, she does not answer appropriately even though the interlocutor gives several cues to the correct forms throughout the interview. We may thus conclude that the findings about SLI in Turkish-German successive bilinguals are comparable to the outcome of SLI in monolinguals in the area of case morphology.

Babur (2007) points out that normally developing Turkish-German bilingual children produce verbal suffixes correctly at the age of about three years. All children use different verb+tense/aspect and modality+person combinations without any mistakes (4–5).

(4) **Hamura** **böyle** **yapıyon.** L1_Naz, 2;5
dough-dat so do-continous-2.p.sg.
'You make the dough in that way.'

(5) **Pisikleti** **buldum.** L2_ND-Far, 3;1
bicycle-acc find-perfect-1.ps. sg.
'I found the bicycle'.

L2_SLI children, however, show several errors in the verbal domain up to the age of 6;5, cf. Examples (6–7).

(6) **Dimdi** **den** **dayadak.** L2_SLI-Erb, 4;0
now you count-future-ø
TR: Şimdi sen sayacak(sın).
'Now, (you) are going to count'.

(7) **O** **gidiyo,** **uyu** **oğda.** L2_SLI-Dev, 5;5
it(bird) go-continous sleep-ø there
TR: O gidiyo uyuyor orada.
'It goes and sleep(?) there'.

(8) **Timdi** **bit** **gide.** L2_SLI-Ard, 4;1
now we go-E
TR: Şimdi biz gide(?).
'Now we (?) go(?)'.

(9) **Didiyo,** **didiyo,** **düt.** L2_SLI-Ard, 4;1
go-contin.3.p.s go-contin-.3.ps. sg. fall-ø down.
TR: Gidiyo, gidiyo düş(?).
'It is going and going and fall(?) down'.

Both ND and SLI bilingual Turkish-German children are able to add up to five verbal morphemes after a verb stem. Nevertheless, we observed a curious error pattern in the language production of the L2–SLI children in the application of tense–aspect–modality markings in obligatory contexts, cf. Examples (8–9). Besides marking verbs in several person/number contexts correctly, L2–SLI children use some verb stems without any marking for tense–aspect–modality ('bare stems') or with a 'proto-morphological' morpheme –E/-I in third person contexts (Figure 16.1). These forms have been reported by Ketrez and Aksu-Koç (2003) and Ekmekçi (1982) for monolingual Turkish children before their second birthday.

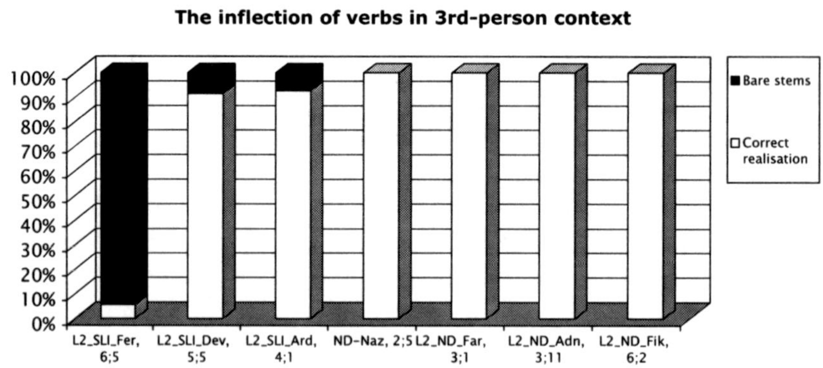

Figure 16.1 The inflection of verbs in third person contexts by bilingual Turkish-German ND and SLI children in Turkish

Furthermore, L2–SLI children omit personal markings in other person/number contexts and realize pronouns instead. In contrast to the L2–SLI-children, none of the normally developing bilingual children in the study omits or substitutes the verbal morphemes. These findings accordingly reveal that the language production of bilingual Turkish-German children with SLI differs qualitatively and quantitatively from unimpaired bilinguals both in the nominal domain and in the verbal domain.

In the following, we will complete the picture of the outcome of SLI in Turkish-German bilinguals by a brief report on findings about the acquisition of German by Turkish-German successive bilinguals with and without SLI.

The Acquisition of German by Successive Bilingual Turkish-German Children

The acquisition of Turkish phonology in bilingual children remains a fertile research area while the acquisition of Turkish phonology is a relatively well-studied topic (Topbaş, 1997, 1999; Topbaş & Yavaş, 2006; also see Chapter 4, this volume). However, a comparison of the sound systems in both languages shows that consonants and vowels in both languages agree to a large extent, except for some specific articulation features. Since sL and cL2 learners acquire Turkish as the first language and no deviation in the application of vowel harmony have as yet been reported, we assume that bilingual children follow the same stages in the acquisition of phonology as known from L1.

In the main, it has been assumed that bilingual children follow the same stages in the acquisition of Turkish phonology. Furthermore, the Turkish data of the Hamburg Project reveal that the error patterns in the Turkish phonology of bilingual children seem to be identical with those of monolingual children. Thus, up to now, interactions between the two systems have been observed as an influence from Turkish to German rather than as a change in L1. During the early acquisition of German by Turkish-German successive bilinguals, for instance, even 3–4-year-old children tend to add an extra vowel between German word-initial consonant clusters – a phenomenon occurring in the language production of adult Turkish learners of German (Özen, 1986; Rollfs, 2001). At the later stages of sL or cL2 acquisition, such productions disappear.

The successive bilingual acquisition of German sentence structure and verbal morphology

German is an OV and a verb-second (V2) language, meaning that the finite verb moves to the second position in main clauses. As soon as monolingual German children produce multiword main clauses (MLUw 2–3), the finite verb is placed in V2, and non-finite verbs remain in verb-final position. The acquisition of the verbal paradigm for lexical verbs coincides with generalized V2, and the correctness rate for SVA (i.e. for finite verbs) exceeds 90%. At this point in acquisition, verb-final utterances decrease. Subject–verb inversion, as in yes–no questions, and subordinate clauses follow this stage (cf. Clahsen, 1982; Clahsen *et al.*, 1993/1994; Rothweiler, 1993; Tracy, 1991).

German children with SLI differ from monolingual unimpaired children in several respects. Following authors such as Clahsen (1991), Clahsen *et al.* (1997), Hamann *et al.* (1998), Leonard (1998) and Wexler (1994, 1996), SLI affects the verbal domain. Morphosyntactic acquisition seems to be impaired. It has been pointed out that children with SLI show no signs of generalized V2 and SVA, as can be seen with unimpaired German monolinguals. Children with SLI prefer short 2–3-word utterances and sentences with finite verbs or non-finite verbs in verb-final position even at the age of 4–5 years. Some of them even produce sentences with infinitives in V2 position.

Recent findings on the unimpaired successive acquisition of German by bilingual children (AO 3–4) reveal that their development of German sentence structure equals L1 acquisition and differs from the outcome of SLI in German monolinguals. As some recent longitudinal case studies show (Kroffke, 2006; Kroffke & Rothweiler, 2006; Rothweiler, 2006, 2007; Thoma & Tracy, 2006), L2–ND children acquire German SVA, V2 movement and subordinate clauses to an extent that is quite comparable to monolinguals. Kroffke (2006) points out that sL children (AO 3–4) show the same coherence in the acquisition of the German SVA paradigm and V2 movement as monolinguals do. Following the same milestones in the acquisition of German sentence structure that have been reported for German L1, the L2–ND children nevertheless vary in their speed of acquisition. It can be concluded, however, that normally developing bilinguals acquire the main features of verbal placement and sentence structure within 8–20 months of exposure to German. Furthermore, the AO as well as the grammatical domain investigated has an impact on the expectations for the acquisition process. Several authors have emphasized that an AO of above 3–4 years may lead to parallelisms between child L2 and child aL2, rather than between L1 and successive bilingual acquisition (e.g. Kroffke, 2006; Meisel, 2007; Schwartz, 2004; Unsworth, 2005). Furthermore, the commonalities of sL and L1 German in the acquisition of sentence structure and SVA may not overcast the possibility of variable patterns in acquisition for other morphological domains, such as plural or gender marking, or the acquisition of case morphology (Bast, 2003; Unsworth, 2005).

The outcome of SLI in the L2 of successive bilingual Turkish-German children

Following the hypothesis that unimpaired sL acquisition shares striking commonalities with L1 acquisition, it can be assumed that the outcome of SLI in sL children patterns with the outcome of German monolinguals in the domain of the German sentence structure and the development of V2 and SVA. A longitudinal study on the acquisition of German by three Turkish-German bilingual children in their first two years of second language acquisition (L2–SLI; age range 3;6–6;5) leads to the conclusion that these children are much more heterogeneous in their developmental paths than the normally developing bilinguals (Kroffke, 2006). The L2–SLI children show typical errors in the verbal domain, such as non-finite verbs in the V2 position. In one spontaneous speech sample, one child, for example, produces up to 11% of all verbs in the V2 position as a non-finite verb (infinitive). Additionally, all children produce verbal stems or verbs that do not follow the SVA condition in V2 and, even at later points of acquisition, verb-final utterances comparable to those known from monolingual children with SLI. Even after 30 months of exposure to German, one successive bilingual child with SLI still prefers verb-final utterances. His overall productivity is limited both in Turkish and in German. A correlation between the acquisition of the complete verbal paradigm and the verbal placement or sentence structure was not documented for any of the children. The L2–SLI children thus differ from their normally developing peers both quantitatively and qualitatively.

Conclusion

The study of SLI in bilinguals may be seen as an interface between SLI and bilingual language acquisition. The findings on SLI in (successive) bilingual Turkish-German children presented here have to be regarded as fragmentary. They may be seen, however, as first steps to a better understanding of the assessment and the outcome of SLI in bilinguals. Tools like Turkish SALT or TELD-3:Turkish offer a broad database for the comparison of language profiles. Their data corpus, however, consists mostly of monolingual data. If the various factors that influence the language development of bilingual Turkish-German children are considered, it would be desirable to extend the databases with a bilingual corpus in order to induce an in-group comparison. The findings from the Hamburg Project reveal that Turkish-German bilingual children with SLI (AO 3–4) produce language-specific errors in their acquisition of both Turkish and German. According to the hypothesis that SLI affects the same grammatical areas both in monolingual and in bilingual children (e.g. Genesee *et al.*, 2005), further investigations and more detailed studies of SLI in monolingual Turkish children will lead to a better understanding of the outcome of SLI in Turkish. Furthermore, a careful interdisciplinary assessment should include all possible resources and a reconstruction and evaluation of the development in both languages as well as a parental interview. An integration of linguistic findings about bilingual development to the assessment of children with language difficulties could prevent misdiagnosis. If the assessment process is carefully planned, we will hopefully be able to differentiate slow second language learners without SLI from bilingual children with SLI in the future.

Note

1. This study has been carried out as a part of the research project 'Specific Language Impairment and early second language acquisition: differentiating deviations in morphosyntactic acquisition', directed by Monika Rothweiler. The project is funded by the Deutsche Forschungsgemeinschaft (German Science Foundation, DFG) within the Collaborative Research Centre on Multilingualism (SFB 538, E4).

References

Aarssen, J. (1996) *Relating Events in Two Languages: Acquisition of Cohesive Devices by Turkish-Dutch Bilingual Children at School Age*. Tilburg: Tilburg University.

Abdalla, F. and Crago, M. (2008) Verb morphology deficits in Arabic-speaking children with specific language impairment. *Applied Psycholinguistics* 29, 315–340.

Abraham, S. (1989) Using a phonological framework to describe speech errors of oral trained, hearing impaired school-agers. *Journal of Speech and Hearing Disorders* 54, 600–609.

Acar, C.T. (2008) The Ongoing Reform in Turkish Public Health Sector: Experiences and Future Prospects. On WWW at http://www.hks.harvard.edu/kokkalis/GSW10/Acar,%20Taylan%20GSW10%20submission.pdf.

Acarlar, F. (2005) Developmental characteristics of language sample measures in the acquisition of Turkish. *Turkish Journal of Psychology* 20 (56), 61–74.

Acarlar, F. and Johnston, J.R. (2006) Computer-based analysis of Turkish child language: Clinical and research applications. *Journal of Multilingual Communication Disorders* 4, 78–94.

Acarlar, F., Miller, J. and Johnston, J. (2006) *Systematic Analysis of Language Transcripts (SALT) for Turkish (Version 9)* [Computer software]. Language Analysis Lab, University of Wisconsin-Madison (distributed by the Turkish Psychological Association, 2007, Ankara).

Akdağ, R., Aydın, S. and Demirel, H. (2007) *Health Transformation Program in Turkey 2002–2007: The Progress so Far.* Ankara: Ministry of Health.

Akdaş, F.V. (2003) Türkiye'de Odyoloji. Paper presented at II *Cochlear Implant and Neuro-Otology Symposium*, December 5–6, İstanbul, Turkey.

Akıncı, M.A. (1996) Les pratiques langagières chez les immigrés turcs en France. *Écarts d'Identité* 76, 14–17.

Akıncı, M.A. (2001) *Développement des compétences narratives des enfants bilingues turc-français en France âgés de 5 à 10 ans.* München: LINCOM.

Akıncı, M.A. (2006) Du bilinguisme à la bilittéracie. Comparaison entre élèves bilingues turc-français et élèves monolingues français. *Langage et Société* 116, 93–110.

Akıncı, M.A. (2008) Language use and biliteracy practices of Turkish-speaking children and adolescents in France. In V. Lytra and J.N. Jorgensen (eds) *Multilingualism and Identities Across Contexts: Cross-Disciplinary Perspectives on Turkish-Speaking Youth in Europe.* Copenhagen Studies in Bilingualism, 45 (pp. 85–108). Copenhagen: University of Copenhagen.

Akıncı, M.A. (2009) Fransa'da Türkçe 'nın Anadili ve Yabancı Dil olarak Eğitiml. In D. Yaylı and Y. Bayyurt (eds.) Yabancilara Türkçe Öğretimi: Polítika, Yöntem ve Beceriler, (pp. 204–222). Istanbul: Anı Yayinları.

Akıncı, M.A. and Jisa, H. (2000) Development of Turkish clause linkage in the narrative texts of Turkish-French bilingual children in France. In A. Göksel and C. Kerslake (eds) *Studies on Turkish and Turkic Languages* (pp. 317–324). Wiesbaden: Otto Harrassowitz Verlag.

Akıncı, M.A., Jisa, H. and Kern, S. (2001) Influence of L1 Turkish on L2 French narratives. In L. Verhoeven and S. Strömqvist (eds) *Narrative Development in a Multilingual Context* (pp. 189–208). Amsterdam: John Benjamins.

Akıncı, M.A., De Ruiter, J.J. and Sanagustin, F. (2004) *Le plurilinguisme à Lyon: le statut des langues à la maison et à l'école*, Paris: L'Harmattan.Aksan, D. (1980) *Her Yönüyle Dil: Ana Çizgileriyle Dilbilim 2.* Ankara: Türk Dil Kurumu.

Aksan, D. (1980) Her Yoṅüyle Dil: Ana Gizgileriyle Dilbilim 2. Ankara: Tuṅk Dil Kurumu Yayınları.

Aksu, A. (1978) *The Acquisition of Casual Connectives in Turkish* (Papers and Reports on Child Language Development, No. 15, pp. 129–139). Stanford: Stanford University.

Aksu-Koç, A. (1986) The acquisition of past reference in Turkish. In D.I. Slobin and K. Zimmer (eds) *Studies in Turkish Linguistics* (Vol. 8, pp. 247–264). Amsterdam: John Benjamins.

Aksu-Koç, A-A. (1988a) *The Acquisition of Aspect and Modality: The Case of Past Reference in Turkish.* Cambridge: Cambridge University Press.

Aksu-Koç, A-A. (1988b) Simultaneity in children's narratives: The development of cohesion in discourse. In S. Koç (ed.) *Studies on Turkish Linguistics* (pp. 55–78). Ankara: Middle East Technical University.

Aksu-Koç, A-A. (1994) Development of linguistic forms: Turkish. In R.A. Berman and D.I. Slobin (eds) *Relating Events in Narrative: A Crosslinguistic Developmental Study* (pp. 329–385). Hillsdale, NJ: Lawrence Erlbaum.

Aksu-Koç, A. (1997) Verb inflection in Turkish: A preliminary analysis of the early stage. In U.W. Dressler (ed.) *Studies in Pre- and Proto-Morphology* (pp. 127–139). Vienna: Verlag Der Österreichischen Akademie der Wissenschaften.

Aksu-Koç, A. (1998a) The role of input vs. universal predispositions in the emergence of tense–aspect morphology: Evidence from Turkish. In Y. Shirai and D.I. Slobin (eds) *The Acquisition of Tense–Aspect Morphology.* Special issue of *First Language* 18, 255–280.

Aksu-Koç, A. (1998b) Changes in the basis for children's assertions: The acquisition of –DIr. Paper presented at the *Ninth International Conference on Turkish Linguistics*, Oxford University Press.

Aksu-Koç, A. (2004) Role of the home context in relations between narrative abilities and literacy practices. In D.D. Ravid and H. Bat-Zeev Shyldkrot (eds) *Perspectives on Language and Language Development: Essays in Honor of Ruth A. Berman.* Dodrecht: Kluwer Academic Press.

Aksu-Koç, A. and Slobin, D.I. (1985) The Acquisition of Turkish. In D.I. Slobin (ed.) *The Crosslinguistic Study of Language Acquisition, Vol I: The Data* (pp. 839–878). Hillsdale, NJ: Lawrence Erlbaum.

Aksu-Koç, A. and Alıcı, D.M. (2000) Understanding sources of beliefs and marking of uncertainty: The child's theory of evidentiality. In E.V. Clark (ed.) *Proceedings of the 30th Annual Child Language Conference* (pp. 123–130). Stanford: Center for the Study of Language and Information.

Aksu-Koç, A. and Ketrez, F.N. (2003a) Early verbal morphology in Turkish: Emergence of inflections. In D. Bittner, W. Dressler and M. Kilani-Schoch (eds) *Development of Verb Inflection in First Language Acquisition. A Crosslinguistic Perspective* (pp. 27–52). Berlin: de Gruyter.

Aksu-Koc, A. and Ketrez, F.N. (2003b) Acquisition of noun and verb categories in Turkish. In A.S. Özsoy, D. Akar, M. Nakipoğlu-Demiralp, E. Erguvanlı-Taylan and A. Aksu-Koç (eds) *Studies in Turkish Linguistics*. Istanbul: Bogazici University.

Aksu-Koç, A. and Tekdemir, G. (2004) Interplay between narrativity and mind-reading: A comparison between Turkish and English. In S. Strömqvist and L. Verhoeven (eds) *Relating Events in Narrative: Typological and Contextual Perspectives* 2 (pp. 307–328). Mahwah, NJ: Lawrence Erlabum.

Aksu-Koç, A., Örüng, S. and Cesur, S. (1999) Pathways to literacy in early childhood II: MOCEP predictors of literacy. Paper presented at *Central Asian Literacy Forum*, MOCEF & ILI, Istanbul, Turkey.

Aksu-Koç, A., Taylan, E. and Bekman, S. (2002) Need assessment in early childhood education and an evaluation of children's level of linguistic competence in three provinces in Turkey. Report submitted to Boğaziçi University Research Fund and the Mother Child Education Foundation (Project No. 00 R101).

Aksu-Koç, A., Ketrez, F.N., Laalo, K. and Pfeiler, B. (2007) Agglutinating languages: Turkish, Finnish and Yucatec Maya. Early development of nominal and verbal morphology from a typological perspective. In S. Laaha and S. Gillis (eds) *Typological Perspectives on the Acquisition of Noun and Word Morphology* (pp. 47–59) (Papers in Linguistics 112). Antwerp: Universiteit Antwerpen.

Aksu-Koç, A., Ketrez, F.N. and Can, A. (2008) Emergence of adjectives in early Turkish child speech. Paper presented in *Workshop on Studies in Pre- and Proto-Morphology*, University of Vienna, Vienna.

Aksu-Koç, A., Acarlar, F., Küntay, A., Maviş, I., Sofu, H., Topbaş, S. and Turan, F. (in preparation) *CDI-MacArthur Communicative Inventory: Turkish Version*. İstanbul: Project supported by TÜBİTAK, No. 10.

Allen, S. (1996) Assessing productivity in acquisition data from polysynthetic languages: An Inuktitut example. Paper presented at the *Seventh International Congress for the Study of Child Language*, Istanbul.

Altan, A. (2005) Analysis of the acquisition of complementation in Turkish naturalistic data (Türkçede tümleç yantümcelerinin edinimi). In M. Sarı and H. Nas (eds) *Proceedings of XIXth National Conference on Turkish Linguistics* (pp. 9–30). Şanlıurfa: Harran University.

Altan, A. (2009a) Acquisition of vowel harmony in Turkish. Poster presented at *Old World Conference in Phonology* 4, Rhodes, Greece.

Altan, A. (2009b) Acquisition of a null subject language. To appear in the *Proceedings of the 13th International Conference on Turkish Linguistics*.

Altay, B., Konrot, A. and Pyman, B. (1989) Extra cochlear application of nucleus 22 channel intra cochlear implant: A case report. In B. Fraysse and N. Cochard (eds) *Cochlear Implant: Acquisitions and Controversies* (pp. 263–272). Toulouse: CochlearAG.

Ammerlaan, T., Hulsen, M., Strating, H. and Yağmur, K. (2001) *Sociolinguistic and Psycholinguistic Perspectives on Maintenance and Loss of Minority Languages*. Münster: Waxmann.

Andersson, L.L. (2004) Appropriate and inappropriate interpretation and use of test scores in early intervention. *Journal of Early Intervention* 27 (1), 55–68.

Andersson, L.L. (2005) Determining the adequacy of tests of children's language. *Communication Disorders Quarterly* 26 (4), 207–225.

Aparici, M., Serrat, E., Capdevila, M. and Serra, M. (2003) Acquisiton of complex sentences in Spanish and Catalan speaking children. In K. Nelson, A. Aksu-Koç and C.E. Johnson (eds) *Children's Language: Interactional Contributions to Language Development* (Vol. 11, pp. 1–25). Mahwah, NJ: Lawrence Erlbaum.

Archibald, J. (2002) Immigrant integration: The ongoing process of reform in France and Québec. In S.J. Baker (ed.) *Language Policy: Lessons from Global Models* (pp. 30–58). Monterey: Monterey Institute.

Arslan, Z.C. (1996) A study on the acquisition of phonology by a Turkish child. Unpublished BA thesis, Boğaziçi University, Istanbul.

ASHA (1990) Scope of practice in speech–language pathology. *American Speech–Language–Hearing Association Statement* LC 6-89, 1–2. Ad Hoc Committee, ASHA.

ASHA (1994) The ASHA code of ethics. *American Speech–Language–Hearing Association Statement* LC 36 (Suppl. 13), 1–2. Ad Hoc Committee, ASHA.

ASHA (2004) *Preferred Practice Patterns for the Profession of Speech-Language Pathology* [Preferred Practice Patterns]. On WWW at http://www.asha.org/policy.

ASHA (2005) *Standards for Accreditation of Graduate Education Programs in Audiology and Speech-Language Pathology*. Academic Program Accreditation, CAA Accreditation Manual. On WWW at http://www.asha.org/policy.

Astington, J.W. and Baird, J.A. (2005) Introduction: Why language matters: In J.W. Astington and J.A. Baird (eds) *Why Language Matters for Theory of Mind* (pp. 3–25). Mahwah, NJ: Lawrence Erlbaum.

Atamaz, F. Yağız-On, A. and Durmaz, B. (2007) Ege Afazi Testi: Testin tanımlanması ve normal kişilerdeki performansı. *Türkiye Fiziksel Tıp ve Rehabilitasyon Dergisi*, 53, 5–10.

August, D. and Hakuta, K. (1998) *Educating Language Minority Students*. Washington, DC: National Academy.

Babur, E. (2007) Specific language impairment in the L1 of successive-bilingual children: Evidence for grammatical SLI in Turkish. *ISB6-The Sixth International Symposium on Bilingualism*, May 30 to June 2, Hamburg.

Babur, E. and Chilla, S. (2008) Language profiles of bilingual Turkish children with/without SLI. *Jahrestagung der Deutschen Gesellschaft für Sprachwissenschaft* (DGfS) 30, Bamberg.

Babur, E., Rothweiler, M. and Kroffke, S. (2007) Spezifische Sprachentwicklungsstörung in der Erstsprache Türkisch. *Linguistische Berichte* 212, 377–402.

Backus, A. (2004) Turkish as an immigrant language in Europe. In T.K. Bhatia and W.C. Ritchie (eds) *The Handbook of Bilingualism* (pp. 689–724). Oxford: Blackwell.

Backus, A. and Boeschoten, H. (1998) Language change in immigrant Turkish. In G. Extra, and J. Maartens (eds) *Multilingualism in a Multicultural Context. Case Studies on South Africa and Western Europe* (pp. 221–237). Tilburg: Tilburg University.

Baker, C. (2006) *Foundations of Bilingual Education and Bilingualism*. Clevedon: Multilingual Matters.

Baker, P. and Eversley, J. (2000) *Multilingual Capital: The Languages of London's Schoolchildren and Their Relevance to Economic, Social and Educational Policies*. London: Battlebridge.

Ball, J. and Lewis, M. (2004) Talking points: What can speech and language professionals contribute to Aboriginal early childhood development? In C.St. Aubin (ed.) *Compendium on Aboriginal Early Childhood Development* (pp. 21–40). Ottawa: Canadian Child Care Federation.

Bamford, J.M. and Mentz, D.L. (1979) The spoken language of hearing impaired children: Grammar. In J. Bench and J.M. Bamford (eds) *Speech-Hearing Tests and the Spoken Language of Hearing Impaired Children*. London: Academic Press.

Bamford, J. and Saunders, E. (1991) *Hearing Impairment, Auditory Perception and Language Disability*. London: Whurr.

Banguoğlu, T. (1986) *Türkçenin Grameri*. Ankara: Türk Tarih Kurumu.

Barrie-Blackley, S., Musselwhite, C. and Rogister, S. (1978) *Clinical Oral Language Sampling: A Handbook for Students and Clinicians*. Danville: The Interstate.

Bartsch, K. and Wellman, H.M. (1995) *Children Talk About the Mind*. Oxford: Oxford University Press.
Bast, C. (2003) Der altersfaktor im zweitspracherwerb: Die entwicklung der grammatischen kategorien numerus, genus und kasus in der nominalphrase im ungesteuerten zweitspracherwerb des Deutschen bei russischen lernerinnen. PhD thesis, University of Cologne.
Bastiaanse, R., Jonkers, R. and Moltmaker-Osinga, U. (1995) Aspects of lexical verbs in the spontaneous speech of agrammatic and anomic patients. In R. Jonkers, E. Kaan and A. Wiegel (eds) *Language and Cognition* (Vol. 5, pp. 13–26). Groningen: Groningen University.
Bates, E. (1995) Inducing agrammatic profiles in normals: Evidence for the selective vulnerability of morphology under cognitive resource limitation. *Journal of Cognitive Neuroscience* 7 (2), 228–257.
Bates, E. and Goodman, J.C. (1999) On the emergence of grammar from the lexicon. In B. MacWhinney (ed.) *Emergence of Language*. Hillsdale, NJ: Lawrence Erlbaum.
Bates, E. and MacWhinney, B. (1987) Competition, variation, and language learning. In B. MacWhinney (ed.) *Mechanisms of Language Acquisition*. Hillsdale, NJ: Lawrence Erlbaum.
Bates, E. and Wulfeck, B. (1989) Crosslinguistic studies of aphasia. In B. MacWhinney and E. Bates (eds) *The Crosslinguistic Study of Sentence Processing* (pp. 328–374). New York: Cambridge University Press.
Bates, E., Bretherton, I. and Snyder, L. (1988) *From First Words to Grammar: Individual Differences and Dissociable Mechanisms*. Cambridge: Cambridge University Press.
Bates, E., Devescovi, A. and Wulfeck, B. (2001) Psycholinguistics: A cross-language perspective. *Annual Review of Psychology* 52, 369–396.
Batman-Ratyosyan, N. and Stromswold, K. (1999) What Turkish acquisition tells us about underlying word order and scrambling. *Proceedings of the 23rd Annual University of Pennsylvania Linguistics Conference*, Pennsylvania.
Batman-Ratyosyan, N. and Stromswold, K. (2002) Morphpsyntax is easy, discourse/Pragmatics is hard. *Proceedings of the 26th Annual Boston University Conference on Language Development* 2, 793–804.
Bauman-Waengler, J. (2004) *Articulatory and Phonological Impairments*. Boston: Pearson.
Baykoç-Dönmez, N. and Arı, M. (1992) 12–30 aylık Türk çocuklarında dilin kazanılması. *Gazi Üniversitesi Eğitim Fakültesi Dergisi* 8 (3), 115–161.
Bedore, L.M. and Leonard, L.B. (2001) Grammatical morphology deficits in Spanish-speaking children with specific language impairment. *Journal of Speech, Language and Hearing Research* 44, 905–924.
Behrens, H. (2001) Cognitive–conceptual development and the acuisition of grammatical morphemes. In M. Bowerman and S.C. Levinson (eds) *Languge Acquisition and Conceptual Development*. Cambridge: Cambridge University Press.
Bekman, S., Aksu-Koç, A. and Erguvanlı-Taylan, E. (under review) Effectiveness of an intervention programme for five and six year olds: A summer-school model.
Belgin, E. (2001) Kliniklerimizi tanıyalım. *Medimagazin* 53, 4.
Berman, R.A. and Slobin, D.I. (1994) *Relating Events in Narrative: A Crosslinguistic Developmental Study*. Hillsdale, NJ: Lawrence Erlbaum.
Berman, R.A. and Verhoeven, L. (2002) Cross-linguistic perspectives on the development of text-production abilities in speech and writing. *Special Issue of Written Language and Literacy* 5:1 & 5:2.
Bernreuter, M. (2005) Türkçe-Almanca iki dilli çocuklarda özgün dil bozuklukları: Anadilin çekim morfolojisinde klinik belirtilerin aranmasında ilk adımlar. In S. Topbaş (ed.) *2. Ulusal Dil ve Konuşma Bozuklukları Kongresi Bildiri Kitabı* (pp. 106–135). Ankara: Kök.

Berry, D., Spillane, N., Ward, A.Z. and Thomson, H. (1996) Specialist unit improves outcome after acute stroke. *Nursing Times* 92 (7), 29–32.

Berument, S.K. and Güven, A.G. (in preparation) *TİFALDİ-Turkish Expressive and Receptive Language Test: Receptive Vocabulary Sub-Scale.*

Bethlehem, D., de Picciotto, J. and Watt, N. (2003) Assessment of verbal fluency in bilingual Zulu-English speakers. *South African Journal of Psychology* 33, 236–240.

Billiez, J. (1990) Le double apprentissage français-arabe au Cours Préparatoire. *LIDIL* 2, 17–50.

Bishop, D. (1992a) The biological basis of specific language impairment. In P. Fletcher and D. Hall (eds) *Specific Speech and Language Disorders in Children* (pp. 2–17). London: Whurr.

Bishop, D. (1992b) The underlying nature of specific language impairment. *Journal of Child Psychology and Psychiatry* 33, 3–66.

Bishop, D.V.M. (1997) *Uncommon Understanding: Development and Disorders of Language Comprehension in Children.* Hove: Psychology Press.

Bishop, D., North, T. and Donlan, C. (1996) Nonword repetition as a behavioral marker for inherited language impairment: Evidence from a twin study. *Journal of Child Psychology and Psychiatry* 36, 1–13.

Blake, J. (2000) *Routes to Child Language. Evolutionary and Developmental Precursors.* Cambridge: Cambridge University Press.

Blamey, P.J. (2003) Development of spoken language by deaf children. In M. Marschark and P.E. Spencer (eds) *Deaf Studies, Language, and Education* (pp. 232–246). Oxford: Oxford University Press.

Blamey, P., Barry, J., Bow, C., Sarant, J., Paatsch, L. and Wales, R. (2001) The development of speech production following cochlear implantation. *Clinical Linguistics & Phonetics* 15 (5), 363–382.

Blamey, P.J., Sarant, J.Z. and Paatsch, L.E. (2006) Relationships among speech perception and language measures in hard-of-hearing children. In P.E. Spencer and M. Marschark (eds) *Advances in the Spoken Language Development of Deaf and Hard-of-Hearing Children* (pp. 85–102). Oxford: Oxford University Press.

Blanche-Benveniste, C. (1995) De la rareté de certains phénomènes syntaxiques en français parlé. *French Language Studies* 5, 17–29.

Bleile, K., Kiel, T. and Ireland, L. (2007) Snapshots of the professions around the world. Paper Presented on November 15–19, ASHA, San Diego.

Bley-Vroman, R. (1990) The logical problem of foreign language learning. *Linguistic Analysis* 20, 3–49.

Blom, E., Polišenská, D. and Weerman, F. (2006/2007) Effects of age on the acquisition of agreement inflection. *Morphology* 16, 313–336.

Bloom, L. and Lahey, M. (1978) Speech perception and sensorineural hearing loss. In M. Ross and T.G. Giolas (eds) *Auditory Management of Hearing-Impaired Children.* Baltimore: University Park Press.

Bloom, L., Hood, L. and Lightbrown, P. (1975) Structure and variation in child language. *Monograph of the Society in Child Development* 40 (2), 160.

Bloom, L., Rocissano, L. and Hood, L. (1976) Child–adult discourse: Developmental interaction between information processing and linguistic knowledge. *Cognitive Psychology* 8, 55–65.

Bloom, L., Tackeff, J. and Lahey, M. (1984) Learning to complement constructions. *Journal of Child Language* 11, 24–34.

Blumenthal, M. and Julien, M.M.R. (2000) Diagnostiek van spraak- en taalproblemen bij meertalige kinderen. Geen diagnose zonder anamnese meertaligheid. *Logopedie en Foniatrie* 1, 13–17.

Boeschoten, H. (1990) The acquisition of modality in Turkish. In H. Boeschoten and L. Verhoeven (eds) *Studies on Modern Turkish* (pp. 231–241). Tilburg: Tilburg University.

Boeschoten, H. (2000) Convergence and divergence in migrant Turkish. In K. Mattheier (ed.) *Dialect and Migration in a Changing Europe* (pp. 145–154). Frankfurt am Main: Lang.

Boeschoten, H. and Broeder, P. (1999) Zum interferenzbegriff in seiner anwendung auf die zweisprachigkeit Türkischer immigranten. In L. Johanson and J. Rehbein (eds) *Türkisch und Deutsch im Vergleich* (pp. 1–21). Wiesbaden: Harrassowitz.

Bollard, P.M., Chute, P.M., Popp, A. and Parisier, S.C. (1999) Specific language growth in young children using the Clarion cochlear implant. *Annals of Otology, Rhinology and Laryngology* 108, 119–123.

Boothe, L.L., Lasky, E.Z. and Kricos, P.B. (1981) Comparison of the language abilities of deaf children and young adults. *Journal of Rehabilitation of the Deaf* 15 (3), 10–16.

Boothroyd, A. and Boothroyd-Turner, D. (2002) Post-implant audition and educational attainment in children with prelingually-acquired profound deafness. *Annals of Otology, Rhinology and Laryngology* 111, 79–84.

Boothroyd, A., Geers, A.E. and Moog, J.S. (1991) Practical implications of cochlear implants. *Ear and Hearing* 12 (Suppl. 4), 81–89.

Bornstein, M. and Haynes, O. (1998) Vocabulary competence in early childhood: Measurement, latent construct, and predictive validity. *Childhood Development* 69, 654–671.

Bortolini, U., Caselli, M.C. and Leonard, L. (1997) Grammatical deficits in Italian-speaking children with specific language impairment. *Journal of Speech, Language, and Hearing Research* 40, 809–820.

Bortolini, U., Arfe, B., Caselli, M.C., Degasperi, L., Deevy, P. and Leonard, L.B. (2006) Clinical markers for specific language impairment in Italian: The contribution of clitics and non-word repetition. *International Journal of Language and Communication Disorders* 41 (6), 695–712.

Botting, N. and Conti-Ramsden, G. (2003) Autism, primary pragmatic difficulties and specific language impairment: Can we distinguish them using psycholinguistic markers? *Development Medicine and Child Neurology* 45, 515–524.

Boutard, C., Claire, I. and Gretchanovsky, L. (1997) *Vol du PC*. Isbergues: Orthoédition.

Bowerman, M. (1973) *Early Syntactic Development: A Cross Linguistic Study with Special Reference to Finnish*. Cambridge: Cambridge University Press.

Brabant, J. (1992) Une insertion économique problématique. *Hommes et Migrations* 1153, 34–38.

Brannon, J.B. (1964) Visual feedback of glossal motions and influence on the speech of deaf. Unpublished PhD thesis, Northwestern University.

Brannon, J.B. (1968) Linguistic word classes in the spoken language of normal, hard-of-hearing and deaf children. *Journal of Speech and Hearing Research* 11, 279–287.

Brannon, J.B. and Murry, T. (1966) The spoken syntax of normal, hard-of-hearing, and deaf children. *Journal of Speech and Hearing Research* 9, 604–610.

Broschart, J. (1991) Noun, verb and participation. A typology of the noun/verb-distinction. In H. Seiler and N. Premper (eds) *Partizipation: Das Sprachliche Erfassen von Sachverhalten* (pp. 65–137). Tübingen: Narr.

Brodsky, P., Waterfall, H. and Edelman, S. (2007) Characterizing motherese: On the computational structure of child-directed language. In D.S. McNamara and

J.G. Trafton (eds) *Proceedings of the 29th Meeting of the Cognitive Science Society* (pp. 833–838). Austin, TX: Cognitive Science Society.

Brown, R. (1973) *A First Language*. Cambridge, MA: Harvard University Press.

Calbour, C. (2006) Une orthophonie pluri-ethnique. De Babel à moi-même. Paper presented at *Sixth CPLOL European Congress*, Berlin, Germany. On WWW at http://www.orthophonistes.fr/upload/100920071914calbour.pdf. Accessed 10.6.2009.

Campbell, T., Dollaghan, C., Needleman, H. and Janosky, J. (1997) Reducing bias in language assessment: Processing-dependant measures. *Journal of Speech, Language and Hearing Research* 40, 519–525.

Caramazza, A. and Berndt, R. (1978) Semantic and syntactic processes in aphasia: A review of the literature. *Psychological Bulletin* 85, 898–918.

Caramazza, A. and Berndt, R. (1985) A multicomponent view of agrammatic Broca's aphasia. In M.L. Kean (ed.) *Agrammatism* (pp. 27–63). Orlando: Academic Press.

Caselli, C., Bates, E., Casadio, P., Fenson, J., Fenson, L., Sanderl, L. and Weir, J. (1995) A cross-linguistic study of early lexical development. *Cognitive Development* 10, 159–199.

Catts, H., Fey, M., Zhang, X. and Tomblin, B. (1999) Language basis of reading and reading disabilities: Evidence from a longitudinal investigation. *Scientific Studies of Reading* 3 (4), 331–361.

Cazden, C.B. (1968) The acquisition of noun and verb inflections. *Child Development* 39 (1), 433–448.

Cerquiglini, B. (2003) *Les Langues de la France*. Paris: Presses Universitaires de France.

Chapey, R. (ed.) (1986) *Language Intervention Strategies in Adult Aphasia* (2nd edn). Baltimore, MD: Williams and Wilkins.

Chapey, R. (1994) *Language Intervention Strategies in Adult Aphasia*. Baltimore: Williams & Wilkins.

Chapman, R.S. and Hesketh, L.J. (2000) The behavioral phenotype of individuals with Down syndrome. *Mental Retardation and Developmental Disabilities Research Reviews* 6, 84–95.

Chapman, R.S., Seung, H-K., Schwartz, S-E. and Kay-Raining Bird, E. (1998) Language skills of children and adolescents with Down syndrome II: Production deficits. *Journal of Speech, Language and Hearing Research* 41, 861–873.

Chen, S. and Bates, E. (1998) The dissociation between nouns and verbs in Broca's and Wernicke's aphasia: Findings from Chinese. *Aphasiology* 12 (1), 5–36.

Chevrie-Muller, C. (2007) Exploration du langage oral. In C. Chevrie-Muller and J. Norbona (eds) *Le Langage de l'Enfant, Aspects Normaux et Pathologiques* (3rd edn, pp. 87–129). Paris: Elsevier.

Chevrie-Muller, C. and Plaza, M. (2001) *Nouvelles Épreuves pour l'Examen du Langage* (N-EEL), Paris: ECPA.

Chevrie-Muller, C., Simon, A.M., Le Normand, M.T. and Fournier, S. (1985a/b) *Batterie d'évaluation psycholinguistique, Partie A (BEPL-A) & Partie B (BEPL-B)*, Paris: ECPA.

Chevrie-Muller, C., Simon, A.M. and Fournier, S. (1997) *Batterie Langage Oral et Ecrit, Mémoire, Attention (L2MA)*. Paris: ECPA.

Chiat, S. (2001) Mapping theories of developmental language impairment: Premises, predictions and evidence. *Language and Cognitive Processes* 16 (2/3), 113–142.

Chin, S.B. (2002) Aspects of stop consonant production by pediatric users of cochlear implants. *Language, Speech, and Hearing Services in Schools* 33, 38–51.

Chin, S.B. (2003) Children's consonant inventories after extended cochlear implant use. *Journal of Speech and Hearing Research* 46, 849–862.

Chin, S.B. and Pisoni, D.B. (2000) A phonological system at 2 years after cochlear implantation. *Clinical Liguistics & Phonetics* 14 (1), 53–73.

Chin, S.B., Finnegan, K.R. and Chung B.A. (2001) Relations among types of speech intelligibility in pediatric users of cochlear implants. *Journal of Communication Disorders* 33, 187–205.

Choi, D. (1995) The development of epistemic sentence-ending modal forms and functions in Korean children. In J. Bybee and S. Fleischman (eds) *Modality in Grammar and Discourse* (pp. 165–204). Amsterdam: John Benjamins.

Choudhury, N. and Benasich, A.A. (2003) A family aggregation study: The influence of family history and other risk factors on language development. *Journal of Speech, Language and Hearing Research* 46, 261–272.

Cindark, I. and Arslan, S. (2004) Deutschlandtürkisch? On WWW at http://www.ids-mannheim.de/prag/soziostilistik/Deutschlandtuerkisch.pdf. Accessed 08.07.2004.

Clahsen, H. (1982) *Spracherwerb in der Kindheit: Eine Untershcung zur Entwicklung der Syntax bei Kleinkindern.* Tübingen: Narr.

Clahsen, H. (1991) *Child Language and Developmental Dysphasia: Linguistic Studies of the Acquisition of German.* Philadelphia: John Benjamins.

Clahsen, H. and Muysken, P. (1986) The availability of universal grammar to adult and child learners: A study of the acquisition of German word order. *Second Language Research* 2, 93–119.

Clahsen, H., Penke, M. and Parodi, T. (1993/1994) Functional categories in early child German. *Language Acquisition* 3 (4), 395–429.

Clahsen, H., Bartke, S. and Göllner, S. (1997) Formal features in impaired grammars: A comparison of English and German SLI children. *Journal of Neurolinguistics* 10 (2/3), 151–171.

Clancy, P., Jacobsen, T. and Silva, M. (1976) The acquisition of conjunction: A cross-linguistic study. *Papers & Reports on Child Language Development* 12, 71–80.

Clancy, P., Lee, H. and Zoh, M. (1986) Processing strategies in the acquisition of relative clauses: Universal principles and language specific realizations. *Cognition* 24, 224–262.

Clark, M. (1985) *Developing the Spoken Language Skills of Hearing Impaired Children: Laying the Foundations.* Manchester: MUTV.

Clark, M. (1986a) *Developing the Spoken Language Skills of Hearing Impaired Children: Building on the Foundations.* Manchester: MUTV.

Clark, M. (1986b) *Developing the Spoken Language Skills of Hearing Impaired Children: Sounds All Around.* Manchester: MUTV.

Clark, M. (1989) *Language through Living for Hearing Impaired Children.* London: Hodder & Stoughton.

Clark, E. (1993) *The Lexicon in Acquisition.* Cambridge: Cambridge University Press.

Clark, M. (2007) *A Practical Guide to Quality Interaction with Children Who Have a Hearing Loss.* San Diego: Plural.

Clark, M. and Tüfekçioğlu, U. (1994) Developing a comprehensive service for the hearing impaired in Turkey. *Journal of the British association of the Teachers of the Deaf* 18 (3), 82–85.

Clements, G.N. and Keyser, S. (1983) *CV Phonology: A Generative Theory of the Syllable.* Cambridge, MA: MIT Press.

CoHE – Turkish Council of Higher Education (2008) The Turkish Higher Educational System. On WWW at http://www.yok.gov.tr/English.

Cohen, A.D. (1989) Attrition in the production lexicon of two Portuguese third language speakers. *Studies in Second Language Acquisition* 11, 135–149.

Colozzo, P., Garcia, R., Curran, M., Gillam, R. and Johnston, J. (2006) Narrative assessment in SLI: Exploring interactions between content and form. Paper presented at the *Symposium for Research in Child Language Disorders*. University of Wisconsin, Madison.

Condouris, K., Meyer, E. and Tager-Flusberg, H. (2003) The relationship between standardized measures of language and measures of spontaneous speech in children with autism. *American Journal of Speech-Language Pathology* 12, 349–358.

Connor, C.M., Craig, H.K., Raudenbush, S.W., Heavner, K. and Zwolan, T.A. (2006) The age at which young deaf children receive cochlear implants and their vocabulary and speech production growth: Is there an added value for early implantation? *Ear & Hearing* 27 (8), 628–644.

Conti-Ramsden, G. (2003) Processing and linguistic markers in young children with specific language impairment (SLI). *Journal of Speech-Language Hearing Research* 46, 1029–1037.

Conti-Ramsden, G., Botting, N. and Faragher, B. (2001) Psycholinguistic markers for specific language impairment (SLI). *Journal of Child Psychology and Psychiatry* 42 (6), 741–748.

Conti-Ramsden, G. and Hesketh, A. (2003) Risk markesr for SLI: A study of young language-learning children. *International Journal of Language and Communication Disorders* 38 (3), 251–263.

Cooper, R.L. (1967) The ability of deaf and hearing children to apply morphological rules. *Journal of Speech and Hearing Research* 10, 77–82.

CPLOL (1988–1998) *10 Years of Activities*. Standing Liaison Committee of Speech and Language Therapists or Logopedists of European Union. Version 24/01/99.

CPLOL (2007) *Revision of the Minimum Standards for Education Completed by the Education Commission*. Standing Liaison Committee of European Union Speech and Language Therapists and Logopedists. 12 May 2007, Adopted at the General Assembly, Riga. On WWW at http://www.cplol.org.

Crago, M. and Westernoff, F. (2002) *Position Paper on Speech-Language Pathology and Audiology in the Multicultural, Multilingual Context*. On WWW at http://www.caslpa.ca/english/resources/position.asp. Accessed 25.12.2007.

Crain, S. and Thornton, R. (1998) *Investigations in Universal Grammar*. Cambridge, MA: MIT Press.

Creese, A., Lytra-Baraç, T. and Yağcıoğlu, D. (2007) Investigating multilingualism in Turkish complementary schools in London. ESRC Report, University of Birmingham.

Crunelle, D., Taillant, A. and Tiberghien, C. (2004) *Sacré Nestor*. Isbergues: Orthoédition.

Crutchley, A. (1999) Bilingual children with SLI attending language units: Getting the bigger picture. *Child Language Teaching and Therapy* 15, 201–217.

Crutchley, A., Conti-Ramsden, G. and Botting, N. (1997) Bilingual children with specific language impairment and standardised assessments: Preliminary findings from a study of children in language units. *International Journal of Bilingualism* 1, 117–134.

Crystal, D. (1982) *Profiling Linguistic Disability*. London: Edward Arnold.

Crystal, D. (1989) *Grammatical Analysis of Language Disability* (2nd edn). London: Cole and Whurr.

Cummins, J. (1976) The influence of bilingualism on cognitive growth: A synthesis of research findings and explanatory hypotheses. *Working Papers on Bilingualism* 9, 1–43.

Cummins, J. (1977) Cognitive factors associated with the attainment of intermediate levels of bilingual skills. *Modern Language Journal* 61, 3–12.
Cummins, J. (1979) Linguistic interdependence and the educational development of bilingual children. *Review of Educational Research* 49 (2), 222–251.
Cummins, J. (1984) Minority students and learning difficulties: Issues in assessment and placement. In M. Paradis and Y. Lebrun (eds) *Early Bilingualism and Child Development* (pp. 47–68). Lisse: Swets and Zeitlinger.
Cummins, J. (1991) Interdependence of first and second-language proficiency in bilingual children. In E. Bialystok (ed.) *Language Processing in Bilingual Children* (pp. 70–89). Cambridge: Cambridge University Press.
Çapan, S. (1988) Acquisition of verb inflections by Turkish children: A case study. In S. Koç (ed.) *Proceedings of Studies on Turkish Linguistics* (pp. 275–286). Ankara: ODTU Pub.
Çeliker, Z.P. and Ege, P. (2005) İşitmeİ engelli çocukların konuşmalarının anlaşılabilirliğini etkileyen faktörler. *Ankara Üniversitesi Eğitim Bilimleri Fakültesi Özel Eğitim Dergisi* 6 (11), 19–32.
Çıtav, N. (2004) Anadili Türkçe olan akıcı tip afazik olguların dil özelliklerinin işitsel anlama, tekrarlama ve adlandırma açısından değerlendirilmesi. MSc thesis, Anadolu University.
Dabène, L. and Billiez, J. (1987) Le parler des jeunes issues de l'immigration. In G. Vermès and J. Boutet (eds) *France, Pays Multilingue: Pratiques des langues en France* T.2 (pp. 62–77). Paris: L'Harmattan.
Dale, P.S. and Henderson, V.L. (1987) An evaluation of the test of early language development as a measure of receptive and expressive language. *Language, Speech, and Hearing Services in Schools* 18, 179–187.
Damian, M.F. (2000) Semantic negative priming in picture categorization and naming. *Cognition* 76, 45–55.
Dasinger, L. and Küntay, A. (1998) Introducing referents in elicited discourse: Finnish vs. Turkish. In A. Aksu-Koç, E. Erguvanlı-Taylan, A.S. Özsoy and A. Küntay (eds) *Perspectives on Language Acquisition* (pp. 263–276). Istanbul: Boğaziçi University.
Davidoff, J. and Masterson, J. (1996) *Transitivity*. On WWW at Dissertations ub.rug.nl/FILES/faculties/arts/1998/r.jonkers/c4.pdf.
Davies, A. (1993) The prevalence of deafness. In J. Ballantyne, M.C. Martin and A. Martin (eds) *Deafness* (5th edn, pp. 1–14). London: Whurr.
Davis, G.A. (2000) *Aphasiology, Disorders and Clinical Practice*. Boston: Allyn & Bacon.
Davis, H. and Silverman, S.R. (1978) *Hearing and Deafness* (4th edn). New York: Holt, Rinehart & Winston.
De Bleser, R. and Kauschke, C. (2003) Acquisition and loss of nouns and verbs: Parallel or divergent patterns? *Journal of Neurolinguistics* 16 (2), 213–229.
De Bots, K. and Weltens, B. (1995) Foreign language attrition. *Annual Review of Applied Linguistics* 15, 151–166.
Decool-Mercier, N. (2008) Les anaphores dans les textes d'enfants bilingues Turc-Français et monolingues Français scolarisés au CM2: Fonctionnement des anaphores et cohésion textuelle. MA dissertation, Université de Rouen, Rouen.
De Groot, A. (1992) Determinants of word translation. *Journal of Experimental Psychology: Learning, Memory and Cognition* 18, 1001–1018.
De Jong, J. (1999) Specific language impairment in Dutch: Inflectional morphology and argument structure. PhD thesis, Rijksuniversiteit Groningen.
De Jong, J. (2008) Bilingualism and language impairment. In M. Ball, N. Mueller and S. Howard (eds) *The Handbook of Clinical Linguistics*. Oxford: Blackwell.

De Jong, J. and Cavus, N. (2007) Grammatical morphology in Turkish-Dutch children with SLI. Paper presented to the *European Study Group on Child Language Disorders*, Cork.

Dell, G.R., Chang, F. and Griffin, Z.M. (1999) Connectionist models of language production: Lexical access and grammatical encoding. *Cognitive Science* 23, 517–542.

Demircan, Ö. (1979) *Türkiye Türkçesinin Ses Düzeni, Türkiye Türkçesinde Sesler.* Ankara: TDK.

Demircan, Ö. (1996) *Türkçenin Sesdizimi.* İstanbul: Der.

Deprez, C. (1994) *Les Enfants Bilingues: Langues et Familles.* Paris: CREDIF Essais-Didier.

Deprez, C., Filhon, A. and Heran, F. (2002) La dynamique des langues en France au fil du XXème siècle. *Population et sociétés* 376, INED.

Devescovi, A. and Caselli, M.C. (2007) Sentence repetition as a measure of early grammatical development in Italian. *International Journal of Language and Communication Disorders* 42 (2), 187–208.

De Villiers, J.G. and De Villiers, P.A. (1973) Across-sectional study of the acquisition of grammatical morphemes in child speech. *Journal of Psycholinguistic Research* 2, 267–278.

De Villiers, J.G. and De Villiers, P.A. (2000) Linguistic determinism and the understanding of false beliefs. In P. Mitchell and K.J. Riggs (eds) *Children's Reasoning and the Mind* (pp. 191–228). UK: Psychology-Press.

De Villiers, J.G., Tager-Flusberg, H.B., Hakuta, K. and Cohen, M. (1979) Children's comprehension of relative clauses. *Journal of Psycholinguistic Research* 8, 499–518.

De Weck, G. (1991) *La Cohésion dans les Textes d'Enfants. Étude du Développement des Processus Anaphoriques.* Neuchâtel: Delachaux & Niestlé.

DfES (2005) *Ethnicity and Education: The Evidence on Minority Ethnic Pupils.* Nottingham: DfES.

Diessel, H. (2004) *Acquisition of Complex Sentences. Cambridge Studies in Linguistics No: 105.* Cambridge: Cambridge University Press.

Diken, İ.H. (2007) *Okul öncesi çocuklar için doğal ortamlarda öğretim teknikleri.* Ankara: Maya Akademi.

Diken, Ö., Topbaş, S. and Diken, İ.H. (in press) The validity and reliability of Maternal Behavior Rating Scale (MBRS) and Child Behavior Scale (CBRS). *Özel Eğitim Dergisi.*

Dirim, İ. and Auer, P. (2004) *Türkisch Sprechen nicht nur die Türken. Über die Unschärfebeziehung Zwischen Sprache und Ethnie in Deutschland.* Berlin: de Gruyter.

Dodd, B. (1995) *Differential Diagnosis and Treatment of Children with Speech Disorder.* London: Whurr.

Dowson, P.W., Blamey, P.J., Dettman, S.J., Rowland, L.C., Barker, E.J., Tobey, E.A., Busby, P.A., Cowan, R.C. and Clark, G.M. (1995) A clinical report on speech production of cochlear implant users. *Ear & Hearing* 16, 551–561.

Driessen, G., van der Slik, F. and de Bot, K. (2002) Home language and language proficiency: A large-scale longitudinal study in Dutch primary schools. *Journal of Multilingual and Multicultural Development* 23 (3), 175–194.

Dressler, W.U. and Peltzer-Karpf, A.M. (1995) The theoretical relevance of pre- and protomorphology in language acquisiton. *Yearbook of Morphology* 1994, 99–122.

Dromi, E. and Berman, R. (1982) A morphological measure of early language development: Data from modern Hebrew. *Journal of Child Language* 9, 403–424.

Dromi, E., Leonard, L., Adam, G. and Zadunaisky-Ehrlich, S. (1999) Verb agreement morphology in Hebrew-speaking children with specific language impairment. *Journal of Speech, Language, and Hearing Research* 42, 1414–1431.

Druks, J. and Carroll, E. (2005) The crucial role of tense for verb production. *Brain and Language* 94 (1), 1–18.

Duchan, J.F. (1982) The elephant is soft and mushy: Problems in assessing children's language. In N. Lass, L. McReynolds, J. Northern and D. Yoder (eds) *Speech, Language and Hearing: Pathologies of Speech and Language* (Vol. 2, pp. 741–760). Philadelphia: W.B. Saunders.

Dunn, L.M. and Dunn, L.M. (1997) *Peabody Picture Vocabulary Test. Turkish version.* Ciecle Pines, MN: American Guidance Service.

Dunn, M., Flax, J., Sliwinski, M. and Aram, D. (1996) The use of spontaneous language measures as criteria for identifying children with specific language impairment: An attempt to reconcile clinical and research incongruence. *Journal of Speech & Hearing Research* 39, 643–654.

Eadie, P.A., Fey, M.E., Douglas, J.M. and Parsons, C.L. (2002) Profiles of grammatical morphology and sentence imitation in children with specific language impairment and Down syndrome. *Journal of Speech, Language and Hearing Research* 45, 720–732.

Easterbrooks, S. R. and Baker, S. (2002) *Language Learning in Children Who Are Deaf or Hard of Hearing*. Boston: Allyn & Bacon.

Echardour, A. and Maurin, E. (1993) La main d'œuvre étrangère. In INSEE (ed.) *Données Sociales 1993* (pp. 504–513). Paris: Hachette.

Edmonds, L. and Kiran, S. (2004) Confrontation naming and semantic relatedness judgements in Spanish/English bilinguals. *Aphasiology* 18 (5–7), 567–579.

Ege, P. and Erdem, R. (2008) The relationship between syntactic and semantic development in normal and mentally-retarded Turkish children. Paper presented at the *Second International Conference on Special Education*, Marmaris, Turkey.

Ege, P., Acarlar, F. and Güleryüz, F. (1998) The relationship between age and mean length of utterance in acquisition of Turkish. *Turkish Journal of Psychology* 13 (41), 19–31.

Ege, P., Acarlar, F. and Güleryüz-Turan, F. (2004) *Ankara Artikülasyon Testi (AAT)*. (Ankara Articulation Test). Ankara: Ankara University.

Eisenberg, S., Fersko, T. and Lundgren, C. (2001) The use of MLU for identifying language impairment in preschool children: A review. *American Journal of the Speech–Language Pathology* 10, 323–342.

Ekinci, D. (2007) Türkçe konuşan işitme engelli çocukların ad durum eklerini kullanım becerilerinin incelenmesi. MA thesis, Anadolu University, Eskişehir.

Ekmekçi, Ö.F. (1979) Acquisition of Turkish: A longitudinal study on the early language development of a Turkish child. PhD thesis, University of Texas, Austin.

Ekmekçi, Ö.F. (1982) Language development of a Turkish child: A speech analysis in terms of length and complexity. *Journal of Human Sciences* 1 (1), 103–112.

Ekmekçi, Ö.F. (1986) The significance of word-order in the acquisition of Turkish. In D.I. Slobin and K. Zimmer (eds) *Studies in Turkish Linguistics* (pp. 265–272). Amsterdam: John Benjamins.

Ekmekçi, Ö.F. (1987) Creativity in the language acquisition process: A Turkish case study. In H. Boeschoten and L. Verhoeven (eds) *Studies on Modern Turkish* (pp. 203–210). Tilburg: Tilburg University.

Ekmekçi, Ö.F. (1988) Coinage of words in child's lexicon in acquiring Turkish. *Studies in Turkish Linguistics* (pp. 79–93). Ankara: Middle East Technical University.

Ekmekçi, Ö.F. and Can, C. (2000) Head parameter setting in the acquisition of Turkish as a first language. In A. Göksel and C. Kerslake (eds) *Studies in Turkish and Turkic Languages* (pp. 275–282). Wiesbaden: Harrassowitz Verlag.

Elman, R.J., Ogar, J. and Elman, S.H. (2000) Aphasia: Awareness, advocacy, and activism. *Aphasiology* 14, 455–459.

Enç, M. (1986) Topic switching and pronominal subjects in Turkish. In D.I. Slobin and K. Zimmer (eds) *Studies in Turkish Linguistics* (pp. 265–272). Amsterdam: John Benjamins.

Ergenç, İ. (1989) *Türkiye Türkçesinin Görevsel Sesbilimi: Sesbirimlere Genel Bakış*. Ankara: Engin.

Erguvanlı-Taylan, E. (1984) *The Function of Word Order in Turkish Grammar.* Berkeley: University of California.

Estabrooks, W. (ed.) (1992) *Do You Hear That?* Washington, DC: AGB Association for the Deaf and Hard of Hearing.

Estabrooks, W. (ed.) (1994) *Hear and Listen! Talk and Sing!* Washington, DC: AGB Association for the Deaf and Hard of Hearing.

Estabrooks, W. (ed.) (2000) *The Baby is Listening*. Washington, DC: AGB Association for the Deaf and Hard of Hearing.

Estabrooks, W. (ed.) (2004) *Listen to This!* (Vol. 1). Washington, DC: AGB Association for the Deaf and Hard of Hearing.

Estabrooks, W. (2006a) *Auditory–Verbal Therapy and Practice.* NW: Alexander Graham Bell.

Estabrooks, W. (ed.) (2006b) *Listen to This!* (Vol. 2). Washington, DC: AGB Association for the Deaf and Hard of Hearing.

Evans, J. and Craig, H. (1992) Language sample collection and analysis: Interview compared to freeplay assessment contexts. *Journal of Speech and Hearing Research* 35, 343–353.

Extra, G. and Verhoeven, L. (1999) *Bilingualism and Migration.* Berlin: Mouton de Gruyter.

Extra, G. and Yagmur, K. (2004) *Urban Multilingualism in Europe: Immigrant Minority Languages at Home and School.* Clevedon: Multilingual Matters.

Fawcett, S., Merinda, P. Smith, V. and Johnston, J. (2001) Measuring progress in early autism: Formal and informal measures. Paper presented to the *American Speech–Language–Hearing Association*, Chicago.

Fayol, M. (1997) *Des Idées au Texte: Psychologie Cognitive de La Production Verbale, Orale et Écrite.* Paris: Universitaires de France.

Fazio, B.B., Johnston, J.R. and Brandl, L. (1993) Relation between mental age and vocabulary development among children with mild mental retardation. *American Journal on Mental Retardation* 97, 541–546.

Felsher, L. and Ross, E. (1994) Knowledge and attitudes of occupational therapists, physiotherapists and speech therapists regarding the role of the speech therapist in the hospital stroke rehabilitation team. *The South African Journal of Communication Disorders* 41, 49–63.

Fenson, L., Dale, P.S., Reznick, J.S., Bates, E., Thal, D.J. and Pethick, S.J. (1994) Variability in early communicative development. *Monographs of the Society for Research in Child Development, Serial* 242 (59), 5.

Ferrand, P. (2000) *Protocole d'Evaluation Rapide.* Isbergues: Orthoédition.

Fey, M. (1986) *Language Intervention with Young Children.* San Diego: College Hill.

Finkbeiner, M., Gollan, T.H. and Caramazza, A. (2006) Lexical access in bilingual speakers: What's the (hard) problem? *Bilingualism: Language and Cognition* 9 (2), 153–166.

Flessas, J. and Lussier, F. (2003) *Epreuves Verbales d'Aptitudes Cognitives* (EVAC), Paris: ECPA.

Fletcher, P., Leonard, L.B., Stokes, S.F. and Wong, A.M.Y. (2005) The expression of aspect in Cantonese-speaking children with specific language impairment. *Journal of Speech, Language and Hearing Research* 48, 231–246.

Francis, N. (2000) The shared conceptual system and language processing in bilingual children: Findings from literacy assessment in Spanish and Náhuatl. *Applied Linguistics* 21 (2), 170–204.

Friedmann, N. and Szterman, R. (2005) Syntactic movement in orally trained children with hearing impairment. *Journal of Deaf Studies and Deaf Education* 11 (1), 56–75.

Frost, L. and Bondy, A. (2002) *The Picture Exchange Communication System Training Manual (PECS)* (2nd edn). Newark, DE: Pyramid Educational Products, Inc.

Fry, D.B. (1978) The role and primacy of the auditory channel in speech and language development. In M. Ross and T.G. Giolas (eds) *Auditory Management of Hearing-Impaired Children* (pp. 15–45). Baltimore: University Park Press.

Furth, H. (1966) *Thinking without Language*. London: Collier-Macmillan.

Gadet, F. and Varro, G. (2006) Le 'scandale' du bilinguisme. Langues en contact et plurilinguismes. *Langage et Société* 116, 9–28.

Gardner, H., Froud, K., McClelland, A. and van der Lely, H.K.J. (2006) Development of the Grammar and phonology screening (GAPS) test to assess key markers of specific language and literacy difficulties in young children. *International Journal of Language and Communication Disorders* 41 (5), 513–540.

Gautier-Kızılyürek, S. (2007) Les enseignements de langue et culture d'origine en France: chronique d'une mort annoncée ? Le cas de la langue Turque. In F. Baider (ed.) *Emprunts Linguistiques, Empreintes Culturelles* (pp. 141–158). Paris: l'Harmattan.

Gavruseva, E. (1998) Left-branch violations in child L2 English. In A. Greenhill, M. Hughes, H. Littlefield and H. Walsh (eds) *Proceedings of the 22nd Boston Conference on Language Development* (pp. 235–245). Somerville, MA: Cascadilla.

Gayraud, F., Jisa, H. and Viguié, A. (2001) Utilisation des outils cohésifs comme indice de sensibilité au registre: Une étude développementale. *AILE* 14, 3–24.

Geers, A.E. (1990) Performance aspects of mainstreaming. In M. Ross (ed.) *Hearing Impaired Children in the Mainstream*. (pp. 119–130). Maryland: York Press.

Geers, A.E. (2004) Speech, language, and reading skills after early cochlear implantation. *Archives of Otolaryngology – Head and Neck Surgery* 130, 634–638.

Geers, A.E. (2006) Spoken language in children with cochlear implants. In P. E. Spencer and M. Marschark (eds) *Advances in the Spoken Language Development of Deaf and Hard-of-Hearing Children* (pp. 244–270). Cary, NC: Oxford University Press.

Geers, A.E. and Moog, J.S. (1978) Syntactic maturity of spontaneous speech and elicited imitations of hearing impaired children. *Journal of Speech and Hearing Disorders* 23, 380–391.

Geers, A.E. and Moog, J.S. (1992) Speech perception and production skills of students with impaired hearing from oral and total communication education settings. *Journal of Speech, Language and Hearing Research* 35, 1384–1393.

Geers, A.E. and Tobey, E. (1992) Effects of cochlear implants and tactile aids on the development of speech production skills in children with profound hearing impairment. *Volta Review* 94 (5), 135–163.

Geers, A., Moog, J. and Brenda, S. (1984) Acquisition of spoken and signed English by profoundly deaf children. *Journal of Speech and Hearing Disorders* 49, 378–388.

Geers, A.E., Nicholas, J.G. and Sedey, A.L. (2003) Language skills of children with early cochlear implantation. *Ear and Hearing* 24 (1), 46–58.

Geisinger, K.F. (1994) Cross-cultural normative assessment: Translation and adaptation issues influencing the normative interpretation of assessment instruments. *Psychological Assessment* 6 (4), 304–312.

Gencan, T.N. (2007) *Dilbilgisi*. Ankara: Tek Ağaç.
Genesee, F., Paradis, J. and Crago, M. (2004) *Dual Development and Language Disorders: A Handbook on Bilingualism and Second Language Learning*. Baltimore: Brookes.
Gierut, J.A. (1989) Maximal opposition approach to phonological treatment. *Journal of Speech and Hearing Disorders* 54, 9–19.
Giles, H., Bourhis, R.Y. and Taylor, D.M. (1977) Towards a theory of language in ethnic group relations. In H. Giles (ed.) *Language, Ethnicity and Intergroup Relations* (pp. 307–348). London: Academic Press.
Girgin, C. (1999) *Türkçe Konuşan Doğal Işitsel Sözel Yöntemle Eğitim Gören Işitme Engelli Kız Çocukların Konuşma Anlaşılırlığı ile Süre ve Perde Özellikleri Ilişkisi*. Eskişehir: Anadolu University, No. 116.
Girgin, Ü. (1997) Eskişehir ili ilkokulları 4. ve 5. sınıf işitme engelli öğrencilerinin okumayı öğrenme durumlarının çözümleme ve anlama düzeylerine göre değerlendirilmesi. PhD thesis. Eskişehir: Anadolu University.
Girgin, C. (2000) Speech intelligibility of Turkish hearing impaired children. ISEC: International Special Education Congress, 24–28 July, University of Manchester, Manchester.
Girgin, M.C. (2006) History of higher education provision for the deaf in Turkey and current applications at the Anadolu University. *The Turkish Online Journal of Educational Technology-TOJET* 5, 3–2.
Girgin, Ü. and Karasu, H.P. (2007) Kaynaştırmadaki işitme engelli öğrencilerin yazılı anlatım beceri düzeylerinin değerlendirilmesi. *Anadolu Üniversitesi Sosyal Bilimler Dergisi* 1, 467–488.
Girgin, M.C. and Ozsoy, B. (2008) The relationship between formant frequency and duration characteristics of vowels and speech intelligibility in Turkish hearing impaired children. *World Applied Sciences Journal* 4 (6), 891–899.
Gold, T. (1980) Speech production in hearing impaired children. *Journal of Communication Disorders* 13 (6), 397–418.
Göksan, B. (2005) İskemik beyin hastalıklarında ikincil önleyici tedavi. In A. Siva, S. Saip and D. Kaynak (eds) *Nörolog olmayanlar icin Nöroloji*. Sürekli Tıp Egitimi Etkinlikleri Sempozyum Dizisi, 42. Istanbul University.
Göksel, A. and Kerslake, C. (2005) *Turkish. A Comprehensive Grammar*. London: Routledge.
Göksun, T., Küntay, A.C. and Naigles, L.R. (2008) Turkish children use morphosyntactic bootstrapping in interpreting verb meaning. *Journal of Child Language* 35, 291–323.
Goldstein, B.A. (2004) Bilingual language development and disorders: Introduction and overview. In B.A. Golstein (ed.) *Bilingual Language Development and Disorders in Spanish-English Speakers* (pp. 3–19). Baltimore: Brookes.
Gollan, T.H., Montoya, R.I. and Werner, G.A. (2002) Semantic and letter fluency in Spanish-English bilinguals. *Neuropsychology* 16 (4), 562–576.
Gonzo, S. and Saltarelli, M. (1983) Pidginazation and linguistic change in emigrant languages. In R.W. Andersen (ed.) *Pidginization and Creolization as Language Acquisition* (pp. 181–197). Rowley: Newburry House.
Goodglass, H. and Kaplan, E. (1972) *The Boston Diagnostic Aphasia Examination*. Philadelphia, PA: Lea & Febiger.
Goodglass, H. and Kaplan, E. (1983) *The Assessment of Aphasia and Related Disorders*. Philadelphia, PA: Lea & Febiger.
Gopnik, M. (1996) Impairments in tense in familial language disorder. PhD thesis, McGill University.
Gordon, J.K. and Dell, G.S. (2003) Learning to divide the labor: An account of deficits in light and heavy verb production. *Cognitive Science* 27, 1–40.
Gregory, E. & Williams, A. (2000) *City Literacies: Learning to Read across Generations and Cultures*. London: Routledge.

Grimault, N., Garnier, S. and Collet, L. (2000) Relationship between amplification fitting age and speech perception performance in school-age children. In R.C. Seewald (ed.) *A Sound Foundation through Early Amplification* (pp. 191–199). NY: Phonak AG.

Grogan, M.L., Barker, E.J., Dettman, S.J. and Blamey, P.J. (1995) Phonetic and phonological changes in the connected speech of children using a cochlear implant. *Annals of Otology, Rhinology, and Laryngology* 166, 390–393.

Grosjean, F. (1982) *Life with two Languages: An Introduction to Bilingualism.* Cambridge: Cambridge University Press.

Grunwell, P. (1985) *PACS: Phonological Analysis of Child Speech.* Windsor: NFER-NELSON.

Gürel, A. (2000) Missing case inflection: Implications for second language acquisition. In S. Howell, A. Fish and T. Keith-Lucas (eds) *Proceedings of the 24th Annual Boston University Conference on Language Development* (pp. 379–390). Somerville, MA: Cascadilla.

Gutierrez-Clellen, V.F. (2000) Language sample analysis in Spanish-speaking children: Methodological considerations. *Language, Speech and Hearing Services in Schools* 31 (1), 88–98.

Güven, A.G. and Berument, S.K. (in preparation) *TİFALDİ-Turkish Expressive and Receptive Language Test: Expressive Vocabulary Sub-Scale.*

Haig, G. (2003) From lexical class to syntactic function: A sketch of Turkish word structure. In S. Özsoy, A.S. Özsoy, D. Akar, M. Nakipoğlu-Demiralp, E. Erguvanlı-Taylan and A. Aksu-Koç (eds) *Studies in Turkish Linguistics* (pp. 59–68). Istanbul: Bogaziçi University.

Håkansson, G. and Nettelbladt, U. (1993) Developmental sequences in L1 (normal and impaired) and L2 acquisition of Swedish syntax. *International Journal of Applied Linguistics* 3 (2), 131–157.

Hakansson, G. and Nettelbladt, U. (1996) Similarities between SLI and L2 children: Evidence from the acquisition of Swedish word order. In C.E. Johnson and J.H.V. Gilbert (eds) *Children's Language* (Vol. 9, pp. 135–151). Mahwah, NJ: Lawrence Erlbaum.

Halliday, M.A.K. (1981) *Learning How to Mean.* London: Edward Arnold.

Halliday, M.A.K. and Hasan, R. (1976) *Cohesion in English.* London: Longman.

Hamann, C., Penner, Z. and Lindner, K. (1998) German impaired grammar: The clause structure revisited. *Language Acquisition* 7 (2–4), 193–245.

Hamers, J.F. and Blanc, M. (1983) *Bilinguisme et Bilingualité.* Bruxelles: Pierre Mardaga.

Hammill, D.D. and Newcorner, P.L. (2008) *Test of Language Development (TOLD-4).* Austin: Pro-ED.

Hansegård, N.E. (1968) *Tvåspråkighet eller Halvspråkighet?* Stockholm: Aldus series 253.

Hansson, K., Nettelbladt, U. and Leonard, L. (2000) Specific language impairment in Swedish: The status of verb morphology and word order. *Journal of Speech, Language, and Hearing Research* 43, 848–864.

Harrison, D.R. (1981) The effects of parent guidance on educational management in Leicestershire. *Report of Proceedings for Conference for Heads of Schools and Services for the Deaf*, Manchester.

Hart, B. and Risley, T.R. (1995) *Meaningful Differences in the Everyday Experience of Young American Children.* New York: Brooks.

Haugen, E. (1977) Norm and deviation in bilingual communities. In P.A. Hornby (ed.) *Bilingualism: Psychological, Social and Education Implications.* New York: Academic Press.

Haznedar, B. (1997) L2 acquisition by a Turkish-speaking child: Evidence of L1 influence. In E. Hughes, M. Hughes and A. Greenhill (eds) *Proceedings of the*

21st Boston University Conference on Language Development. Somerville, MA: Cascadilla.

Haznedar, B. (2003) Missing surface inflection in adult and child L2 acquisition. In J.M. Liceras, H. Zobl and H. Goodluck (eds) *Proceedings of the Sixth Generative Approaches to Second Language Acquisition Conference* (*GASLA 2002*) (pp. 140–149). Somerville, MA: Cascadilla.

Heilmann, J., Miller, J.F., Nockerts, A. and Andriacchi, K. (2006) Agreement and reliability of language sample analysis revisited. Paper presented to the *Symposium on Research and Child Language Disorders*, Madison, WI.

Helloin, M-C., Lenfant, M. and Thibault, M-P. (2002) *Une Batterie Cognitive d'Examen du Langage Oral et écrit* (EXALANG 5–8). Mont-Saint-Aignan: Motus.

Helloin, M.C., Lenfant, M. and Thibault, M.P. (2006) *Une Batterie Cognitive d'Examen du Langage Oral* (EXALANG 3–6). Mont-Saint-Aignan: Motus.

Hélot, C. (2007) *Du Bilinguisme en Famille au Plurilinguisme à l'Ecole*. Paris: L'Harmattan.

Herkenrath, A. and Karakoç, B. (2002) Zum erwerb von verfahren der subordination bei Türkisch-Deutsch bilingualen kinder: Transkripte und quantitative aspekte. *Hamburg Working Papers in Multilingualism* 37.

Herkenrath, A., Karakoç, B. and Rehbein, J. (2003) Interrogative elements as subordinators in Turkish: Aspects of Turkish-German bilingual children's language use. In N. Müller (ed.) *(Non) Vulnerable Domains in Bilingualism* (Hamburg Studies on Multilingualism 1) (pp. 221–269). Amsterdam: John Benjamins.

Hernandez, A.E. and Kohnert, K. (1999) Aging and language switching in bilinguals. *Aging, Neuropsychology and Cognition* 6, 69–83.

Hess-Gabriel, B. (1979) *Zur Didaktik des Deutschunterrichts für Kinder Türkischer Muttersprache*. Tübingen: Narr.

Hick, R.F., Botting, N. and Conti-Ramsden, G. (2005) Short-term memory and vocabulary development in children with down syndrome and children with specific language impairment. *Developmental Medicine & Child Neurology* 47, 532–538.

Hickmann, M. (2004) Le développement de la cohésion dans la narration orale chez l'enfant: perspectives inter-langues. *Cahiers d'Acquisition et de Pathologie du Langage* 24, 13–31.

Hillenbrand, J., Getty, L.A., Clark, M.J. and Wheeler, K. (1997) Acoustic characteristics of American English vowels. *Journal of Acoustical Society of America* 5 (1), 3099–3111.

Hillis, A.E. and Caramazza, A. (1994) Theories of lexical processing and rehabilitation of lexical deficits. In M.J. Riddoch and G.W. Humphries (eds) *Cognitive Neuropsychology and Cognitive Rehabilitation*. Hillsdale, NJ: Lawrence Erlbaum.

Hoff, E. (2006) How social contexts support and shape language development. *Developmental Review* 26, 55–88.

Howell, J. and Dean, E. (1995) *Treating Phonological Disorders in Children: Metaphon-Theory to Practice* (2nd edn). London: Whurr.

Hresko, W., Reid, D. and Hammill, D. (1999) *Test of Early Language Development—Third Edition: Examiner's Manual (TELD-3)*. Austin, TX: Pro-ED.

Huang, R., Hopkins, J. and Nippold, M.A. (1997) Satisfaction with standardized language testing: A survey of speech–language pathologists. *Language, Speech and Hearing Services in Schools* 28, 12–23.

Hudgins, C.V. and Numbers, F.C. (1942) An investigation of the intelligibility of the speech of the deaf. *Genetic Psychology Monoghraphs* 25, 289–392.

Hudson, B.W. (2007) *Evaluating and Enhancing Children's Phonological Systems: Research and Theory to Practice.* Greenville, SC: Thinking Pub.

Hughes, D., McGillivray, L. and Schmidek, M. (1997) *Guide to Narrative Language.* Eau Claire, WI: Thinking.

Human Development Report (HDI) (2007–2008) Country Fact Sheet. On WWW at http://hdrstats.undp.org/countries/country_fact_sheets/cty_fs_TUR.html.

Hyltenstam, K. and Abrahamsson, K. (2003) Maturational Constraints in SLA. In C.J. Doughty and M.H. Long (eds) *The Handbook of Second Language Acquisition* (pp. 539–588). Malden, Oxford: Blackwell.

IALP News (1998) Guidelines for initial education in Logopedics. (Speech/ LanguagePathology/Therapy, Orthophony etc). The Education Committee-(International Association of Logopedics and Phoniatrics, 140894 RL disk 4). *Folia Phoniatrica et Logopaedica* 50, 230–234.

Indredavik, B., Bakke, F., Slordahl, S.A., Rokseth, R. and Haheim, L.L. (1999) Stroke unit treatment: 10-year follow-up. *Stroke* 30, 1524–1527.

Indredavik, B., Bakke, F., Solberg, R., Rokseth, R., Haheim L.L. and Holme, I. (1991) Benefits of a stroke unit: A randomized controlled trial. *Stroke* 22, 1026–1031.

Ingram, D. (1981) *Procedures for the Phonological Analysis of Children's Language.* Baltimore: University Park Press.

Inhelder, B. (1968) *The Diagnosis of Reasoning in the Mentally Retarded.* New York: Chandler.

Inizan, A. (1998) *Analyse du savoir lire de 8 ans à l'âge adulte* (ANALEC), Editions du Centre de Psychologie Appliquée (ECPA), Paris.

Inizan, A. (2000) *Batterie prédictive de l'apprentissage de la lecture* (BP/BL), Editions du Centre de Psychologie Appliquée (ECPA), Paris.

Insalaco, D., Ozkurt, E. and Santiago, D. (2007) The perceptions of students in the allied health professions towards stroke rehabilitation teams and the SLP's role. *Journal of Communication Disorders* 40 (3), 196–214.

INSEE (1997) *Les Immigrés en France, Contours et Caractères.* Paris: INSEE.

Irtis-Dabbagh, V. (2003) *Les Jeunes Issus de l'Immigration de Turquie en France: État des Lieux, Analyses et Perspectives,* Paris: L'Harmattan.

Jakobson, R. (1971) *Studies on Child Language and Aphasia.* Mouton: Paris

Jisa, H. (1987) Sentence connectors in French children's monologue performance. *Journal of Pragmatics* 11, 607–621.

Johnston, J.R. (1985) Fit, focus and functionality: An essay on early language intervention. *Child Language Teaching and Therapy* 1 (2), 125–134.

Johanson, L. (1988) Zur entwicklung Türkeitürkischer varietäten in Nordwesteuropa. *Turkish in North-West Europe Newsletter* 1, 3–8.

John, J.E. and Howarth, J.N. (1965) The effect of time distortions on the intelligibility of deaf children's speech. *Language and Speech* 8 (2), 127–134.

Johnston, J. (1993) Definition and diagnosis of language development disorders. In G. Blanken, J. Dittmann, H. Grimm, J. Marshall and C-W. Wallesch (eds) *Linguistic Disorders and Pathologies: An International Handbook* (pp. 574–585). Berlin: de Gruyter .

Johnston, J. (2001) An alternate MLU calculation: Magnitude and variability of effects. *Journal of Speech, Language, and Hearing Research* 44, 156–164.

Johnston, J.R. (2004) Fearless and bold in following ideas wherever they lead. The Elizabeth Bates Memorial Lecture. *25th Symposium on Research in Child Language Disorders*, Wisconsin.

Johnston, J. (2006) *Thinking about Child Language: Research to Practice.* New York: Thinking.

Johnston, J. and Schery, T. (1976) The Use of grammatical morphemes by children with communication disorders. In D. Morehead and A. Morehead (eds) *Normal and Deficient Child Language*. Baltimore: University Park Press.

Johnston, J. and Kamhi, A. (1984) The same can be less: Syntastic and semantic aspects of the utterances of language impaired children. *Merrill-Palmer Quarterly* 30, 65–86.

Johnston, J., Miller, J., Curtiss, S. and Tallal, P. (1993) Conversations with language impaired children: Asking questions. *Journal of Speech and Hearing Research* 36, 973–978.

Joint Committe on Infant Hearing (2007) Year 2007 Position statement: Principles and guidelines for early hearing detection and intervention programs. *The Volta* Review 107 (2), 141–189.

Jonkers, R. (2000) Verb finding problems in Broca's aphasia: The influence of transitivity. In R. Bastiaanse and Y. Grodzinsky (eds) *Grammatical Disorders in Aphasia: A Neurolinguistic Perspective* (pp. 105–123). London: Whurr.

Jonkers, R. and Bastiaanse, R. (1998) How selective are selective word class deficits? Two case studies of action and object naming. *Aphasiology* 12, 245–256.

Kastoryano, R. (2003) *Les Turcs d'Europe et leur désir d'Europe", Cemoti, 36.* On WWW at http://cemoti.revues.org/document1497.html.

Kauschke, C., Lee, H. and Pae, S. (2007) Similarities and variation in noun and verb acquisition: A crosslinguistic study of children learning German, Korean, and Turkish. *Language and Cognitive Processes* 22 (7), 1045–1072.

Keenan, E.L. and Comrie, B. (1977) Noun phrase accessibility and universal grammar. *Linguistic Inquiry* 8, 63–99.

Keim, I. (2007) *Die "Türkischen Powergirls". Lebenswelt und Kommunikativer Stil einer Migrantinnengruppe in Mannheim.* Tübingen: Narr 39.

Kelly, D. and Rice, M. (1986) A strategy for language assessment of young children: A combination of two approaches. *Language, Speech and Hearing Services in Schools* 17, 83–94.

Kemp, K. and Klee, T. (1997) Clinical language sampling practices: Results of a survey of speech-language pathologists in the United States. *Child Language Teaching and Therapy* 21, 161–172.

Kempe, V., Brooks, P.J. and Gillis, S. (2007) Diminutives provide multiple benefits for language acquisition. In I. Savickiene and W.U. Dressler (eds) *The Acquisition of Diminutives.* Amsterdam: John Benjamins.

Kennedy, M. (2007) Principles of assessment. In R. Paul and P.W. Cascella (eds) *Introduction to Clinical Methods in Communication Disorders* (2nd edn, pp. 39–83). New Jersey: Brookes.

Kern, S. (2003) Le compte-rendu parental au service de l'évaluation de la production lexicale des enfants français entre 16 et 30 mois. *Glossa* 8, 48–62.

Kern, S. (2004) Développement du langage chez le jeune enfant: Le compte-rendu parental au service de l'évaluation de la production lexicale des enfants Français entre 16 et 30 mois. *Les cahiers de la SBLU (Société Belge des Logopèdes Universitaires)* 17, 5–12.

Ketrez, F.N. (2007) Revisiting the Turkish relatives. *Journal of Turkish Linguistics* 1, 1–17.

Ketrez, F.N. (1999a) Early verbs and the acquisition of Turkish argument structure. MA thesis, Boğaziçi University, Istanbul.

Ketrez, F.N. (1999b) Kişi eklerinin edinimi. In Y. Aksan ve M. Aksan (eds) *XII. Dilbilim Kurultayı Bildirileri* (pp. 163–174). Ankara: Şafak.

Ketrez, F.N. (2000) Eylem öğe yapılarının ediniminde eden-özne ilişkisi [agent-subject relation in the acquisition of argument structure]. In A.S. Özsoy and

E.E. Taylan (eds) *XIII. Ulusal Dilbilimi Kurultay Bildirileri.* Istanbul: Bogazici University.
Ketrez, F.N. (2003) Variation in Turkish mother's style. In S. Özsoy, D. Akar, M. Nakipoğlu-Demiralp, E. Erguvanlı-Taylan and A. Aksu-Koç (eds) *Studies in Turkish Linguistics* (pp. 447–453). Istanbul: Boğazici University.
Ketrez, F.N. (2004) A case-study on the accusative case in Turkish. Paper presented at WECOL '04, USC, LA, (to appear in the proceedings volume).
Ketrez, F.N. (2005) Children's scope of indefinite objects. PhD thesis, University of Southern California, Los Angeles.
Ketrez, F.N. (2007) Alignment versus linearity constraints in a Turkish child's speech. *Dilbilim Araştırmaları* 2007, 77–88.
Ketrez, F.N. and Aksu-Koç, A. (2007) The (scarcity of) diminutives in early child speech. In I. Savickiene and W.U. Dressler (eds) *The Acquisition of Diminutives.* Amsterdam: John Benjamins.
Ketrez, F.N. and Aksu-Koç, A. (2009) Early nominal morphology in Turkish: Emergence of case and number. In U. Stephany and M. Voeykova (eds) *Development of Noun Inflection in First Language Acquisition: A Cross Linguistic Perspective.* Berlin: Mouton de Gruyter.
Khomsi, A. (1987) *Epreuve d'évaluation des stratégies de compréhension en situation orale* (O-52). Paris: ECPA.
Khomsi, A. (1999) *Epreuve d'évaluation de la compétence en lecture. Lecture de mots et compréhension – Révisée* (LMC-R), Editions du Centre de Psychologie Appliquée (ECPA), Paris.
Khomsi, A. (2001) *Evaluation du Langage Oral* (ELO). Paris: ECPA.
Khomsi, A. (2002) *Bilan de lecture informatisé* (BLI), Editions du Centre de Psychologie Appliquée (ECPA), Paris.
Kılıç, M.A. (2003) Türkiye Türkçesi'ndeki ünlülerin sesbilgisel özellikleri. In A.S. Özsoy, E. Erguvanlı-Taylan, A. Aksu-Koç, D. Akar and M. Nakipoğlu (eds) *Studies in Turkish Linguistics.* Istanbul: Boğaziçi University.
Kılıç, M.A., Okur, E., Yıldırım, İ., Öğüt, F., Denizoğlu, İ., Kızılay, A., Oğuz, H., Kandoğan, T., Doğan, M., Akdoğan, Ö., Berkiroğlu, N., Öztarakçı, H. (2008.). Ses Handikap Endeksi Tùrkçe versiyonunun guvenirliği ve gegerliliği. KBB İhtisas Derg, 18(3): 139–147.
Kılıç, M.A. and Öğüt, F. (2004) A high rounded vowel in Turkish: Is it a central or back vowel? *Speech Communication* 43, 143–154.
Kilani, S. and Dressler, W.U. (2002) The emergence of inflectional paradigms in two French Corpora: An illustration of general problems of pre- and proto-morphology. In M. Voeikova and W.U. Dressler (eds) *Pre- and Protomorphology: Early Phases of Morphological Development in Nouns and Verbs.* München: Lincom Europa.
Kim, Y.J. (1989) Theoretical Implications of complement structure acquisition in Korean. *Journal of Child Language* 16, 21–31.
Kipp, S., Clyne, M. and Pauwels, A. (1995) *Immigration and Australia's Language Resources,* Canberra: Australian Government Publishing Service.
Kırcaali-İftar, G. (2003) *Otistik Özellik Gösteren Çocuklara İletişim Becerilerinin Kazandırılması (PECS).* İstanbul: Ya-Pa.
Kiran, S. (2007) Semantic complexity in the treatment of naming deficits. *American Journal of Speech Language Pathology* 16 (February), 1–12.
Klatter-Folmer, J. (1996) Turkse kinderen en hun schoolsuccess. PhD thesis, Tilburg University.
Klee, T. (1985) Clinical language sampling: Analysing the analyses. *Child Language Teaching and Therapy* 1, 182–198.
Klee, T. (1992) Developmental and diagnostic characteristics of quantitative measures of children's language production. *Topics of Language Disorders* 12 (2), 28–41.

Klee, T. and Paul, R. (1981) A comparison of six structural analysis procedures: A case study. In J. Miller (ed.) *Assessing Language Production in Children*. Austin: Pro-ED.

Klee, T. and Fitzgerald, M.D. (1985) The relation between grammatical development and mean length of utterance in morphemes. *Journal of Child Language* 12, 251–269.

Klee, T., Schaffer, M., May, S., Membrino, I. and Mougey, K. (1989) A comparison of the age-MLU relation in normal and specifically language-impaired preschool children. *Journal of Speech and Hearing Disorders* 54, 226–233.

Klee, T., Stokes, S.F., Wong, A.M., Fletcher, P. and Gavin, W.J. (2004) Utterance length and lexical diversity in Cantonese-speaking children with and without specific language impairment. *Journal of Speech, Language, and Hearing Research* 47, 1396–1410.

Kohnert, K.J., Hernandez, A.E. and Bates, E. (1998) Bilingual performance on the boston naming test: Preliminary norms in Spanish and English. *Brain and Language* 65 (3), 422–440.

Konrot, A. (1981) A new phoneme of 'voiced velar stop erosion'? Phonetic explanation for the phonological status of the so-called 'soft g' in Turkish. *University of Essex Department of Language and Linguistics Occasional Papers* 34, 12–24.

Konrot, A. (1994a) Özel eğitim alanına öğretmen yetiştirmede bir uygulama. [A Model in Training Special Education Teachers in Turkey]. *Özel Eğitim Dergisi* 1 (1), 47–53.

Konrot, A. (1994b) First Lecture from Prof. Dr. Ahmet Konrot. *Anadolu University Bulletin* 8 (pp. 14–16).

Konrot, A. (2004) Avrupa Birliği'nde konuşma ve dil terapisti yetiştirme, Türkiye'deki mevcut durum ve öneriler. *II. National Speech and Language Pathology Congress Book* (pp.18–26). Eskişehir: Anadolu University.

Kopkallı, H. (1993) A phonetic and phonological analysis of final devoicing in Turkish. PhD thesis, University of Michigan.

Kopkallı-Yavuz, H. (2000a) Acoustic analysis of voicing contrast in Turkish stops. In A. Göksel and C. Kerslake (eds) *Studies on Turkish and Turkic Languages. Turcologica* 46. Bodenheim: Harrassowitz Verlag Wiesbaden.

Kopkallı-Yavuz, H. (2000b) *Türkçedeki /v/'nin sebilimsel ve sesbilgisel özellikleri*. In A.S. Özsoy and E. Erguvanlı-Taylan (eds) *XIII. Dilbilim Kurultay Bildirileri*. İstanbul: Boğaziçi University.

Kopkallı-Yavuz, H. (2001) Türkçe'deki /a/'nın sesbilimsel özellikleri. *Dilbilim Araştırmaları 2001*. İstanbul: Boğaziçi University.

Kopkallı-Yavuz, H. (2003a) Turkish Consonants. In Z. Balpınar (ed.) *Turkish Phonology, Morphology and Syntax*. Eskişehir: Anadolu University.

Kopkallı-Yavuz, H. (2003b) Turkish Vowels. In Z. Balpınar (ed.) *Turkish Phonology, Morphology and Syntax*. Eskişehir: Anadolu University.

Kopkallı-Yavuz, H. (2003c) Phonological processes in Turkish. In Z. Balpınar (ed.) *Turkish Phonology, Morphology and Syntax*. Eskişehir: Anadolu University.

Kopkallı-Yavuz, H. and Topbaş, S. (2000) Children's preferences in early phonological acquisition: How does it reflect sensitivity to the ambient language? In A. Göksel and C. Kerslake (eds) *Studies on Turkish and Turkic Languages* (pp. 291–298). Wiesbaden: Harrassowitz Verlag.

Kopkallı-Yavuz, H., Topbaş, S., Koçak, İ. and Cangökçe-Yaşar, Ö. (2008a) A phonetic analysis of Turkish 'r'. Paper presented at *The 12th Congress of the International Clinical Phonetics and Linguistics Association*, June 25–28, İstanbul, Turkey.

Kopkallı-Yavuz, H., Koçak, İ., Topbaş, S. and Cangökçe-Yaşar, Ö. (2008b) "Soft g" in Turkish: A phonetic analysis. Paper presented at *The 12th Congress of the*

International Clinical Phonetics and Linguistics Association. June 25–28, 2008. İstanbul, Turkey.

Kornfilt, J. (1997) *Turkish Grammar.* London: Routledge.

Kretschmer, R.R. and Kretschmer, L.W. (1978) Language and deafness. In R.R. Kretschmer and L.W. Kretschmer (eds) *Language Development and Intervention with the Hearing Impaired* (pp. 85–142). Baltimore: University Park Press.

Kroffke, S. (2006) Erstsprache, Zweitsprache, Spezifische Sprachentwicklungsstörung? Eine Untersuchung des Erwerbs der deutschen Hauptsatzstruktur durch sukzessiv-bilinguale Kinder mit türkischer Erstsprache. PhD thesis, University of Hamburg.

Kroffke, S. and Rothweiler, M. (2006) Variation im frühen Zweitspracherwerb des Deutschen durch Kinder mit türkischer Erstsprache. In M. Vliegen (ed.) *Variation in Sprachtheorie und Spracherwerb. Akten des 39. Linguistischen Kolloquiums in Amsterdam* (pp. 145–154). Frankfurt: Peter Lang.

Kroffke, S. and Meyer, B. (2007) Verständigungsprobleme in bilingualen Anamnesegesprächen. In S. Kameyama and B. Meyer (eds) *Mehrsprachigkeit am Arbeitsplatz* (Forum Angewandte Linguistik Bd. 48) (pp. 149–183). Frankfurt: Peter Lang.

Kroll, J. and Curley, J. (1988) Lexical memory in novice bilinguals: The role of concepts in retrieving second language words. In P.M. Gruneburg and R. Sykes (eds) *Practical Aspects of Memory* (Vol. 2). New York: Wiley.

Kroll, J.F. and Stewart, E. (1994) Category interference in translation and picture naming: Evidence for asymmetric connections between bilingual memory representations. *Journal of Memory and Language* 33, 149–174.

Kuczaj, S.A. and Maratsos, M.P. (1975) What children can say before they will? *Merrill-Pulmer Quarterly* 21, 89–111.

Kumin, L. (1996) Speech and language skills in Down syndrome. *Mental Retardation and Developmental Disabilities Research Reviews* 2, 109–115.

Kükürt-Özge, D. (2004) Comprehension of Turkish relative clauses in Broca's aphasia and children. MA thesis, Middle Eastern Technical Uniersity, Ankara.

Küntay, A.C. (1999) How do Turkish preschoolers anchor referents in conversational extended discourse? *Psychology of Language and Communication* 3 (1), 83–92.

Küntay, A.C. (2002) Development of the expression of indefiniteness: Presenting new referents in Turkish picture-series stories. *Discourse Processes* 33 (1), 77–101.

Küntay, A. and Slobin, D.I. (1994) Nouns and verbs in Turkish child directed speech. In D. MacLaughlin and S. McEwan (eds) *Proceedings of the 19th Annual Boston University Conference on Language Development (BUCLD)* (pp. 323–334). Boston, MA: Boston University.

Küntay, A. and Slobin, D.I. (1996) Listening to a Turkish mother: Some puzzles for acquisition. In D.I. Slobin, J. Gerhardt, A. Kyratzis and J. Guo (eds) *Social Interaction, Social Context, and Language: Essays in Honor of Susan Ervin-Tripp* (pp. 265–286) Hillsdale, NJ: Lawrence Erlbaum.

Küntay, A. and Slobin, D.I. (1999) The acquisition of Turkish as a native language: A research review. *Turkic Languages* 3 (2), 151–188.

Küntay, A. and Slobin, D.I. (2001) Discourse behavior of lexical categories in Turkish child directed speech: Nouns vs. verbs. *Proceedings for the VIIIth Congress for the International Association for the Study of Child language* (pp. 928–946). New York: Cascadilla.

Küntay, A. and Slobin, D.I. (2001) Discourse behavior of lexical categories in Turkish child-directed speech: Nouns vs. verbs. In M. Almgren, A. Barreña, I.I.M. Ezeizabarrena and B. MacWhinney (eds) *Research on Child Language*

Acquisition: Proceedings for the Eighth Conference of the International Association for the Study of Child Language (pp. 928–946). New York: Cascadilla.

Küntay, A. and Slobin, D.I. (2002) Putting interaction back into child language: Examples from Turkish. *Psychology of Language and Communication* 6, 5–14.

Küntay, A.C. and Ahtam, B. (2004) Annelerin çocuklarıyla geçmiş hakkındaki konuşmalarının anne eğitim düzeyiyle ilişkisi. (Effect of maternal education on Turkish mothers' styles of reminiscing with their children). *Türk Psikoloji Dergisi* 19 (54), 19–31.

Küntay, A.C. and Özyürek, A. (2006) Learning attentional contrasts in using demonstratives in conversation: What do language-specific strategies in Turkish reveal? *Journal of Child Language* 33, 303–320.

Ladefoged, P. (1989) Representing phonetic structure. *UCLA Working Papers in Phonetics* WPP, No. 73.

Ladefoged, P. and Maddieson, I. (1997) *The Sounds of the World's Languages*. Great Britain: Blackwell.

Lahey, M. (1988) *Language Disorders and Language Development*. New York: Macmillan.

Lahey, M., Liebergott, J., Chesnick, M., Menyuk, P. and Adams, J. (1992) Variability in children's use of grammatical morphemes. *Applied Psycholinguistics* 13, 373–398.

Langhorne, P., Williams, B.O., Gilchrist, W. and Howie, K. (1993) Do stroke units save lives? *Lancet* 342, 395–398.

Lapointe, S.G. (1985) A theory of verb form use in the speech of agrammatic aphasics. *Brain and Language* 24, 100–155.

Laughton, J. and Hasenstab, S.M. (2000) Auditory learning, assessment, and intervention with school-age students who are deaf and hard-of-hearing. In J.G. Alpiner and P.A. McCarthy (eds) *Rehabilitative Audiology: Children and Adults* (pp. 178–225). Baltimore: Lippincott.

Law, Z.W.Y. and So, L.K.H. (2006) Phonological abilities of hearing impaired Cantonese-speaking children with cochlear implants or hearing aids. *Journal of Speech, Language, and Hearing Research* 49, 1342–1353.

Laws, G. and Bishop, D.V.M. (2003) A comparison of language in adolescents with Down syndrome and children with specific language impairment. *Journal of Speech, Language and Hearing Research* 46, 1324–1339.

Leadholm, B.J. and Miller, J.F. (1992) *Language Sample Analysis: The Wisconsin Guide*. Madison, WI: Wisconsin Department of Public Instruction.

Lecocq, P. (1996) *Une épreuve de compréhension syntaxico-sémantique* (E.CO.S.SE), Presses Universitaires du Septentrion, Villeneuve d'Ascq.

Le Dorze, G. and Brassard, C. (1999) A description of the consequences of aphasia on aphasic persons and their relatives and friends, based on the WHO model of chronic diseases. *International Journal of Language and Communication Disorders* 34, 291–309.

Lee, L. (1974) *Developmental Sentence Scoring*. Evanston: Northwestern University.

Lee, H.T. and Law, A. (2000) Evidential final particles in child Cantonese. In E.V. Clark (ed.) *The Proceedings of the 30th Annual Child Language Conference* (pp. 131–138). Stanford: Center for the Study of Language and Information.

Lefavrais, P. (2005) *Alouette-R*, Editions du Centre de Psychologie Appliquée (ECPA), Paris.

Légé, Y. and Dague, P. (1976) *Test de vocabulaire en images* (VOCIM), Paris: ECPA.

Lenneberg, E. (1967) *Biological Foundations of Language*. New York: Wiley.

Leonard, L.B. (1989) Language learnability and specific language impairment in children. *Applied Psycholinguistics* 10, 179–202.

Leonard, L.B. (1998) *Children with Specific Language Impairment*. Cambridge, MA: MIT Press.

Leonard, L.B. (2000) Specific language impairment across languages. In D.V.M. Bishop and L.B. Leonard (eds) *Speech and Language Impairments in Children*. Hove: Psychology.

Leonard, L.B. (2002) SLI across several languages: Some new findings. Plenary paper presented at the *Conference of the International Association for the Study of Child Language*, Madison, WI.

Leseman, P. and van Tuijl, C. (2001) Home support for bilingual development of Turkish 4–6 year-old immigrant children in the Netherlands: Efficacy of a home-based educational program. *Journal of Multilingual and Multicultural Development* 22 (4), 309–324.

Lewis, G. (1967) *Turkish Grammar*. Oxford: Oxford University Press.

Limber, J. (1973) The genesis of complex sentences. In T.E. Moore (ed.) *Cognitive Development and the Acquisition of Language* (pp. 169–185). New York: Academic Press.

Linares, N. (1983) Rules for calculating mean length of utterance in morphemes for Spanish. In D.R. Omark and J.G. Erickson (eds). *The Bilingual Exceptional Child*. San Diego: College Hill Press.

Ling, D. (1976) *Speech and the hearing Impaired Child: Theory and Practice*. Washington, DC: The A.G.B. Association.

Long, S., Fey, M. and Channel, R. (2000) *Computerized Profiling (CP; Version 9.26)* (Computer software, Windows only). Cleveland, OH: case Western Reserve University. On WWW at http://www.computerized profiling.org/.

Lüdi, G. and Py, B. (2003) *Etre bilingue* (2nd edn). Berne: Peter Lang.

Lüdi, G. (2001) L'enfant bilingue: Chance ou surcharge? On WWW at http://www.romsem.unibas.ch/sprachenkonzept/Annexe_8.html.

Lund, N.J. and Duchan, J.F. (1993) *Assessing Children's Language in Naturalistic Contexts* (3rd edn). Englewood Cliffs, NJ: Prentice-Hall.

Lust, B., Flynn, S. and Foley, C. (1996) What children know about what they say? Elicited imitation as a research method for assessing children's syntax. In D. McDaniel, C. McKlee and H. Smith Cairns (eds) *Methods for Assessing Children's Syntax* (pp. 55–76). Cambridge, MA: MIT Press.

Luzzatti, C. and Chierchia, G. (2002) On the nature of selective deficits involving nouns and verbs. *Rivista di Linguistica* 14 (1), 43–71.

MacLachlan, B.G. and Chapman, R.S. (1988) Communication breakdowns in normal and language learning-disabled children's conversation and narration. *Journal of Speech and Hearing Disorders* 53, 2–7.

MacWhinney, B. (1996) The CHILDES system. *American Journal of Speech Language Pathology* 5, 5–14.

MacWhinney, B. (2000) *The CHILDES Project: Tools for Analyzing Talk*. Mahwah, NJ: Lawrence Erlbaum.

Maeder, C. (2006) *Test de Compréhension Syntaxique* (T.C.S.), Isbergues: Orthoédition.

Mahon, M., Crutchley, A. and Quinn, T. (2003) Editorial: New directions in the assessment of bilingual children. *Child Language Teaching and Therapy* 19 (3), 237–243.

Mahoney, G. (2008) *The Maternal Behavior Rating Scale-revised (MBRS)*. (Available from the author: Mandel School of Applied Social Sciences, Case Western Reserve University, Cleveland, Ohio, US).

Mahoney, G. and Wheedon, C.A. (1999) The effect of teacher style on interactive engagement of pre-school aged children with special learning needs (Child Behavior Rating Scale-CBRS). *Early Childhood Research Quarterly* 14 (1), 51–68.

Malvern, D., Richards, B., Chipere, N. and Duran, P. (2004) *Lexical Diversity and Language Development: Quantification and Assessment*. New York: Palgrave Macmillan.

Manço, U. (2004) Turcs d'Europe: une présence diasporique unique par son poids démographique et sa complexité sociale. In A. Manço (éd.) *Turquie: vers de Nouveaux Horizons Migratoires?* (pp. 153–177). *Paris*: L'Harmattan.

Maratsos, M. (1982) The child's construction of grammatical categories. In E. Wanner and L.R. Gleitman (eds) *Language acquisition: The State of the Art*. Cambridge: Cambridge University Press.

Marchman, V.A. and Bates, E. (1994) Continuity in lexical and morphological development: A test of the critical mass hypothesis. *Journal of Child Language* 21, 339–366.

Marchman, V.A., Martinez-Sussmann, C. and Dale, P.S. (2004) The language specific nature of grammatical development: Evidence from bilingual language learners. *Developmental Science* 7, 212–224.

Markides, A. (1970) The speech of deaf and partially-hearing children with special reference to factors affecting intelligibility. *The British Journal of Disorders of Communication* 5, 126–140.

Markides, A. (1983) *The Speech of Hearing Impaired Children*. Manchester: Manchester University Press.

Marschark, M. and Spencer, P.E. (2005) Spoken language development of deaf and hard-of-hearing children: Historical and theoretical perspectives. In P.E. Spencer (ed.) *Advances in the Spoken Language Development of Deaf and Hard-of-Hearing Children* (pp. 3–21). North Carolina: Oxford University Press.

Marton, K., Schwartz, R.G., Farkas, L. and Katsnelson, V. (2006) Effect of sentence length and complexity on working memory performance in Hungarian children with specific language impairment (SLI): Across-linguistic comparison. *International Journal of Language and Communication Disorders* 41 (6), 653–673.

Maurin, N. (2006) *Test de Langage Oral Complexe pour collégiens (TLOCC)*. Isbergues: Orthoédition.

Mavis, İ. (2004) Describing the use of Turkish morphology in two aphasic patients and observing their spontaneous recovery: A case study. In A.S. Özsoy, D. Akar, M. Nakipoğlu-Demiralp, E.E. Taylan and A. Aksu-Koç (eds) *Studies in Turkish Linguistics* (pp. 247–259). Istanbul: Boğaziçi University.

Maviş, İ. (2005) Language characteristics of fluent aphasic patients in Turkish. *Journal of Multilingual Communication Disorders* 3 (2), 75–89.

Maviş, İ. (2007) Perspectives on public awareness of stroke and aphasia among Turkish patients in a neurology unit. *Clinical Linguistics and Phonetics* 21 (1), 55–70.

Maviş, İ. (2008) The regression hypothesis revisited: Evidence from Turkish. *Clinical Linguistics & Phonetics* 22 (10), 783–794.

Maviş, İ. and Ege, P. (2002) The emergence of voice morphology in Turkish speaking children. Poster presentation at *Symposium of IASCL*, July, Madison, WI.

Maviş, İ. and ve D. Özbabalık. (2006) Yaşlılıkta nörolojik temelli iletişim sorunları ve dil ve konuşma terapisi. *Anadolu Üniversitesi Sosyal Bilimler Dergisi* 6 (1), 1–18.

Maviş, İ. and Tunçer, M. (2007) Afazili ve sağlıklı yetişkinlerden resim betimleme yöntemi ile alınan dil örneklerinin karşılaştırılması. *Dilbilim Araştırmaları 2007* (pp. 33–45). İstanbul: Boğaziçi University.

Maviş, İ. and Toğram, B. (2009) *Afazide Dil Değerlendirme Testi* (*ADD*). (Language Assessment Test for Aphasia in Turkish–ADD). Ankara: Detay.

Maviş, İ., Doğramacı, Ö. and Diken, İ. (2005) Birincil bakıcıların felçli ve afazili bireylerin sözel olmayan davranışlarına ilişkin görüşleri. *Türk Serebrovasküler Hastalıklar Dergisi* 11 (3), 97–106.

Maviş, İ., Colay, K., Topbaş, S. and Tanrıdağ, O. (2007) Gülhane Afazi Testi-2: Standardizasyon ve geçerlik-güvenirlik çalışması. *Türkiye Nöroloji Dergisi* 13 (2), 25–35.

Mawhood, L., Howlin, P. and Rutter, M. (2000) Autism and developmental receptive language disorder-A comparative follow-up in early adult life, I: Cognitive and language outcomes. *Journal of Child Psychology and Psychiatry and Allied Disciplines* 41, 547–559.

Mayer, M. (1969) *Frog, Where Are You?* New York: Dial book for Young Readers.

McCarthy, D. (1930) *The Language Development of the Preschool Child.* Minneapolis: University of Minnesota Institute of Child Welfare Monograph Series IV.

McCauley, R.J. (1996) Familiar strangers: Criterion-referenced measures in communication disorders. *Journal of Language, Speech and Hearing Services in Schools* 27, 122–131.

McCauley, R.J. (2001) *Assessment of Language Disorders in Children.* Mahwah, NJ: Lawrence Erlbaum.

McCauley, R.J. and Swisher, L. (1984) Use and misuse of norm-referenced tests in clinical assessment: A hypothetical case. *Journal of Speech and Hearing Disorders* 49, 338–348.

McFadden, T.U. (1996) Creating language impairments in typically achieving children: The pitfalls of "Normal" normative sampling. *Language, Speech and Hearing Services in Schools* 27, 3–9.

McGarr, N. and Osberger, M.J. (1978) Pitch deviancy and intelligibility of deaf speech. *Journal of Communication* 3, 237–247.

Meisel, J.M. (1997) The acquisition of the syntax of negation in French and German: Contrasting first and second language development. *Second Language Research* 13, 227–263.

Meisel, J.M. (2004) The bilingual child. In T.K. Bhatia and W.C. Ritchie (eds) *The Handbook of Bilingualism* (pp. 91–113). Oxford: Blackwell.

Meisel, J.M. (2007) *Exploring the Limits of the LAD: A Collection of Four Papers.* Hamburg: Working Papers in Multilingualism 80.

Meltzoff, A.N. (2002) Imitation as a mechanism of social cognition: Origins of empathy, theory of mind and representation of action. In U. Goswami (ed.) *Blackwell Handbook of Childhood Cognitive Development.* Oxford: Blackwell Publishing.

Menn, L. and Obler, L.K. (1990) *Agrammatic Aphasia: Cross-Language Narrative Sourcebook.* Amsterdam/Philadelphia: John Benjamins.

Menyuk, P. (1963) A preliminary evaluation of grammatical capacity in children. *Journal of Verbal Learning and Verbal Behavior* 2, 429–539.

Merrell, A.W. and Plante, E. (1997) Norm-referenced test interpretation in the diagnostic process. *Speech–Language–Hearing Association* 28, 50–58.

Miceli, G., Silveri, M.C., Villa, G. and Caramazza, A. (1984) On the basis for the agrammatics' difficulty in producing main verbs. *Cortex* 20, 207–220.

Miller, J.F. (1981) *Assessing Language Production in Children: Experimental Procedures.* Austin: Pro-Ed.

Miller, J.F. (1991) Quantifying productive language disorders. In J. Miller (ed.) *Research on Child Language Disorders: A Decade of Progress.* Boston, MA: College Hill.

Miller, J.F. (1992) Computational approaches to the analysis of language impairment. In P. Fletcher and B. MacWhinney (eds) *The Handbook of Child Language* (pp. 545–572). London: Blackwell.

Miller, J.F. (1999) Profiles of language development in children with Down syndrome. In J.F. Miller, M. Leddy and L.A. Leavitt (eds) *Improving the Communication of People with Down Syndrome* (pp. 11–39). Baltimore: Paul Brookes.

Miller, J.F. (2004) Using language sample analysis to document language status and monitor change. Paper presented to the *British Columbia Association of Speech Language Pathologists and Audiologists*, Kelowna, B.C., October.

Miller, J.F. and Chapman, R.S. (1981) The relation between age and mean length of utterance in morphemes. *Journal of Speech and Hearing Research* 24, 154–161.

Miller, J.F. and Chapman, R.S. (1984–2000) *Systematic Analysis of Language Transcripts* (Vols 1–6). Madison: University of Wisconsin, Language Analysis Lab.

Miller, J.F. and Chapman, R. (1993) *SALT: Systematic Analysis of Language Transcripts* [Computer software]. Baltimore: University Park Press.

Miller, J.F. and Iglesias, A. (2003–2007) *Systematic Analysis of Language Transcripts* (Vols 7–9). Madison: University of Wisconsin, Language Analysis Lab.

Miller, J.F., Heilmann, J., Nockerts, A. and Andriacchi, K. (2006) Standardizing language sample analysis. Paper presented to the *Symposium on Research in Child Language Disorders*, Madison, WI.

Miyamoto, R.T., Kirk, K.I., Todd, S.L., Robbins, A.M. and Osberger, M.J. (1995) Speech perception skills of children with multichannel cochlear implants or hearing aids. *Annals of Otology, Rhinology and Laryngology* 166 (Suppl.), 334–337.

Miyamoto, R.T., Svirsky, M.A. and Robbins, A.M. (1997) Enhancement of expressive language in prelingually deaf children with cochlear implants. *Acta Otolaryngologica* 117 (2), 154–157.

MoFA – Turkish Ministry of Foreign Affairs (2008) *Report*. Online document retrieved October 24, 2008, from http://www.disisleri.gov.tr.

MoH – Turkish Ministry of Health (2004) *Report of Public Health*. Ankara: SB-HM-2004/1.

Mohammad, S. and Hirst, G. (2005) *Distributional Measures as Proxies for Semantic Relatedness*. Netherlands: Kluwer Academic Press.

Monaco AP (SLIC) (2007) Multivariate linkage analysis of specific language impairment (SLI). *Annals of Human Genetics* 71 (5), 660–673.

MoNE – Turkish Ministry of National Education (2006) *National Report for the Handicapped, 2002* [*Özürlüler için ülke raporu, 2002*]. T.C. Başbakanlık Özürlüler İdaresi Başkanlığı. Ankara, Turkey.

MoNE – Turkish Ministry of National Education (2007) *Milli Eğitim İstatistikleri: Örgün Eğitim 2006–2007* [*National Education Statistics, Formal Education 2006–2007*]. Ankara: MEB.

MoNE – Turkish Ministry of National Education (2009) *Özel Eğitim ve Rehabilitasyon Merkezi Dil ve Konuşma Güçlüğü Destek Eğitim Programı* [*Private Special Education and Rehabilitation Centers Supportive Education Program for Speech and Language Disorders*]. Ankara: MEB.

Mordecai, D. and Palin, M. (1982) *Lingquest 1 & 2* (computer program). East Moline, IL: Lingquest Software.

Moyle, M.J. Weismer, S.E., Evans, J.L. and Lindstrom, M.J. (2007) Longitudinal relationships between lexical and grammatical development in typical and late-talking children. *Journal of Speech, Language, and Hearing Research* 50, 508–528.

Naigles, L.R. (1990) Children use syntax to learn verb meanings. *Journal of Child Language* 17, 357–374.

Nakipoğlu-Demiralp, M. and Ketrez, N. (2007) Children's overregularizations and irregularizations of the Turkish aorist. In D. Bamman, T. Magnitskaia and C. Zaller (eds) *BUCLD 30: Proceedings of Boston University Conference on Language Development* 2 (pp. 399–410). Somerville, MA: Cascadilla.

Nap-Kolhoff, E. (2009) Second language acquisition in early childhood: A longitudinal multiple case study of Turkish-Dutch children. Unpublished PhD dissertation, Tilburg University, The Netherlands.

Nelson, N.W. (1998) *Childhood Language Disorders in Context: Infancy through Adolescence.* Boston: Allyn & Bacon.

Newcomer, P.L. and Hammill, D.D. (1977) *Test of Language Development. (TOLD-4).* Austin, TX: Pro-ED.

Newcomer, P.L. and Hammill, D.D. (2008) *Test of Language Development, Fourth Edition (TOLD-4): Primary and Intermediate.* Austin, TX: Pro-ED.

Nice, M.M. (1925) Length of sentences as a criterion of a child's progress in speech. *Journal of Educational Psychology* 16, 370–379.

Nicholas, J.G. (2000) Age differences in the use of informative/heuristic communicative functions in young children with and without hearing loss who are learning spoken language. *Journal of Speech, Language, and Hearing Research* 43, 380–394.

Nicholas, L.E. and Brookshire, R.H. (1993) Quantifying connected speech of adults with aphasia, *Journal of Speech and Hearing Research* 36, 338–350.

Nicholas, J.G. and Geers, A.E. (2006) Effects of early auditory experience on the spoken language of deaf children at 3 years of age. *Ear and Hearing* June, 286–298.

Nicholas, J.G. and Geers, A.E. (2007) Will they catch up? The role of age at cochlear implantation in the spoken language development of children with severe to profound hearing loss. *Journal of Speech and Language Research* 50, 1048–1062.

Nikolopoulos, T.P., Dyar, D., Archbold, S. and O'Donoghue, G.M. (2004) Development of spoken language grammar following cochlar implantation in prelinguallly deaf children. *Archives of Otolaryngology – Head and Neck Surgery* 130, 629–633.

OECD (2007) Reviews of National Policies for Education. Basic Education in Turkey. Background Report. On WWW at http:// www.oecd.org/edu/reviews/national policies. Accessed 10.01.2009.

O'Hara, M. and Johnston, J. (1997) Syntactic bootstrapping in children with specific language impairment. *European Journal of Disorders of Communication* 32, 147–164.

Oller, D.K., Jensen, H.T. and Lafayette, R.H. (1978) The relatedness of phonological processes of a hearing impaired child. *Journal of Communication Disorders* 11, 97–105.

O'Neill, D.K. (2005) Talking about "new" information: The given/new distinction and children's developing theory of mind. In J.W. Astington and J.A. Baird (eds) *Why Language Matters Why Language Matters for Theory of Mind* (pp. 84–105). Mahwah, NJ: Lawrence Erlbaum.

Orgassa, A. (2009) Specific language impairment in a bilingual context: The acquisition of Dutch inflection by Turkish-Dutch learners. Doctoral dissertation, University of Amsterdam.

Orgassa, A. and Weerman, F. (2008) Dutch gender in specific language impairment and second language acquisition. *Second Language Research* 24(3), 333–364.

Osberger, M.J., Miyamoto, R.T., Zimmermen-Phillips, S., Kemink, J.L., Stroer, B.S., Firszt, J.B. and Novak, M.A. (1991) Independent evaluation of the speech perception abilities of children with the Nucleus 22-channel cochlear implant system. *Ear & Hearing* 12 (4), 66–80.

Owens, R. (1999) *Language Disorders: A Functional Approach to Assessment and Intervention.* Boston: Allyn & Bacon.

Öğüt, F., Kılıç, M.A., Engin, E.Z. and Midilli, R. (2006) Voice onset times for Turkish stop consonants. *Speech Communication* 48, 1094–1099.

Özcan, H.F. (1996) Is the two-stage modal of grammatical development universal? A study on the morphological agreement in the development of L1. Paper presented at the *VIIth International Conference on Child Language*, Boğaziçi University, İstanbul.

Özcan, H.F. (1997) Pronominalizations in the narratives of Turkish-speaking children. In E.V. Clark (ed.) *The Proceedings of the 28th Annual Child Language Research Forum* (pp. 243–258). Stanford, CA: Center for the Study of Language and Information.

Özcan, H.F. (1998) Definite and indefinite nouns in the discourse of Turkish-speaking children. In L. Johanson (ed.) The Mainz meeting. *Proceedings of the Seventh International Conference on Turkish Linguistics* (pp. 552–567) (Turcologica 32). Wiesbaden: Harrassowitz.

Özcan, H.F. (2000) Production of relative clauses in the acquisition of Turkish: The role of parallel function hypothesis. In A. Göksel and C. Kerslake (eds) *Studies in Turkish and Turkic Languages* (pp. 307–313). Wiesbaden: Harrassowitz Verlag.

Özcan, H.F. and Topbaş, S. (1996) A semantic analysis of conjunctions in the acquisition of Turkish. *VIIth International Congress for the Study of Child Language*, 14–19 July, Boğaziçi University, İstanbul.

Özcan, H.F. and Topbaş, S. (2000) Structural and semantic analysis of verbs in the acquisition of Turkish. In I. Barriere, G. Morgan, S. Chiat and B. Woll (eds) *Current Research in Language and Communication Science* (Vol. 1, pp. 57–67). London: City University.

Özdemir, G. (2000) Beyin krizi nedir? Hakkında bilmek istedikleriniz. *Association of Turkish CV Disorders* 3, Eskişehir.

Özen, E. (1986) Phonetische Probleme türkischsprachiger Deutschlerner. *Deutsch Lernen* 3, 11–55.

Özge, D. (2007) Comprehension of Turkish relative clauses in children and adults with agrammatic aphasia. Poster presented at the *British Aphasiology Society Biennal International Conference*. Edinburgh.

Özge, D., Marinis, T. and Zeyrek, D. (in press) Comprehension of subject and object relative clauses in monolingual Turkish children. In S. Ay, A. Özgur, E. İclal, S. Gökmen, S. İşsever and D. Peçenek (eds) *Proceedings of the Fourteenth International Conference of Turkish Linguistics (ICTL)*. Harrasowitz Verlag.

Özsoy, S.A. (1988) On Complementation in Turkish: Possessed Impersonal Infinitives. In S. Koç (ed.) *Studies in Turkish Linguistics*. METU, Ankara.

Özsoy, Y. (1971) *Konuşma Özürlü Çocuklar ve Eğitimi*. Ankara: Ankara University 21.

Özsoy, Y. (1982) *Eskişehir Konuşma Değerlendirme Testi*. Eskişehir: Anadolu University.

Özyürek, A. and Kita, S. (2000) Attention manipulation in the situational use of Turkish demonstratives. Paper presented at the *Linguistic Society of America Conference*, Chicago.

Paradis, M. (2001) The need for awareness of aphasia symptoms in different languages. *Journal of Neurolinguistics* 14, 85–94.

Paradis, J. (2005) Grammatical morphology in children learning English as a second language: Implications of similarities with specific language impairment. *Language, Speech and Hearing Services in Schools* 36, 172–187.

Paradis, J. (2007) Bilingual children with specific language impairment: Theoretical and applied issues. *Applied Psycholinguistics* 28, 512–564.

Paradis, J. and Crago, M. (2000) Tense and temporality: A comparison between children learning a second language and children with SLI. *Journal of Speech and Hearing Disorders* 43 (4), 834–848.

Paradis, J. and Crago, M. (2001) The morphosyntax of specific language impairment in French: An extended optional default account. *Language Acquisition* 9, 269–300.

Paradis, J. and Crago, M. (2003) What can SLI Tell us about transfer in SLA? In J.M. Liceras, H. Zobl and H. Goodluck (eds) *Proceedings of GASLA 2002 Conference* (pp. 219–226). Somerville, MA: Cascadilla.

Parker, M.D. and Brorson, K. (2005) A comparative study between mean length of utterance in morphemes (MLUm) and mean length of utterance in words (MLUw). *First Language* 25 (3), 365–376.

Parr, S., Byng, S., Gilpin, S. and Ireland, C. (1997) *Talking about Aphasia: Living with Loss of Language after Stroke*. Buckingham: Open University.

Paul, R. (2001) *Language Disorders from Infancy through Adolescence: Assessment and Intervention*. (2nd edn) St. Louis, MO: Mosby-Year Book.

Peng, S.C., Spencer, L.J. and Tomblin, J.B. (2004) Speech intelligibility of pediatric cochlear implant recipients with 7 years of device experience. *Journal of Speech, Language, and Hearing Research* 47, 1227–1236.

Pert, S. (2003) Developing an expressive language assessment for children in Rochdale with a Pakistani heritage background. *Child Language Teaching and Therapy* 19 (3), 267–289.

Petek-Salom, G. (2001) Des gendres et des brus importés de Turquie par les familles. *Hommes et Migrations* 1232, 41–50.

Peters, A.M. and Menn, L. (1993) False starts and filler syllabus: Ways to learn grammatical morphemes. *Languages* 69 (4), 742–777.

Peterson, G.E. and Barney, H.L. (1952) Control methods used in a study of the identification of vowels. *Journal of Acoustical Society of America* 24, 175–184.

Peterson, C. and McCabe, A. (1983) *Developmental Psycholinguistics: Three Ways of Looking at a Child's Narrative*. New York: Plenum Press.

Pfaff, C.W. (1994) Early bilingual development of Turkish children in Berlin. In G. Extra and L. Verhoeven (eds) *The Cross-linguistic Study of Bilingual Development* (pp. 75–97). Amsterdam: Koninklijke Academie van Wetenschappen.

Plante, E. and Vance, R. (1994) Selection of preschool language tests: A data-based approach. *Speech–Language–Hearing Services in Schools* 25, 15–24.

Plante, E. and Vance, R. (1995) Diagnostic accuracy of two tests of preschool language. *Journal of Speech–Language Pathology* 4, 70–76.

Potter, M., So, K., von Eckardt, B. and Feldman, L. (1984) Lexical and conceptual representation in beginning and proficient bilinguals. *Journal of Verbal Learning and Verbal Behavior* 23, 23–381.

Power, D.J. and Quigley, S.P. (1973) Deaf children's acquisition of the passive voice. *Journal of Speech and Hearing Research* 16, 5–11.

Pressnell, L.M. (1973) Hearing impaired children's comprehension and production of syntax in oral language. *Journal of Speech and Hearing Research* 16 (1), 12–21.

Prévost, P. (2003) Truncation and missing inflection in initial child L2 German. *Studies in Second Language Acquisition* 25, 65–97.

Quigley, S.P. and King, C.M. (1980) Syntactic performance of hearing impaired and normal hearing individuals. *Applied Psycholinguistics* 1, 329–356.

Quigley, S.P., Smith, N.L. and Wilbur, R.B. (1974a) Comprehension of relativized sentences by deaf students. *Journal of Speech and Hearing Research* 17, 325–341.

Quigley, S.P., Montanelli, D.S. and Wilbur, R.B. (1976a) Some aspects of the verb system in the language of deaf students. *Journal of Speech and Hearing Research* 19, 536–550.

Quigley, S.P., Wilbur, R.B. and Montanelli, D.S. (1974b) Question formation in the language of deaf students. *Journal of Speech and Hearing Research* 17, 699–713.

Quigley, S.P., Wilbur, R.B., Power, D.J. and Montanelli, D.S. (1976b) Complement structures in the language of deaf students. *Journal of Speech and Hearing Research* 19, 448–457.

Quigley, Wilbur, Power, Montanelli and Steinkamp (1976c) *Syntactic Structures in the Language of Deaf Children.* Urbana, Ill.: Institute for Child Behavior and Development, quoted in Quigley and King (1980).
Quigley, S.P., Power, D.J. and Steinkamp, M.W. (1977) The language structure of deaf children. *Volta Review* 79 (2), 73–84.
Quigley, S., Steinkamp, M., Power, D.J. and Jones, B. (1978) *Test of Syntactic Abilities.* Beaverton, Ore: Dormac.
Radford, A. (1990) *Syntactic Theory and the Acquisition of English Syntax.* Oxford, MA: Blackwell.
Ramos, M. and Ramos, J. (2007) *Test of Early Language Development—3: Spanish.* Austin, TX: Pro-ED.
Rapin, I. (1996) *Preschool Children with Inadequate Communication.* London: MacKeith.
Rapin, I. and Allen, D. (1998) The semantic-pragmatic deficit disorder: Classification issues. *International Journal of Language and Communication Disorders* 33 (1), 82–90.
Ravid, D.D. and Levie, R. (under review) Adjectives in later language development: Text-embedded analyses.
Redmond, S.M. (2004) Conversational profiles of children with ADHD, SLI and typical development. *Clinical Linguistics and Phonetics* 18 (2), 107–125.
Rehbein, J. (2001) Turkish in European Societies. *Lingua e Stile* XXXVI/2, 317–334.
Rehbein, J. and Karakoç, B. (2004) On contact-induced language change of Turkish aspects: Languaging in bilingual discourse. In C.B. Dabelsteen and J.N. Jørgensen (eds) *Languaging and Language Practices* (pp. 125–149). Copenhagen: Copenhagen Studies in Bilingualism 36.
Rescorla, L. (1989) The Language Development Survey: A screening tool for delayed language in toddlers. *Journal of Speech and Hearing Disorders* 54, 587–599.
Rice, M. L. and Wexler, K. (1996) A phenotype of specific language impairment: Extended optional infinitives. In M.L. Rice (ed.) *Towards a Genetics of Language.* Mahwah, NJ: Lawrence Erlbaum.
Rice, M.L. and Warren, S.F. (eds) (2004) *Developmental Language Disorders: From Phenotypes to Etiologies.* Mahwah, NJ: Lawrence Erlbaum.
Rice, M.L., Warren, S.F. and Betz, S.K. (2005) Language symptoms of developmental language disorders: An overview of autism, Down syndrome, Fragile X, specific language impairment, and Williams syndrome. *Applied Psycholinguistics* 26, 7–27.
Richter, B., Eibele, S., Laszig, R. and Lohle, E. (2002) Receptive and expressive skills of 106 children with a minimum of 2 years' experience in hearing with a cochlear implant. *International Journal of Pediatric Otorhinolaryngology* 64, 111–125.
Riegel, M., Pellat, J.C. and Rioux, R. (1994) *Grammaire Méthodique du Français: Linguistique Nouvelle.* Paris: PUF.
Rispens, E. (2004) Syntactic and phonological processing in developmental dyslexia. Retrieved July 15, 2005, from http://www.ub.rug.nl/eldoc/dis/arts/j.e.rispens/
Rispoli, M. and Hadley, P. (2001) The leading-edge: The significance of sentence disruptions in the development of grammar. *Journal of Speech Language and Hearing Research* 44, 1131–1143.
Roberts, P.M. and Le Dorze, G. (1997) Semantic organization, strategy use, and productivity in bilingual semantic verbal fluency. *Brain and Language* 59 (3), 412–449.
Roberts, S. and Leonard, L. (1997) Grammatical deficits in German and English: A crosslinguistic study of children with specific language impairment. *First Language* 17, 131–150.
Roberts, P.M., Garcia, L.J., Desrochers, A. and Hernandez, D. (2002) English performance of proficient bilingual adults on the Boston Naming Test. *Aphasiology* 16 (4–6), 635–645.
Roberts, J., Rice, M. and Tager-Flusberg, H. (2004) Tense marking in children with autism. *Applied Psycholinguistics* 25, 429–448.

Rollins, R.P. and Snow, C.E. (1998). Shared attention and grammatical development in typical children and children with autism. *Journal of Child Language* 25, 653–673.

Rondal, L.A., Ghiotto, M., Bredart, S. and Bachelet, J.F. (1987) Age relation, reliability and grammatical validity of measures of utterance length. *Journal of Child Language* 14, 433–446.

Ronjat, J. (1913) *Le Développement du Langage Observé Chez un Enfant Bilingue*. Paris: Champion.

Rosenbaum, F. (1997) *Approche Transculturelle des Troubles de la Communication: Langage et Migration* (collection orthophonie). Paris: Masson.

Rossari, C. (2000) *Connecteurs et Relations de Discours: Des Liens Entre Cognition et Signification*. Nancy: Presses Universitaires de Nancy.

Rosselli, M., Ardila, A., Araujo, K., Weekes, V.A., Caracciolo, V., Padilla, M. and Ostrosky-Solí, F. (2000) Verbal fluency and repetition skills in healthy older Spanish-English bilinguals. *Applied Neuropsychology* 7 (1), 17–24.

Rothweiler, M. (1993) *Der Erwerb von Nebensätzen im Deutschen: Eine Pilotstudie*. Tübingen: Niemeyer.

Rothweiler, M. (2006) The acquisition of V2 and subordinate clauses in early successive acquisition of German. In C. Lleó (ed.) *Interfaces in Multilingualism: Acquisition, Representation and Processing* (pp. 91–113). Amsterdam: John Benjamins.

Rothweiler, M. (2007) Multilingualism and language impairments. In P. Auer and L. Wei (eds) *Multilingualism* (pp. 229–246). Berlin: de Gruyter.

Rothweiler, M., Babur, E. and Kroffke, S. (2007) Spezifische sprachentwicklungsstörung im kontext kindlicher mehrsprachigkeit: Ergebnisse zur kasusmorphologie in der erstsprache Türkisch. *Sprache, Stimm, Gehör* 31, 1–7.

Rothweiler, M., Chilla, S. and Babur, E. (2010) Specific language impairment in Turkish: Evidence from Turkish-German successive bilinguals. *Clinical Linguistics & Phonetics* Early online, 1–16.

Saben, C.B. and Ingham, J.C. (1991) The effects of minimal pairs treatment on the speech sound production of two childrens with phonologic disorders. *Journal of Speech, Language-Hearing Research* 34, 1023–1040.

Saffran, E.M., Berndt, R.S. and Schwartz, M.F. (1989) The quantitative analysis of agrammatic production: Procedure and data. *Brain and Language* 37, 440–479.

Salameh, E.K. (2006) Linguistic and cultural factors affecting assessement and intervention for bilingual children with language impairment. Paper presented at the *CPLOL Congress*, Berlin.

Santelli, E. (2007) Familles d'origine maghrébine et orthophonie: le vécu de la prise en charge. In L. Tain (ed.) *Le Métier d'Orthophoniste: Langage, Genre et Profession* (pp. 219–233). Rennes: Editions ENSP.

Sarachan-Deily, A.B. (1982) Hearing impaired and hearing readers' sentence processing errors. *The Volta Review* 84, 81–95.

Savaşır, I. (1986) Habits and abilities in Turkish. In D.I. Slobin and K. Zimmer (eds) *Studies in Turkish Linguistics* (pp. 137–146). Amsterdam: John Benjamins.

Savaşır, I. and Gee, J. (1982) The functional equivalents of the middle voice in child language. *Proceedings of the 8th Annual Meeting of the Berkeley Linguistics Society*. Berkeley: University of California.

Savaşır, I. and Şahin, N. (1995) Wechsler Çocuklar İçin Zeka Ölçeği (WISCR) El Kitabı. Ankara.: Türk Psikologlar Derneği Yayınları.

Scarborough, H. (1990) The index of productive syntax. *Journal of Psycholinguistic Research* 11, 1–22.

Scarborough, H., Wycoff, J. and Davidson, R. (1986) A reconsideration of the relation between age and mean utterance length. *Journal of Speech and Hearing Research* 29, 394–399.

Scarborough, H.S., Rescorla, L., Tager-Flusberg, H., Fowler, A.E. and Sudhalter, V. (1991) The relation of utterance length of grammatical complexity in normal and language disordered groups. *Applied Psycholinguistics* 12, 23–45.

Schirmer, B.R. (1985) An analysis of the language of young hearing-impaired children in terms of syntax, semantics, and use. *American Annals for the Deaf* 130 (1), 15–19.

Schlichting, L. (2002) *Taalscreening bij Marokkaanse en Turkse kinderen met de tweetalige Lexiconlijsten*. Amsterdam: JIP.

Schlichting, L. (2006) *Lexiconlijsten; Instrument om de Taalontwikkeling te Onderzoeken bij Jone Marokkaanse en Turkse Kinderen in Nederland*. Amsterdam: JIP.

Schneider, P., Hayward, D. and Dube, R. (2006) Storytelling from pictures using the Edmonton narrative norms instrument. *Journal of Speech–Language Pathology and Audiology* 30, 224–238.

Schöler, H., Fromm, W. and Kany, W. (eds) (1998) *Spezifische Sprachentwicklungsstörung und Sprachlernen. Erscheinungsformen, Verlauf, Folgerungen für Diagnostik und Therapie*. Heidelberg: Programm Ed. Schindele.

Schwartz, B.D. (2004) On child L2 development of syntax and morphology. *Lingue e Linguaggio* 3, 97–132.

Scott, C.M. and Stokes, S.L. (1995) Measures of syntax in school-age children and adolescents, *Language, Speech and Hearing Services in Schools* 26, 309–319.

Segal, E., Duchan, J. and Scott, P. (1991) Role of interclausal connectives in narrative structuring: Evidence from adults' interpretations of simple stories. *Discourse Processes* 14, 27–54.

Segalowitz, N. and de Almeida, R.G. (2002) Conceptual representation of verbs in bilinguals: Semantic field effects and a second-language performance paradox. *Brain and Language*.

Selen, N. (1979) *Söyleyiş Sesbilimi, Akustik Sesbilim ve Türkiye Türkçesi*. Ankara: TDK.

Semel, E.M., Wiig, E. and Secord, W. (1989) *CELF-R Screening Test*. San Antonio, TX: Psychological Corporation.

Serry, T.A. and Blamey, P.J. (1999) A 4-year investigation into phonetic inventory development in young cochlear implant users. *Journal of Speech, Language and Hearing Research* 42, 141–154.

Seyfried-Culbertson, D.N. and Kricos, P.B. (2002) Language and speech of the deaf and hard of hearing. In R.L. Schow and M.A. Nerbonne (eds) *Introduction to Audiological Rehabilitation* (4th edn, pp. 183–224). Boston: Allyn & Bacon.

Sezer, E. (1986) An autosegmental analysis of compensatory lengthening in Turkish. In L. Wetzels and E. Sezer (eds) *Studies in Compensatory Lengthening*. Riverton: Foris.

Sezer, E. (1991) On non-final stress in Turkish. *Journal of Turkish Studies* 5, 61–69.

Sheldon, A. (1974) The role of parallel function in the acquisition of relative clauses in English. *Journal of Verbal Learning and Verbal Behavior* 13, 272–281.

Shirai, Y. and Andersen, R.W. (1995) The acquisition of tense-aspect morphology: A prototype Account. *Language* 71, 743–762.

Shriberg, L.D. (1993) Four new speech and prosody-voice measures for genetics research and other studies in developmental phonological disorders. *Journal of Speech and Hearing Research* 36, 105–140.

Shriberg, L.D. and Kwiatkowski, J. (1982) Phonological disorders III. A procedure for assessing severity of involvement. *Journal of Speech and Hearing Disorders* 47, 256–270.

SIG in Bilingualism (2007) *Good Practice for Speech and Language Therapists Working with Clients from Linguistic Minority Communities*. London: RCSLT.

Simmons-Mackie, N., Code, C., Armstrong, E., Stiegler, L. and Elman, R.J. (2002) What is aphasia? Results of an international survey. *Aphasiology* 16, 837–848.

SIS – Turkish State Institute of Statistics (2002) *Turkey Disability Survey*, Ankara: DIE/SIS.
Skutnabb-Kangas, T. and Toukomaa, P. (1976) *Teaching Migrant Children's Mother tongue and Learning the Language of the Host Country in the Context of the Socio-cultural Situation of the Migrant Family*. Tampere: Tukimuksia Research Reports.
Slobin, D.I. (1982) Universal and particular in the acquisition of language. In E. Wanner and L.R. Gleitman (eds) *Language Acquisition: The State of the Art* (pp. 128–172). Cambridge, Cambridge University Press.
Slobin, D.I. (1985) Crosslinguistic evidence for the language-making capacity. In D.I. Slobin (ed.) *The Crosslinguistic Study of Language Acquisition 2: Theoretical Issues* (pp. 1157–1256). Hillsdale, NJ: Lawrence Erlbaum.
Slobin, D.I. (1986) The Acquisition and use of relative clauses in Turkic and Indo-European languages. In D.I. Slobin and K. Zimmer (eds) *Studies in Turkish Linguistics* (pp. 277–298). Amsterdam/Philadelphia: John Benjamins.
Slobin, D. (1991) Aphasia in Turkish: Speech production in Broca's and Wernicke's patients. *Brain and Language* 41, 149–164.
Slobin, D.I. (1993) Converbs in Turkish child language: The grammaticalization of event coherence. In M. Haspelmath and E. König (eds) *Converbs (Adverbial Participles, Gerunds) in Crosslinguistic Perspective*. Berlin/New York: Mouton de Gruyter.
Slobin, D.I. (1994) Passives and alternatives in children's narratives in English, Spanish, German and Turkish. In B. Fox and P.J. Hoppper (eds) *Voice, Form and Function* (pp. 341–364). Amsterdam: John Benjamins.
Slobin, D.I. (1995) Converbs in Turkish child language: The grammaticalization of event coherence. In M. Haspelmath and E. König (eds) *Converbs in Cross-Linguistic Perspective: Structure and Meaning of Adverbial Verb Forms – Adverbial Participles, Gerunds* (pp. 349–371). Berlin/New York: Mouton de Gruyter.
Slobin, D.I. and Welsh, C.A. (1973) Elicited imitation as a research tool in developmental psycholinguistics. In C.A. Ferguson and D.I. Slobin (eds) *Studies of Child Language Development* (pp. 485–497). New York, NY: Holt, Rinehart & Winston.
Slobin, D.I. and Bever, T.G. (1982) Children use canonical sentence schemas: Crosslinguistic study of word order and inflections. *Cognition* 12, 229–265.
Slobin, D.I. and Talay, A. (1986) Development of pragmatic uses of subject proouns in Turkish child language. In A. Aksu-Koç and E. Erguvanlı-Taylan (eds) *Proceedings of the Turkish Linguistics Conference* (pp. 207–227). Istanbul: Boğaziçi University.
Słodowicz, S. (2007) Complement control in Turkish. *ZAS Papers in Linguistics* 47, 125–157.
Smith, C.R. (1975) Interjected sounds in deaf children's speech. *Journal of Communication Disorders* 8, 123–128.
Sofu, H. (1995) Acquisition of Lexicon in Turkish. PhD thesis, Çukurova University.
Sofu, H. (1998) Farklı sosyo-ekonomik katmanlardan çocukların dil ediniminde kişi ve zaman eklerinin kullanımı. *XII. Dilbilim Kurultayı Bildirileri*. Ankara: Ankara Univ.
Spaulding, T.J., Plante, E. and Farinella, K.A. (2006) Eligibility criteria for language impairment: Is the low end of normal always appropriate? *Speech–Language–Hearing Association* 37, 61–72.
Spencer, P.E. and Marschark, M. (2003) Cochlear implants. In M. Marschark and P.E. Spencer (eds) *Deaf Studies, Language, and Education* (pp. 434–450). US: Oxford University Press.

Spencer, L.J., Barker, B.A. and Tomblin, J.B. (2003) Exploring the language and literacy outcomes of pediatric cochlear implant users. *Ear & Hearing* 24, 236–247.

Springer, L., Huber, W., Schlenck, K-J. and Schlenck, C. (2000) Agrammatism: deficit or compensation? Consequences for aphasia therapy. *Neuropsychological Rehabilitation* 10, 279–309.

SPSS (1997) *SPSS Base 7.5 Applications Guide*. Chicago, IL: SPSS Inc.

St. Louis, K., Topbaş, S. and Özdemir, S. (2008) Turkish stuttering association: A model project to bring stuttering self-help to Turkey. *Perspectives on Fluency and Fluency Disorders* 18, 119–123.

Stark, R.E. and Tallal, P. (1981) Selection of children with specific language impairment. *Journal of Speech and Hearing Disorders* 46, 114–122.

Steenge, J. (2006) *Bilingual Children with Specific Language Impairment: Additionally Disadvantaged?* Nijmegen: EAC, Research Centre on Atypical Communication.

Steib, F. (2006) La prise en charge des enfants Turcophones: Quel accompagnement parental? MA dissertation, Université Louis Pasteur, Strasbourg.

Stoel-Gammon, C. (2001) Down syndrome phonology: Developmental patterns and intervention strategies. *Down Syndrome Research and Practice* 7 (3), 93–100.

Stokes, S.F. and Fletcher, P. (2003) Aspectual forms in Cantonese children with specific language impairment. *Linguistics* 41, 381–405.

Stokes, S.F., Wong, A.M.Y., Fletcher, P. and Leonard, L.B. (2006) Nonword repetition and sentence repetition as clinical markers of specific language impairment: The case of Cantonese. *Journal of Speech, Language, Hearing Research* 49, 219–236.

Svirsky, M.A., Robbins, A.M., Kirk, K.I., Pisoni, D.B. and Miyamoto, R.T. (2000) Language development in profoundly deaf children with cochlear implants. *Psychological Science* 11 (2), 153–158.

Tabors, P. and Snow, C. (1994) English as a second language in preschools. In F. Genesee (ed.) *Educating Second Language Children: The Whole Child, the Whole Curriculum, the Whole Community* (pp. 103–125). New York, NY: Cambridge University Press.

Tanrıdağ, O. (1993) *Afazi*. Ankara: GATA.

Tardiff, T. (1994) Nouns are not always learned before words, but why? Evidence from Mandarin Chinese. Poster presented at the *Stanford Child Language Research Forum*, Stanford University, CA.

Taylan, E.E. (1998) What determines the choice of nominalizer in Turkish nominalized complement clauses. In B. Caron (ed.) *Proceedings of the 18th International Congress of Linguistics* (pp. 220–230). Oxford: Pergamon.

Taylan, E.E. and Aksu-Koç, A. (1998) Function of relative clauses in narrative discourse. In L. Johanson (ed.) *Proceedings of the Seventh International Conference on Turkish Linguistics* (pp. 271–285). Wiesbaden: Harrasowitz Verlag.

Taylan, E.E. and Aksu-Koç, A. (2003) Çocukta dilbilgisi yetisinin değerlendirilmesi üzerine bir çalışma (An attempt at the evaluation of linguistic competence in the child). Paper presented at the *XVIIth Linguistics Conference*. Eskişehir: Anadolu University.

Templin, M. (1957) *Certain Language Skills in Children: Their Development and Inter-Relationships*. Minneapolis, MN: University of Minnesota.

Thoma, D. and Tracy, R. (2006) Deutsch als frühe Zweitsprache: Zweite Erstsprache? In B. Ahrenholz (ed.) *Kinder mit Migrationshintergrund*. Fillibach, Ort: Verlag.

Thomason, S. and T. Kaufman (1988) *Language Contact, Creolization, and Genetic Linguistics*, Berkeley: University of California Press.

Thordardottir, E.T. and Weismer, S.E. (1998) Mean length of utterance and other language sample measures in early Icelandic. *First Language* 18, 1–32.

Thordardottir, E.T. and Weismer, S.E. (2002) Content mazes and filled pauses in narrative language samples of children with specific language impairment. *Brain and Cognition* 48 (2–3), 587–592.

Thornton, R. (1995) Referentiality and Wh-movement in child English: Juvenile D-Linkuency. *Language Acquisition* 4, 139–175.

Tinelli, A. (2004) De l'exil à l'orthophonie, ou la possible trajectoire linguistique des enfants d'origine Turque: Réflexion sur les difficultés langagières des enfants de migrants Turcs. Published MA dissertation, Université Louis Pasteur, Strasbourg.

Tobey, E.A. and Hasenstab, S. (1991) Effects of a nucleus multichannel cochlear implant upon speech production in children. *Ear & Hearing* 12 (Suppl.), 48–54.

Tobey, E.A., Pancamo, S., Staller, S.J., Brimacombe, J.A. and Beiter, A.L. (1991) Consonant production in children receiving a multichannel cochlear implant. *Ear & Hearing* 12, 23–31.

Tobey, E., Geers, A. and Brenner, C. (1994) Speech production results: Speech feature acquisition. *The Volta Review* 96 (5), (monograph), 109–129.

Toğram, B. (2008) Sağlıklı ve inmeli bireylere uygulanan 'Afazide dil değerlendirme aracı'nın geçerlik, güvenirlik ve standardizasyon çalışması (Validity, reliability, and standardization study of language assessment tool for aphasia administered to healthy people and people with aphasia due to stroke). PhD thesis, Anadolu University.

Tomasello, M. (1992) *First Verbs: A Case Study of Early Lexical Development*. Cambridge: Cambridge University Press.

Tomasello, M. (2003) The key is social cognition. In D. Gentner and S. Goldin-Meadow (eds) *Language in Mind* (pp. 47–58). Cambridge, MA: MIT Press.

Tomasello, M. and Brooks, P. (1999) Early syntactic development. In M. Barrett (ed.) *The Development of Language* (pp. 161–190). Hove, England: Psychology.

Tomasello, M., Kruger, A.C. and Ratner, H.H. (1993) Cultural learning. *Behavioral and Brain Sciences* 16, 495–511.

Tomblin, J.B., Spencer, L., Flock, S., Tyler, R. and Gantz, B. (1999) A comparison of language achievement in children with cochlear implants and children using hearing aids. *Journal of Speech, Language and Hearing Research* 42, 497–511.

Tomblin, J.B., Spencer, L.J. and Gantz, B.J. (2000) Language and reading acquisition in children with and without cochlear implants. *Advances in Otorhinolaryngology* 57, 300–304.

Tompkins, C.A., Jackson, S.T. and Schulz, R. (1990) On prognostic research in adult neurologic disorders. *Journal of Speech, Language and Hearing Research* 33, 398–401.

Topbaş, S. (1989) The frequency effect and the acquisition of /k/, /t/ ve /tʃ/ sounds in Turkish. MSc thesis, City University, London.

Topbaş, S. (1996) Sesbilgisi açısından dil edinim süreci. *Dilbilim Araştırmaları* 96, 295–309.

Topbaş, S. (1997) Phonological acquisition of Turkish children: Implications for phonological disorders. *European Journal of Disorders of Communication* 32, 377–396.

Topbaş, S. (1999) Dil ve Konuşma Sorunlu Çocukların Sesbilgisel Çözümleme Yöntemi ile Değerlendirilmesi ve Konuşma Dillerindeki Sesbilgisel Özelliklerin Betimlenmesi. PhD thesis, 1994, Anadolu University, Eskişehir.

Topbaş, S. (2004/5) *Türkçe Sesletim Sesbilgisi Testi* (*SST*) [Turkish Articulation and Phonology Test]. Ankara: Ministry of National Education, 4. Akşam Sanat Okulu.

Topbaş, S. (2006a) A Turkish perspective on communication disorders. *Logopedics Phoniatrics Vocology* 31, 76–88.

Topbaş, S. (2006b) Does the speech of Turkish-speaking phonologically disordered children differ from that of children speaking other languages? *Clinical Linguistics & Phonetics* 20 (7), 509–522.

Topbaş, S. (2006c) Linguistic deficits in Turkish-speaking language impaired children. Paper presented at the *ASHA Convention*, San Diego.

Topbaş, S. (2007a) Turkish speech acquisition. In S. McLeod (ed.) *The International Guide to Speech Acquisiton* (pp. 566–579). New York: Thompson Learning.

Topbaş, S. (2007b) Özgül dil bozuklukları ve Türkçe Erken Dil Gelisim Testi uygulamaları. Presented on the *4. National Congress of Speech and Language Disorders*, May 3–5, Istanbul/Turkey.

Topbaş, S. (2008) Speech-language pathology in Turkey and the world. Paper presented at *SKYBUD*, December, Istanbul.

Topbaş, S. and Ball, M.J. (in preparation) LARSP: Turkish. In M.J. Ball, D. Crystal and P. Fletcher (eds) *Assessing Grammar: The Languages of LARSP*. London, UK: Multilingual Matters.

Topbaş, S. and Özcan, H. (1995) Anlatılarda bağlaç kullanımı: Normal ve özel eğitim gereksinimli öğrenciler arasında bir karşılaştırma. *IX. Dilbilim Kurultayı Bildiriler Kitabı*. Bolu: Abant İzzet Baysal University.

Topbaş, S. and Özcan, F.H. (1997) Pronominals and their pragmatic functions in the acquisition of Turkish. In K. İmer and N.E. Uzun (eds) *Proceedings of the Eighth International Conference on Turkish Linguistics* (pp. 139–148). Ankara: Ankara University.

Topbaş, S. and Konrot, A. (1998) Variability in phonological disorders: Can we search for systematicity? Evidence from Turkish-speaking children. In W. Ziegler and K. Deger (eds) *Clinical Phonetics and Linguistics* (pp. 79–87). London: Whurr Publishers.

Topbaş, S. and Kopkallı-Yavuz, H. (1998) The onset of a linguistic system: Is there evidence from the acquisition of final devoicing in Turkish? In A. Sorace, C. Heycock and R. Shillcock (eds) *Proceedings of GALA '97-Generative Approaches to Language Acquisition* (pp. 284–289). Edinburgh: Edinburgh University Press.

Topbaş, S. and Yavaş, M. (2006) Phonological acquisition and disorders in Turkish. In Z. Hua and B. Dodd (eds) *Phonological Development and Disorders in Children: A Multilingual Perspective* (pp. 233–265). Clevedon, Multilingual Matters.

Topbaş, S. and Güven, S. (2007) *Test of Early Language Development (TELD-3): Turkish Version*. Eskişehir: DILKOM, Anadolu University.

Topbaş, S. and Güven, S. (2008) Specific language impairment in Turkish. *Abstract Proceedings of 12th ICPLA Congress*, Istanbul, Turkey.

Topbaş, S., Maviş, I. and Başal, M. (1997) Acquisition of bound morphemes: Nominal case morphology in Turkish. In K. İmer and N.E. Uzun (eds) *Proceedings of the 8th* International Conference on Turkish Linguistics (pp. 127–137). Ankara: Ankara University.

Topbaş, S., Maviş, İ. and Özdemir, S. (2003) Mothers intentional communicative language to Turkish children with delayed and normal language development. In S. Özsoy, D. Akar, M. Nakipoğlu-Demiralp, E.E. Taylan and A. Aksu-Koç (eds) *Studies in Turkish Linguistics* (pp. 469–478). Istanbul: Boğaziçi University.

Topbaş, S., Özdemir, S., Maviş, İ. and St. Louis, K. (2009) *Project e-ÖZYARDEP: Expanding community based self-help through internet for stuttering in Turkey*. Ankara: TÜBİTAK-SOBAG, Project No. 107K093.

Topbaş, S., Güven, S., Maviş, İ., Ege, P., Emeksiz, Z. and Kopkallın-Yavuz, H. (in preparation) Test of Language Development-4: Turkish (TOLD-4:T). Eskisehir: Ongoing Project supported by TÜBİTAK, No. 109K001.

Tough, J. (1981) *Listening to Children Talking*. London: Ward Locke Educational.

Tözün, I. (2005) *Talking Turkey: The Language, Culture and Identity of Turkish Speaking Children in Britain*. Stoke on Trent: Trentham Books.

Tracy, R. (1991) *Sprachliche Strukturentwicklung Linguistische und Cognitions Psychologische Aspekte einer Theorie des Erstspracherwerbs*. Tübingen: Gunter Narr.

Tsimpli, I. and Mastropavlou, M. (2004) Feature-interpretability in child and adult L2 acquisition, and SLI. Ms thesis, University of Thessaloniki.

Tufan, İ. and Arun, Ö. (2006) *Türkiye Özürlüler Araştırması 2002 İkincil Analizi*. Ankara: TÜBİTAK-SOBAG Projesi, No. 104K077.

Tuncer, M. and Maviş, İ (2008) Perceptions of allied health professionals in Turkey towards stroke rehabilitation teams and SLP's role. 2008 ASHA Convention, Chicago.

Tur-Kaspa, H. and Dromi, E. (1998) Spoken and written language assessment of orally trained children with hearing loss: Syntactic structures and devations. *Volta Review* 100 (3), 7–11.

Tüfekçioğlu, U. (1988) The development of an auditory oral program in Turkey. In I.G. Taylor (ed.) *The Education of the Deaf: Current Perspectives* (Vol. 2, pp. 1014–1019). New York: Croom Helm.

Tüfekçioğlu, U. (1989) Farklı iki eğitim ortamında sözlü eğitim alan işitme engelli çocukların konuşma dillerinin karşılaştırılması [A comparison of the spoken language of hearing impaired children receiving oral education in two different educational settings]. PhD thesis, Anadolu University, Eskişehir.

Tüfekçioğlu, U. (1992) *Kaynaştırmadaki İşitme Engelli Çocuklar*. Eskişehir: Anadolu University.

Tüfekçioğlu, U. (1996) Comparative results of the spoken language analysis of hearing impaired children attending two different programs in Turkey. In K. Verch (ed.) *Hard of Hearing, Deafened, Born Deaf: Ways and Aids to Self-Realization* (pp. 1–14). Rendsburg, Germany: IOR-The International Organization of the Rehabilitation for Hearing Impaired.

Tüfekçioğlu, U. (1998) *Farklı Eğitim Ortamlarındaki İşitme Engelli Öğrencilerin Konuşma Dillerinin İncelenmesi*. Eskişehir: Anadolu University.

Tüfekçioğlu, U. (2000) Quality versus Inclusion. *ISEC: International Special Education Congress*. University of Manchester. On WWW at http://www.isec2000.org.uk.

Tüfekçioğlu, U. (2008a) Speech production of hearing impaired Turkish children in an auditory-oral program. Unpublished manuscript, İÇEM, Anadolu University, Eskişehir.

Tüfekçioğlu, U. (2008b) Tense–Aspect–Modality in the spoken language productions of hearing impaired Turkish children. Unpublished manuscript, İÇEM, Anadolu University, Eskişehir.

Tüfekçioğlu, U. (2008c) Coordinating conjunctions in the spoken language productions of hearing impaired Turkish children. Unpublished manuscript, İÇEM, Anadolu University, Eskişehir.

Tüfekçioğlu, U. (2008d) Verbals used as subordinating conjunctions in the spoken language productions of hearing impaired Turkish children. Unpublished manuscript, İÇEM, Anadolu University, Eskişehir.

Tüfekçioğlu, U. (2009a) *Developing the Test of Syntactic Structures for Turkish (TSST) for Assessing Hearing Impaired Children's Language (work in progress)*. Eskişehir: İÇEM, Anadolu University.

Tüfekçioğlu, U. (2009b) Measuring length of utterances of hearing impaired children with MLU and MSL. Unpublished manuscript, İÇEM, Anadolu University, Eskişehir.

Tüfekçioğlu, U. (2009c) Morpho-syntactic errors in spoken language of hearing impaired Turkish children. Unpublished manuscript, İÇEM, Anadolu University, Eskişehir.

Tüfekçioğlu, U., Erdiken, B., Girgin, C. and Girgin, Ü. (1992) *Engelliler için Eğitim Modelleri Geliştirme Projesi.* Eskişehir: Devlet Planlama Teşkilatı, Anadolu University.

Tüfekçioğlu, U., Girgin, Ü. and Turan, Z. (2009) The case of other hearing impaired children in Turkey. Unpublished manuscript, İÇEM, Anadolu University, Eskişehir.

Türk, O., Şayli, Ö., Özsoy, A.S. and Arslan, L.M. (2005) Türkçe'de ünlülerin formant frekans incelemesi. In İ. Ergenç, S. İşsever, S. Gökmen and Ö. Aydın (eds) *Dilbilim İncelemeleri.* Ankara: Doğan.

Ukrainetz, T. and Blomquist, C. (2002) The criterion validity of four vocabulary tests compared with a language sample. *Child Language Teaching & Therapy* 18, 59–78.

Underhill, R. (1980) *Turkish Grammar* (2nd edn, 1980). Cambridge, MA: MIT Press.

Underhill, R. (1986) Turkish. In D.I. Slobin (ed.) *The Crosslinguistic Study of Language Acquisition.* Hillsdale, NJ: Lawrence Erlbaum.

UNESCO (2008) EFA Global Monitoring Report 2007. *Early Childhood Care and Education.* On WWW at http://unesdoc.unesco.org/images/0017/001776/177609e.pdf

Unsworth, S. (2005) Child L2, adult L2, child L1: Differences and similarities. A study on the acquisition of object scrambling in Dutch. PhD thesis, Utrecht Institute of Linguistics, LOT.

Uzuner, Y. (1997) Okulöncesi Çağda İşitme Engelli Çocuğu Olan Normal İşiten Bir Annenin Grup Oyunu Esnasında Kullandığı Stratejilerin İncelenmesi. MA thesis, Anadolu University.

Uzuner, Y. (1999) *Okulöncesi çağda iki işitme engelli çocuk ve onların normal işiten annelerinin çeşitli bağlamlardaki etkileşimlerinde gerçekleşen iletişim bozukluklarını düzeltmek için annelerin uyguladıkları stratejilerin karşılaştırılması.* Unpublished manuscript, Anadolu University, Eskişehir.

Van den Heuvel, E.T.P., De Witte, L.P., Stewart, R.E., Schure, L.M., Sanderman, R. and Meyboom-de Jong, B. (2002) Long-term effects of a group support program and an individual support program for informal caregivers of stroke patients: Which caregivers benefit the most? *Patient Educaion and Counseling* 47 (4), 291–299.

Van der Heijden, H. (1997) 'Yapmak' eylemininin tekdilli ve ikidilli ortamlardaki edinimi. *XI. Dilbilim Kurultayı Bildirileri* (pp. 271–285). Ankara: Middle East Technical University.

Van der Heijden, H. (1999) Word formation processes in young bilingual children. In G. Extra and L.Verhoeven (eds) *Bilingualism and Migration* (pp. 123–140). Berlin: de Gruyter.

Van der Hulst, H. and van der Weige, J. (1991) Topics in Turkish phonology. H. Boeschoten and L. Verhoeven (eds) *Turkish Linguistics Today.* Leiden: E.J. Brill.

Van der Lely, H.K.J. (1997) *Advanced-Syntactic Test of Pronominal Reference (A-STOP).* (Available from author: Centre for Developmental Language Disorders and Cognitive Neuroscience, University College London, London, UK).

Van der Lely, H.K.J. (2005) Domain-specific cognitive systems: Insight from grammatical-specific language impairment. *Trends in Cognitive Sciences* 9, 53–59.

Van Riper, C. (1963) *Speech Correction: Principles and Methods* (4th edn). Englewood Cliffs, NJ: Prentice-Hall.

Verhoeven, L. and van Balkom, H. (2004) Developmental language disorders: Classification, assessment, and intervention. In L. Verhoeven and H. van Balkom (eds) *Classification of Developmental Language Disorders: Theoretical Issues and Clinical Implications.* London: Lawrence Erlbaum.

Verhoeven, L. and Vermeer, A. (2006) *Taaltoets Alle Kinderen*. Arnhem: Cito.
Verhoeven, L., Narain, G., Extra, G., Konak, Ö.A. and Zerrouk, R. (1995) *Toets Tweetaligheid*. Arnhem: Cito.
Verhoeven, L., Aparici, M., Cahana-Amitay, D., Van Hell, J., Kriz, S. and Vigue-Simon, A. (2002) Clause packaging in writing and speech: A cross developmental analysis. *Written Language and Literacy* 5 (2), 135–162.
Vermeer, A. (2000) Coming to grips with lexical richness in spontaneous speech data. *Language Testing* 17, 65–83.
Vicari, S., Caselli, M.C., Gagliardi, C., Tonucci, F. and Volterra, V. (2002) Language acquisition in special populations: A comparison between Down and Williams syndromes. *Neuropsychologia* 40, 2461–2470.
Vihman, M.M. and Ferguson, C.A. (1986) Phoological development from babbling to speech: Common tendencies and individual differences. *Applied Psycholinguistics* 7, 3–40.
Villanova de, R. (1997) Turkish housing conditions in France: From tenant to owner. In S. Özüekren and R. van Kempen (eds) *Turks in European Cities: Housing and Urban Segregation: Comparative Studies in Migration and Ethnic Relations 4* (pp. 98–121). ERCOMER, Utrecht: Utrecht University.
Vinkler, Z. and Pleh, C. (1995) A case of a specific language impaired child in Hungarian. In M. Kovacevic (ed.) *Language and Language Communication Barriers: Research and Theoretical Perspectives in Three European Languages* (pp. 131–158). Hrvatska: Svehcilisna.
Vion, M. and Colas, A. (2005) Using connectives in oral French narratives: Cognitive constrains and development of narrative skills. *First Language* 25 (1), 39–66.
Volterra, V., Caselli, M.C., Capirci, O., Tonucci, F. and Vicari, S. (2003) Early linguistic abilities of Italian children with Williams Syndrome. *Developmental Neuropsychology* 23 (1 & 2), 33–58.
Watkins, R., Kelly, D., Harbers, H. and Hollis, W. (1995) Measuring children's lexical diversity: Differentiating typical and impaired language learners. *Journal of Speech & Hearing Research* 38 (6), 1349–1355.
Wells, G. (1985) *Language Development in the Preschool Years*. Cambridge: Cambridge University Press.
Wexler, K. (1994) Optional infinitives, head movement and the economy of derivations. In D. Lightfoot and N. Hornstein (eds) *Verb Movement* (pp. 305–350). Cambridge: Cambridge University Press.
Wexler, K. (1996) The development of inflection in a biologically based theory on language acquisition. In M. Rice (ed.) *Toward a Genetics of Language* (pp. 113–144). Mahwah, NJ: Lawrence Erlbaum.
Whong-Barr, M. and Schwartz, B.D. (2002) Morphological and syntactic transfer in child L2 acquisition of the English dative alternation. *Studies in Second Language Acquisition* 22, 579–616.
Wilbur, R.B. (1977) An explanation of deaf children's difficulty with certain syntactic structures of English. *Volta Review* 77, 85–92.
Wilbur, R.B., Quigley, S.P. and Montanelli, D.S. (1975) Conjoined structures in the written language of deaf students. *Journal of Speech and Hearing Research* 18, 319–335.
Willmes, K. and Poeck, K. (1993) To what extend can aphasic syndromes be localized? *Brain* 116, 1527–1540.
Wong-Fillmore, L. (1991) Second language learning in children: A model of language learning in social context. In E. Bialystok (ed.) *Language Processing by Bilingual Children* (pp. 49–69). Cambridge: Cambridge University Press.
World Health Organization (WHO) (2001) ICD-10-mental, behavioral and developmental disorders. Geneva: WHO Division of Mental Healths.

World Health Organization (WHO) (2007a) International classification of Functioning, Disability and Health (ICF), Geneva, Switzerland. On WWW at http://www.who.int/classsifications/icfbrowser/. Accessed 07.01.2009.

World Health Organization (WHO) (2007b) International Statistical Classification of Diseases and Related Problems 10th Revision, Version for 2007, Geneva, Switzerland. On WWW at http://apps.who.int/classifications/apps/icd/icd10online/. Accessed 07.01.2009.

Wright, S. and Kurtoglu-Hooton, N. (2006) Language Maintenance: The case of a Turkish speaking community in Birmingham. *International Journal of the Sociology of the Language* 181, 43–56.

Xanthos, A., Laaha, S., Gillis, S., Stephany, U. and Aksu-Koç, A. (in press) On the role of morphological richness in the early development of noun and verb inflection.

Yagmur, K. and Akıncı, M-A. (2003) Language use, choice, maintenance and ethno-linguistic vitality of Turkish speakers in France: Intergenerational differences. *International Journal of the Sociology of Language* 164, 107–128.

Yalçınkaya, F. and Belgin, E. (in preparation) *Preschool Language Scale (PLS 3): Turkish Version.* Ankara: Hacettepe University.

Yarbay-Duman, T. and Bastiaanse, R. (2009) Time reference through verb inflection in Turkish agrammatic aphasia. *Brain and Language* 108, 30–39.

Yarbay-Duman, T., Aygen, G., Özgirgin, N. and Bastiaanse, R. (2007) Object scrambling and finiteness in Turkish agrammatic production. *Journal of Neurolinguistics* 20, 336–331.

Yarbay-Duman, T., Aygen, G. and Bastiaanse, R. (2008) The production of Turkish relative clauses in agrammatism: Verb inflection and constituent order. *Brain and Language* 105 (3), 149–160.

Yavaş, M. and Topbaş, S. (2004) Liquid development in Turkish: Salience vs. frequency. *Journal of Multlingual Communication Disorders* 2 (2), 110–123.

Yavuzer, G., Küçükdeveci, A., Arasıl, T. and Elhan, A. (2001) Rehabilitation of stroke patients: Clinical profile and functional outcome. *American Journal of Physical Medicine & Rehabilitation* 80, 250–255.

Yolcu-Kamali, B.C. (2004) Comprehension of reversible sentences in Turkish agrammatism. MA thesis, Boğaziçi University, Istanbul.

Yolcu-Kamali, B., Mayr, C., Boeckx, C. and Szczegielniak, A. (2006) *Revisiting Agrammatic Comprehension: The Case of Turkish Left Periphery in Aphasia.* LPIA, Venice, Italy.

Yoshinaga-Itano, C. (2000) Assessment and intervention with preschool children who are deaf and hard-of-hearing. In J.G. Alpiner and P.A. McCarthy (eds) *Rehabilitative Audiology: Children and Adults* (pp. 140–177). Baltimore, MD: Lippincott Williams & Wilkins.

Yoshinaga-Itano, C. (2001) Development of audition and speech: Implications with infants who are deaf or hard of hearing. *The Volta Review* (monograph) 100 (5), 213–234.

Yoshinaga-Itano, C. (2005) Early identification, communication modality, and the development of speech and spoken language skills: Patterns and considerations. In P.E. Spencer (ed.) *Advances in the Spoken Language Development of Deaf and Hard-of-Hearing Children* (pp. 298–327). Cary, NC: Oxford University Press.

Yoshinaga-Itano, C., Sedey, A., Coulter, D. and Mehl, A. (1998) Language of early- and later-identified children with hearing loss. *Pediatrics* 102, 1161–1171.

Yumrutaş, N. (2008) Acquisition of complex sentences. Unpublished manuscript. Department of Western Languages and Literatures. Boğaziçi Univetisty, İstanbul.

Zemva, N. (1999) Aphasic patients and their families: Wishes and limits. *Aphasiology* 13 (3), 219–234.

Zeyrek, D., Hatipoğlu, Ç. and Atalay, N.B. (2007) Türkçe /r/'nin Akustik Özellikleri. Paper presented at *21. Dilbilim Kurultayı*. Mersin, Turkey.

Zimmerman, I., Steiner, V. and Pond, R. (2002) *Preschool Language Scale-4*. San Antonio, TX: Psychological Corp.

Zirotti, J.P. (2006) Enjeux sociaux du bilinguisme à l'école. *Langage et Société* 116, 73–92.

Zorman, M., Valdois, S., Jacquier-Roux, M., Lequette, C. and Pouget, G. (2005) *Outil de dépistage des dyslexies – Version 2 (ODEDYS – version 2)*, free access on web site of Cogni-Sciences. On WWW at http://www.cognisciences.com/article.php3?id_article=37.

Zurif, E. and Caramazza, A. (1976) Psycholinguistic structures in aphasia: Studies in syntax and semantics. In H. and H.A. Whitaker (eds) *Studies in Neurolinguistics* (Vol. 1). New York: Academic Press.

Index